Nutrition: Eating Patterns and Health

Nutrition: Eating Patterns and Health

Edited by Margo Field

SYRAWOOD
PUBLISHING HOUSE
New York

Published by Syrawood Publishing House,
750 Third Avenue, 9th Floor,
New York, NY 10017, USA
www.syrawoodpublishinghouse.com

Nutrition: Eating Patterns and Health
Edited by Margo Field

International Standard Book Number: 978-1-68286-622-1 (Hardback)

Cataloging-in-Publication Data

Nutrition : eating patterns and health / edited by Margo Field.
p. cm.
Includes bibliographical references and index.
ISBN 978-1-68286-622-1
1. Nutrition. 2. Food habits. 3. Health. I. Field, Margo.
RA784 .N88 2018
613.2--dc23

Printed in China.

TABLE OF CONTENTS

PREFACE

Nutrition is the science of understanding and studying the relation of food substances to the growth, health, maintenance, reproduction, etc. of the body. It also includes the study of assimilation, absorption, excretion, biosynthesis, food intake and catabolism. This book includes some of the vital pieces of work being conducted across the world, on various topics related to nutrition and the different diseases caused because of the lack of proper diet. The topics covered in this extensive book deal with the core aspects of nutrition. It aims to equip students and experts with the advanced topics and upcoming concepts in this area.

This book unites the global concepts and researches in an organized manner for a comprehensive understanding of the subject. It is a ripe text for all researchers, students, scientists or anyone else who is interested in acquiring a better knowledge of this dynamic field.

I extend my sincere thanks to the contributors for such eloquent research chapters. Finally, I thank my family for being a source of support and help.

Editor

Three week dietary intervention using apricots, pomegranate juice or/and fermented sour sobya and impact on biomarkers of antioxidative activity, oxidative stress and erythrocytic glutathione transferase activity among adults

Mostafa Gouda[1], Amr Moustafa[2], Laila Hussein[1*] and Mohamed Hamza[3]

Abstract

Background: The beneficial effects of the polyphenol (PP) rich fruits and Lactic acid bacteria fermented foods had been reported as cost-effective strategies for health promotion. Randomized controlled trial was designed to test the hypothesis that daily intake of polyphenol rich pomegranate juice (PGJ) or/ and lactic acid bacteria fermented sobya (FS) improved selected biomarkers of relevance to heath status.

Methods: The design of the human trial consisted of 35 healthy adults, who were distributed to 5 equal groups; The first group served as control and received no supplements; the second group received fresh apricot fruits (200 g); the third (PGJ) (250 g), the fourth a mixture of PGJ (150 g) and FS (140 g) and the fifth group received (FS) (170 g). The supplements were served daily between 5 – 6 pm for 21 days. Blood and urine samples were collected at days zero and 22 of the dietary intervention. The supplements were analyzed chemically for (PP) contents and total antioxidative activities and microbiologically for selected bacteria and yeast counts. The blood samples were assayed for plasma antioxidative activities and for erythrocytic glutathione transferase activity (E-GST). Urine samples were analyzed for the excretions of total PP, antioxidative activity and thiobarbituric acid reactive substances (TBARS). Statistical analysis: Two way analysis of variance (ANOVA) was conducted and included the main effects of treatment, time and treatment x time interaction.

Results: Daily intake of (PGJ) for 3 weeks significantly increased the plasma and urinary anti-oxidative activities and reduced the urinary excretion of (TBARS). Daily intake of (FS) for 3 weeks increased only (E-GST) activity. Daily intake of a mixture of PGJ and (FS) was also effective.

Conclusions: The daily intakes of PGJ and/ or (FS) affected positively selected biomarkers of relevance to health status. These functional foods have potential implication for use as bio-therapeutic foods.
(Continued on next page)

* Correspondence: dr.lailahussein@yahoo.com
[1]Department of Nutrition & Food Sc, National Research Center, Giza, Dokki, Egypt
Full list of author information is available at the end of the article

(Continued from previous page)

Trial registration: The study was approved by the research ethical committee of the Ministry of Health & population, Egypt. The trial registration - the unique identifying number. (REC) decision No 12-2013-9, which complied with the Declaration of Helsinki guidelines (2004). The protocol was fully explained to all subjects and written informed consent was obtained before their participation in the trial.

Keywords: Pomegranate juice, Sobya, Human trial, Antioxidative activity, Oxidative stress, Erythrocytic glutathione-S-transferase

Introduction

Under normal physiological conditions, all cells in the body are exposed chronically to oxidants from both endogenous and exogenous sources; yet the intracellular "redox buffer" mechanism provides significant protection mainly by the antioxidant network [1]. Disturbance in the prooxidant- antioxidant balance in favor of the former leads to what is known as oxidative stress [2]. This oxidative stress and reactive oxygen species (ROS) can cause damage to DNA, proteins and lipids an d end up with an epidemic of non communicable chronic human diseases [3–5]. The prevalence of NCD are at escalating in Egypt due to activation of 64 genes involved in inflammation [6, 7] and other modifiable risk factors [8]. Medical and pharmacologic chemotherapeutic agents were reported to reduce cardio vascular mortality among individuals at risk, but they may induce oxidative stress, which increases to an invasive stage with disease progression [9]. Plant polyphenols possess the ideal chemical structure for free radical scavenging activity and their in vitro antioxidative activities are more effective than tocopherols and ascorbate [10]. Designing effective preventive strategies using naturally occurring phytonutrients aiming at reducing oxidative stress is one of the cost-effective strategies to move people's lifestyle toward healthier behaviors [11].

Pomegranate is a popular fruit grown in Egypt with annual production of approximately 130000 tons [12]. Natural unprocessed pomegranate juice (PGJ) is superior to commercial juices in their polyphenol (PP) contents with mean levels of 421 and 382 mg per 100 ml, respectively. Another investigation reported respective (PP) concentrations of 139 mg gallic acid equivalent (GAE) per 100 ml juice and may reach over 200 mg GAE/ 100 ml, when the other phenolic compounds; anthocyamin, ellagitannins, and tannin punicalagin were included [13]. Dietary pomegranate intake in human trials elevated urinary excretion of the above mentioned phenolic metabolites, which are the bioactive constituents responsible for more than >50 % of the antioxidative capacity activity of the juice [14, 15] and are the biomarkers linked to health promotion [16]. Measurement of GST activity had been recommended for the evaluation of protective treatment in trials considering antioxidant strategies. The expression of the phase II hepatic glutathione *S*-transferase was activated in the liver cells of animals following feeding pomegranate anthocyanins flavonoids. The molecular mechanism was related to activation of antioxidant response element (ARE) upstream of genes that regulate the expression of GST [17].

Specific strains of lactic acid bacteria (LAB) possess also antioxidative ability, scavenge reactive oxygen species and chelate metal ions, which provide protection against oxidative stress and lipid peroxidation [18, 19]. The regular intake of LAB fermented foods such as sourdough [20], water kefir [21, 22] and sour sobya [23] containing specific strains of (LAB) with antioxidative capacity activity, contribute to their health effects. Furthermore, the oral administration of some strains of LAB (*L plantarum*) to humans was capable to break down phenolic acids and hydrolysable tannins into phenolic metabolites that are more easily absorbed in the body and enhancing the gut antioxidative effects [24].

In vivo and ex vivo functional biomarkers such as thiobarbituric acid reactive substances (TBARS) are developed for assessing exposure to antioxidant and to lipid oxidation and oxidative stress status [25].

The objective of the present study is to assess the effectiveness of dietary intervention with apricots (AP), pomegranate juice (PGJ), LAB fermented sour sobya (FS) or mixtures of PGJ and FS by healthy adults on biomarkers of antioxidative capacity activity (AEAC), oxidative stress (TBARS) and phase II glutathione-S-transferase enzyme activity [E- GST].

Subjects and methods

A Randomized controlled trial (RCT) was conducted on 35 healthy Egyptian adults (25 men and 10 women) between the ages of 21– 35 years (mean age 27.8 ± 0.96 years). The study received the approval from the research ethical committee (REC) decision No 12-2013-9, Ministry of Health & population, Egypt, which complied with the Declaration of Helsinki guidelines (2004). The protocol was fully explained to all subjects and written informed consent was obtained before their participation in the trial.

Inclusion criteria were healthy adults aging 21 – 35 years. Exclusion criteria at the time of the screening were: History of diabetes, hypertension, heart disease, endocrine disorders, abnormal blood chemistry profile, fasting LDL-cholesterol concentration > 3.37 mmol/L, fasting triacylglycerol concentration > 3.39 mmol/L, smoking, use of antioxidant, vitamin supplements or having taken part in any dietary intervention trials. Female subjects were neither pregnant nor lactating. The volunteers were instructed to continue to eat their normal diet and not to alter their usual dietary or fluid intake with the exception of the foods and beverages that are high in dietary flavonoids, such as purple grapes, cocoa and chocolate during the entire three week dietary intervention trial. Also As a Muslim country red wine drinking is unknown to almost all of the youths, because its drinking is prohibited by religion. Also Egypt is not a coffee drinking country. Volunteers who met the initial inclusion/exclusion criteria took part in the study and there were no withdrawals.

Participant characteristics are summarized in Table 1. Supplements Apricots (AP) (family *Rosaceae; Prunus Armenia*) and pomegranate (family *Punicaceae; Punica granatum L.*) were purchased in batches from El Obour market. AP were stored immediately in packages each containing 200 g net (AP) and were saved in the refrigerator at 4 °C. Pomegranates were picked by hand, washed and stored in tanks. The fruit was crushed and squeezed in an electric juicer (Brand, Germany) and the juice (PGJ) (approximately 30 % of the fruit weight) was packed immediately in 250 ml or 100 ml portions in air tight polyethylene bottle with screw caps and frozen at -200 °C. Lactic acid bacteria fermented sour sobya (FS) was purchased from the retail market (El Rahmany brand) once weekly and saved in the refrigerator.

Design of the RCT

The volunteers were divided into five groups of equal size and each group consisted of 5 men and 2 women. The first group served as control and received no supplements; the second group received fresh (AP) fruits (200 g); the third (PGJ) (250 g), the fourth a mixture of PGJ (150 g) and FS (140 g) and the fifth group received (FS) (170 g). The portions were reasonable dose to eat or to drink over the course of a day and the volunteers were given instructions to consume the portion between 5 – 7 pm.

Dietary assessment

Three-day food diaries (including two weekdays and one weekend day) were completed by the participants to monitor the subjects' dietary compliances and assess their nutrient intakes. Dietary intake were calculated using a computer-aided nutritional analysis program (Nutri survey, Seoul, Korea).

Venous blood collection

One day before starting the trial and on day 22, Blood was taken into vacutainer tubes containing citrate, under quality control. The plasma was separated from blood by centrifugation in a cooling centrifuged at 3500 rpm for 10 min. Collected plasma were stored at -200 °C until analysis. The red blood cells were washed with cold physiological saline and the packed red blood cells were stored at – 200C.

Urine samples were collected from all volunteers at day zero and day 22 and saved frozen at -20 °C.

Blood and urine collection and storage

Overnight fasted blood samples (3 ml) were collected one day before starting the dietary intervention and after 3 weeks of the dietary intervention (Day 22). All blood samples were collected from the left antecubital vein between 8:00 and 9:00 am in tubes containing sodium citrate. The plasma was separated from blood cells by centrifugation at 3000 rpm for 15 min at 4o C and the separated plasma was stored at -700 C for later biochemical analysis. The red blood cells (RBCs) were washed using cold physiological saline solution and stored at -200C. Urine samples were collected in the early morning after the subjects had fasted 10–12 h both on −1, and +21 d dietary intervention and aliquots (2 mL) were immediately frozen at −20 °C for biochemical analysis.

Table 1 Baseline characteristics of the study subjects

Parameter	Unit	$\bar{x}$ ±SE	Median	Q1	Q3
Age	years	27.8±0.96	27.00	24.00	29.75
BMI	$Kg.m^{-1}$	23.7±0.58	23.57	21.48	25.98
Estimated energy intake	Kcal/d	1969±138.78	1903.0	1555	2262
Plasma Antioxidant activity	AEAC/100ml	3.79±0.33	3.37	2.92	4.27
Erythrocyte GST Activity	IU/g Hb	4.65±0.46	4.09	2.73	6.23
Urinary polyphenols	GAE/mg creat	11.45±2.57	6.96	4.89	12.59
Urinary Antioxidant activity	AEAC/mg creat*	7.21±0.84	6.46	4.04	8.55
Urinary TBA	µg/mg creat	114.75±17.37	83.30	47.76	141.71

$\bar{x}$ ±SE: Mean ± standard Error, * : mmol ascorbic acid equivalent antioxidant capacity / mg creatinine),
GAE : gallic acid equivalent

Laboratory investigations

Determination of total polyphenols

The solid-phase extraction (SPE) Cartridge (60 mg) Strata-C18 (Phenomenex,Torrance,CA, USA); Folin Ciocalteu reagent (Catalog No47641; Sigma, USA). MilliQ ultrapure water (Millipore Iberica, Madrid, Spain). All of the analytical steps were carried out in dim light. The PPs of AP and PGJ were extracted vigorously from 4 g AP or 10 g PGJ with 5 ml distilled water then with 20 ml absolute MetOH. After centrifugation in the cold, the supernatant was aspirated and concentrated in vaccuo to 4 ml [26]. Clean up step on Waters 3 ml HLB (60 mg) cartridges were equilibrated with the successive addition of absolute methanol (1 ml) and H_2O (1 ml). Aliquots of the methanolic fruit extracts (2 ml) were loaded on the activated SPE; washing with the successive addition of H_2O (10 ml) and 5 % aqueous MetOH (1 ml). The PP containing fraction was eluted after the addition of 5 ml absolute MetOH. The elute was concentrated under a stream of nitrogen to 2 ml. Aliquots (20 µl (were taken for the analysis of PP using the Folin Ciocalteau colorimetric method [27] and the results were expressed as gallic acid equivalent (GAE) per g apricot or g PGJ.

Measurement of total polyphenolic compounds in urine

Total polyphenols in the urine samples were assayed after the clean up step by the solid-phase extraction (SPE) as described earlier [28, 29]. Aliquots of the centrifuged urine samples (1 ml) were acidified with normal hydrochloric acid (17 µl) and were loaded onto an activated Waters Cartridge, preconditioned with 1 ml methanol and equilibrated with 1 ml of 1.5 mol/l aqueous formic acid. The SPE cartridge was washed twice with 2 ml of the same formic acid and 2 ml of water-methanol (95:5 by volume) to elute the impurities. Elution of the (PP) was completed with a mixture containing 1 ml of methanol containing 1 ml/l of formic acid (2 %)- methanol- H_2O (2/60/38 v/v/v). Aliquots of the elute (500 µl) were pipetted into Eppendorf vials for the colorimetric determination of the (PP). Successive addition of Folin_Ciocalteu reagent (50 µl), followed by 20 % sodium carbonate (600 µl). The tubes were left in the dark for 60 min and then the absorbance of the developed color was measured at 765 nm against a blank. A blank and standard working solutions of gallic acid (0.215 mg/ml) were run in parallel. Urinary (PP) excretion was expressed as mg GAE per g of creatinine.

Plasma antioxidative activity ascorbic acid equivalents (AEAC)

The assay is based on the measurement of the scavenging ability of antioxidants towards the stable DPPH (1,1-diphenyl-2-picrylhydrazyl) radical compound [30]. Aliquots of plasma samples (100 µl) were mixed with 400 µl methanol and after vortexing the tubes were centrifuged at 10,000 x g for 10 min at 4 °C. Aliquots of the clear protein free supernatant (20 µl) was added to 350 µl DPPH reagent (0.127 mol/L methanol) under vigorous shaking for 30 sec. The tubes were then incubated in the dark at room temperature for 30 min. The control was prepared as above without any extract, and MeOH was used for the baseline correction. Standard solutions of ascorbic acid at increasing concentrations (1- 5 µmol/ l) were freshly prepared and treated as described above. Reduction of the absorbance at 515 nm was measured using a UV-Vis spectrophotometer (Shimadzu-Germany). A standard curve was plotted for the relation between ascorbic acid concentrations and the absorbance at 515 nm. All experiments were carried out in triplicate. The radical scavenging activity (RSA) was expressed as the inhibition percentage using the following formula:

$$\%\,\text{RSA} = ((\text{Abs control - Abs sample}) \times 100) / \text{Abs control}$$

The plasma antioxidative capacity activity was expressed as mmol antioxidative activity ascorbic acid equivalents (AEAC) per 100 ml plasma.

Urinary antioxidative activity ascorbic acid equivalents (AEAC)

This was assessed using the DPPH equivalent, according to an adapted colorimetric procedure [31]. Aliquots of filtered urine samples (100 µl) were mixed thoroughly using a vortex mixer with 3 mL DPPH solution in methanol (0.05 g/L) and the tubes were kept in a water bath at 25 °C in dim light for 30 min for the complete development of the reaction. The absorbance of the yellow color was measured spectrophotometrically against a blank at 517 nm.

Three measurements were conducted for each extract. The control solution contained 100 µl of DI water and 3 mL of DPPH solution in methanol. Standard ascorbic acid of increasing concentrations (2-10 µM/L) was treated in a similar manner and run in parallel. The inhibition of free radical in percent (I %) was calculated according to the formula: $[(A0 - A1) / A0] \times 100$, whereby A0 is the absorbance of the control reaction (containing all reagents except the urine), and A1 is the absorbance of the urine sample. All measurements were carried out in triplicates. Urinary antioxidant activity was expressed as as mmol antioxidative activity ascorbic acid equivalents (AEAC) per mmol creatinine).

Urinary thiobarbituric acid-reacting species (TBARS)

Lipid peroxidation (LP) was measured in the urine samples as malondialdehyde (MDA), which was assayed by the thiobarbituric acid reactive species (TBARS) as described earlier [32]. Briefly, aliquots (200 µl) of urine samples were mixed with 10 µl of 5 % butylated hydroxyl toluene in glacial acetic acid, followed by the addition of 300 μl of 0.5 % aqueous TBA solution. After vortexing, the tubes were incubated at 100o C for 30 min and the absorbance of the developed pink color was recorded spectrophotometrically at 532 nm. Samples were blanked against reference cuvettes containing reagent without urine. The concentration of TBARS was calculated from the absorbance at 532 nm using the molar extinction coefficient of 156000. To control for urine concentration the data were normalized to urine creatinine concentration.

Determination of urinary creatinine

Aliquots of the urine samples (3 μl) were pipetted into a 96-well plate for the determination of creatinine by the alkaline picrat method [33]. Aliquots (60 μl) of aqueous picric acid solution (10 g/l) and a 60 μl aliquot of sodium hydroxide (100 g/l) were added in sequence. After 15 min the intensity of the color was read at 500 nm in the ASYS Expert Plus multi-channel microplate reader (Biochrom Lt, Cambridge, UK). The concentration was calculated using a standard creatinine solution.

Assay of erythrocytic glutathione-S-transferase activity (E-GST).

The principle of the assay is based on the conjugation of 1-chloro-2,4dinitro benzene (CDNB) with glutathione (GSH)

$$\text{CDNB} + \text{GSH} \rightarrow \text{CDNB} - \text{S} - \text{glutathione}$$

Aliquots (20 μl) of the washed erythrocytes were lyzed by mixing with 180 μl stabilizing reagent [34] and the tubes were kept in a thermo flask at -18 °C for 10 minutes. After thawing, 50 μL of the hemolysate was added to enzyme assay mixture containing 0.68 ml of distilled water and 200 μL phosphate buffer (100 mM phosphate buffer, K_2HPO_4/KH_2PO_4; pH = 6.5) and 20 μL CDNB (0.5 mM) pre- incubated at 25oC for 10 minutes. The enzymatic GST assay started immediately at 25 °C by adding 50 μL GSH (1.0 mM). And monitoring the rate of increase in absorbance at 340 nm for 10 minutes at 25 °C against a blank solution containing the reaction mixture, in which; the haemolysate was substituted with distilled water [35]. The specific E-GST activity is μmol glutathione transferred /min at 37 °C/g Hb, which is synonymous to IU/g Hb.

Hemoglobin concentration was determined in the hemolysate by the cyan- methaemoglobin reaction using Drabkin reagent [34] and the results were expressed in g/dL.

Statistical analysis

Values are presented as means and SEM and differences with values <0.05 are considered significant. Two way ANOVA were conducted using the general linear model procedure to assess the differences in the effect of the four dietary supplements (Apricots, pomegranate, mixture of pomegranate – sour sobya or sour sobya) and control on outcome measures. The models included the main effects of treatment, two time points and treatment x time interaction. Fisher's least significant differences were used to account for multiple testing [36]. Pearson correlation was used in the correlation evaluations. All evaluations were performed with excel software (release 16) and MSTAT-C computer package [37].

Results

Table 1 presents the baseline characteristics of the volunteers. At base line all participants excreted urinary total polyphenols, but the inter individual variation was quite high (4.89-12.59 mg GAE / 100 ml urine).

Composition of the four supplements served to the volunteers are presented in Table 2. Dietary supplements 1,2,3,4,5 provided daily 0, 1.52, 24.71, 9.89 and 0 mg

Table 2 Composition of the supplements

Parameter	Unit	Dietary supplements				
		Control	AP*	PGJ*	PGJ* + FS*	FS*
		Portion served	Portion served	Portion served	Portion served	Portion served
Portion Size	g	–	200	250	100 +150	170
Total solids	g	–	27.47	17.75	48	40.01
Carbohydrate	g	–	22	32.75	59	51.1
Dietary Fiber	g	–	4	0.25	48.6	54
Energy	Kcal	–	100	135	290	263
Lactobacillus, diverse	cfu / serving size	–	–	–	4.5×10^9	5.1×10^9
Yeast	cfu /serving size	–	–	–	2.44×10^{10}	2.77×10^{10}
Total Polyphenols	mg* / portion g	–	32±0.24	519.1±8.75	207.65±3.5	–
Antioxidant activity	(AEAC)**	–	5.70±0.74	11.35±2.2	11.37±2.05	7.74±1.33

*: mg gallic acid equivalent (GAE) , Ap: Apricot, PGJ: Pomegranate juice, FS: Fermented sobya;
**: mmol ascorbic acid equivalent antioxidant capacity

total polyphenol per portion. Respective antioxidative activity ascorbic acid equivalents (AEAC) were 0, 5.70 ± 0.74, 11.35 ± 2.2, 11.37 ± 2.05 and 7.74 ± 1.33 as showed in Table 2. The 170 g portion of FS provided 5.1×10^9 cfu total *Lactobaccilli* and 2.77×10^{10} cfu yeasts, while the respective counts were 4.5×10^9 cfu total *Lactobaccilli* and 2.44×10^{10} cfu yeasts in the daily portion of the mixture of PGJ & FS supplement.

The urinary total polyphenol excretion increased by approximately 9- fold excess from baseline level of 5.7 to 55.2 μg/mg creatinine following 3 week dietary intervention with PGJ ($P < 0.01$). The 3 week dietary intervention with the mixture of PGJ - FS increased urinary polyphenol excretion compared to the respective baseline level, but the difference didn't attain significant level ($P > 0.05$). Neither the control group nor the three week dietary intervention with AP change the urinary total polyphenol excretion compared to the respective baseline levels ($P > 0.05$) (Table 3).

The three week dietary intervention with PGJ was associated with significant increase in the mean plasma antioxidative activity ascorbic acid equivalents (AEAC) compared to the respective baseline level ($P < 0.05$) and similar significant increase were obtained in the urinary AEAC ($P < 0.05$) compared with the respective baseline concentrations (Table 3). The three week dietary intervention with a mixture of PGJ and FS was associated with an increase in the plasma (AEAC) compared with the respective baseline level ($P < 0.05$). The 3 week dietary intervention with fermented sobya (FS), increased the plasma AEAC by 23 %, which did not attain significant level ($P > 0.05$), while the urinary increase in AEAC (131 %) compared to the respective baseline levels, but the difference didn't attain significant difference ($0.1 > P > 0.05$) (Table 3). Neither the control group nor the dietary intervention with AP changed the AEAC to any extent and the results were similar to those obtained with the respective base line levels (Table 3).

Urinary excretion of TBARS decreased by 63.5, 41.6 and 48.1 % at the end of the three week dietary intervention with PGJ ($P < 0.05$), mixture of PGJ & FS ($P < 0.05$) and FS ($0.1 > P > 0.05$), respectively compared to the respective baseline levels. Neither the control group nor the three week dietary intervention with apricots reduced the urinary TBARS concentration ($P > 0.05$) (Table 3).

The baseline Erythrocytic glutathione-S- transferase activity (E-GST) activity averaged 4.65 ± 0.46 IU/g Hb. The mean E-GST increased significantly after the 3 week dietary intervention with fermented sobya (FS) compared with the respective base line activity ($P < 0.05$). The increases in the enzymatic activities among the four other groups didn't attain significant level ($P > 0.05$).

Table 4 presents the two way ANOVA showing no significant differences between individuals. The ANOVA test reveals high stastistical significant differences in the other sources of variations, *i.e* dietary supplements, time points and interaction between dietary supplements and time points. Fisher's least significant differences were used to account for multiple testing

Very high positive significant correlation coefficients were obtained between urinary total polyphenols concentration and urinary AEAC ($r = 0.96, P < 0.000$). Inverse significant correlations were also found between the excretions of urinary total polyphenols total polyphenols concentration and urinary TBARS excretion (Table 5).

Discussion

The promotion of a healthy life style with non-pharmacological means is a preventive measure strategy and our work aimed at throwing light on the importance of carrying out dietary intervention trials in human

Table 3 Initial and final mean urinary polyphenols, plasma and urinary antioxidative activity, urinary TBARS and erythrocytic GST activity among subjects receiving different dietary supplements

Parameter	Unit	Control			Apricot			Pomegranate			Pomegranat+Sobya			Sobya		
		Baseline	Final		Baseline	Final		Baseline	Final		Baseline	Final		Baseline	Final	
		$\bar{x}$±SE	$\bar{x}$±SE	P	$\bar{x}$±SE	$\bar{x}$±SE	P	$\bar{x}$±SE	$\bar{x}$±SE	P	$\bar{x}$±SE	$\bar{x}$±SE	P	$\bar{x}$±SE	$\bar{x}$±SE	P
Urinary polyphenol	GAE/mg creat	10.36 ±1.8	8.11 ±2.2		18.47 ±9.7	10.36 ±2.2		5.70 ±1.4	55.23 ±21.7	<0.05	10.40 ±3.2	21.62 ±7.3		11.84 ±6.2	9.86 ±1.8	
Urinary Antioxidant activity	AEAC/mg creat*	9.74 ±2.0	8.13 ±2.7		4.25 ±0.9	7.56 ±2.9		7.18 ±0.9	46.57 ±18.0	<0.05	10.90 ±2.4	20.25 ±3.9		3.89 ±0.9	10.30 ±2.3	
Urinary TBARS	μg/mg creat	83.04 ±12.1	75.17 ±15.3		68.82 ±30.9	50.19 ±7.7		173.93 ±44.8	51.48 ±8.2	<0.05	157.70 ±47.8	40.62 ±8.3	<0.05	82.77 ±27.8	29.97 ±4.4	
Plasma antioxidant	AEAC/ 100 ml	6.36 ±2.81	5.99 ±2.66		4.16 ±0.51	3.90 ±0.86		3.64 ±0.30	5.92 ±0.68	<0.05	2.78 ±0.11	4.49 ±0.58	<0.05	3.70 ±0.33	4.55 ±0.27	
E-GST Activity	IU/g Hb	5.94 ±3.3	5.45 ±4.1		4.64 ±1.2	3.97 ±0.8		4.73 ±1.0	8.34 ±1.0		4.56 ±1.0	6.90 ±1.0		4.26 ±0.5	7.21 ±0.8	<0.05

$\bar{x}$±SE: Mean ± standard Error, * : mmol ascorbic acid equivalent antioxidant capacity / mg creatinine, GAE : gallic acid equivalent; Mean values are significantly different if the P-Values are less than 0.05 ($P<0.05$)

Table 4 Mean squares analysis of variance for E-GST activity, plasma anti-oxidative activity, urinary anti-oxidative activity, urinary TBA and urinary polyphenol excretions under five dietary supplements

Source of variation	df	E-GST	Plasma Antioxidant	Urinary Antioxidant	Urinary TBA	Urinary polyphenol
Replicates	**6**	19.00	0.36	123.16	7508.8	642.51
Dietary Supplement (DS)	**4**	9.04**	13.96**	1052.62**	8423.2*	993.17
Time point (T)	**1**	41.84**	11.87**	2261.58**	71153.3**	1640.05*
Interaction (T × DS)	**4**	13.92**	4.64**	916.08**	10122.7*	1911.84**

* and ** denote significance at 5% and 1% probability level, respectively

beings with the PGJ and probiotic LAB fermented food products. The relationship between the polyphenol rich fruits and LAB fermented supplements and prevention of diseases in man is the topic of numerous investigations during recent years [38].

Antioxidant potency of commonly consumed PGJ was evaluated through several in vitro methodologies. Hundreds of Norwegian dietary plants were screened for antioxidative activity by automated FRAP assay, and pomegranate was the fruit with the highest antioxidative activity ascorbic acid equivalents (AEAC) with mean level of 11.3 mmol /100 g, while the respective value for apricot was 0.52 mmol /100 g [39]. Slightly higher antioxidative activities were reported for fresh PGJ with mean level of 15 AEAC / L, compared to the respective value of 12 – 13 AEAC for frozen PGJ [40].

The antioxidant capacity of PGJs obtained from eight Iranian cultivars were determined by the scavenging activity against (DPPH) showed that the cultivar Izmir 8 was with the highest scores with efficient concentration (EC 50) of 29.8 ± 2.9 ml PJ/ g of DPPH [41]. The above mentioned reported levels are higher than the respective mean level of 4.5 AEAC per Liter PGJ obtained in the present study.

The bioavailability of pomegranate flavonoid is influenced by "LADME" [42]. The concept LADME stands for liberation from the food matrix (bioaccessibility), absorption, distribution, metabolism and excretion [43]. The dietary polyphenols escape absorption in the small intestine and are degraded in the colon under the catalytic action of the enormous number of colonic microbiota amount to 1014 colony forming units.

The first step in polyphenol degradation involves the release of aglycones by microbial glycosidases, which enhances their absorption. Plasma ellagic acid (EA) peaked after one hour of oral ingestion of 180 mL PGJ with mean concentration of 31.9 ng / mL plasma [14]. Identical results were obtained following the daily consumption of capsules (800 mg) containing 330.4 mg pomegranate punicalagins and 21.6 mg EA [44]. According to the authors, the (EA) peak reached 33.8 ± 12.7 ng/mL plasma. This finding presents evidence that pome granate ellagic acid (EA) was absorbed in humans. The increase in pom egranate ellagic acid (EA) was associated with significant increases in plasma AEAC averaging 31.8, 1.62 and 1.43 %, after 0.5, one and two hours post ingestion, respectively [44]. Furthermore, urinary urolithin metabolites persisted for 48 hours after PGJ ingestion [45].

In the present study, the three week dietary intervention with PGJ was quite appropriate to raise and maintain the body pools of phenols. The high AEAC of plasma and urine of our subjects is in good agreement with other studies reporting high plasma antioxidant capacity in human volunteers after PGJ consumption [44].

It is suggested that the gastrointestinal tract plays an important role in the first-pass metabolism of dietary flavonoids [46], whereby, during phase I metabolism, intestinal bacteria reductases convert pomegranate flavonoids into the urolithins and enabling reuptake [47]. Urolithin A and urolithin B are the PGJ metabolites detected in the plasma of volunteers following 5 day intakes of one liter of PGJ daily containing 4.37 g/L punicalagins and 0.49 g/L anthocyanins [48]. Their persistence in plasma and tissues suggest that they account for some of the health benefits of PGJ [14]. Specific strains of L. plantarum possess enzyme tannase (tannin acyl -hydrolase) and are able to degrade hydrolyzable tannins and tannic acid, to the monomeric antioxidant derivatives gallic acid and pyrogallol [49]. Eubacterium ramulus is one of the key colonic bacteria implicated in the biotransformation of the polyphewnolic

Table 5 Correlation coefficients between Percentage change(%) of biochemical plasma antioxidative, urinary polyphenol, urinary antioxidant and urinary thiobarbituric acid

Biochemical parameter	Unit	Urinary polyphenol	Urinary antioxidant activity	Urinary TBARS
Urinary polyphenol	GAE/mg creat	1	0.93***	-0.31*
Urinary antioxidant activity	AEAC/mg creat*	0.93***	1	-0.28*
Urinary TBARS	µg/mg creat	-0.31*	-0.28*	1

*:P<0.05;**:P<0.01;***:P<0.001; (AEAC) *: mmol ascorbic acid equivalent antioxidant capacity/creatinine

compounds quercetin, apigenin and naringenin [50]. In phase II metabolism, polyphenols and their reductive metabolites are then conjugated with glucuronic acid and sulfate. by intestinal microsomes [47].

Erythrocytic glutathione-S-transferase (E-GST) designated GST3 or GSTı belongs to phase II metabolizing enzyme superfamily involved in the cellular detoxification of both xenobiotic and endobiotic compounds [51]. This enzyme serves to scavenge free radicals that are produced from oxidative stress by actively transporting GSH- xenobiotic conjugates. Induction of E-GST by expression had been implicated in protection of blood stream and other target cells from genotoxic insults [52]. One study reported no changes in the activities of E-GST following treatment with pomegranate polyphenols, although the concentrations of the lipid peroxidation marker malondialdehyde was reduced [53]. Our results are in agreement with this report, since the increase in E-GSH activity was not significant following the 3 week dietary intervention with PGJ, yet the reduction in lipid peroxidation marker malondialdehde was tremendous. Significant increase in the E –GST activity was found only after the three week dietary intervention with fermented sobya ($t = 2.27$, $P < 0.05$). This finding suggests that the sobya micro-organisms (LAB and/ or yeast) potentially modulated the expression of GST genes related to biotransformation. This finding supports the important role of fermented products in primary chemo- prevention. Reinforcing the activity of GST protects target cells [54]. Similar finding was reported with the complex fermentation of inulin-type fructans which favourably modulate the expression of genes related to biotransformation in carcinoma cells [55].

Urinary excretion of either free aglycones or conjugated polyphenols in humans are the valid biological markers of exposure and are more affordable approach in epidemiological studies and in metabolic studies [56, 57]. Repeated consumption of PP rich food sources resulted in the urinary excretion of 111 metabolites and about 160 aglycone metabolites originating from various classes of dietary polyphenols and maximum excretion rates occurred 3-4 days after juice ingestion [58, 59]. More than 80 urinary polyphenol metabolites could be identified nowadays with high predicting ability of food intake (food metabolome) within the population of 4 European countries [57]. The development of novel analytic methods is now essential to measure large sets of polyphenols biomarkers and evaluate the role of these metabolites in disease prevention. The biomarkers are indicator of responses to dietary intervention that can aid in understanding the prediction of treatment [60]. In the present study, daily intake of 250 ml PGJ totaling 5.25 liters per 21 days increased the mean urinary polyphenol excretion ($P < 0.05$) from 6 GAE at day 0 to 55 GAE/mg creatinine at day 22. All other supplements failed to increase urinary PP excretion to a significant level ($P > 0.05$). In both laboratory and clinical studies, the pomegranate combats numerous pathological changes associated with cardiovascular disease [61, 62]. Pomegranate fights cardiovascular disease by reducing oxidative stress, inhibiting the oxidation of potentially harmful LDL [63], quenching free radicals and supporting the synthesis and activity of nitric oxide [64, 65]. Oxidation protection actions of dietary polyphenols include reactive species scavenging, enzyme modulation to interference with cell signaling and oxidative stability [66]. The chemo preventive action of PGJ was attributed to the modulation of cellular signaling processes including nuclear factor-kappa-B (NF-κB) and activator protein-1(AP-1) DNA binding [67]. Separation of individual polyphenols from the crude PGJ were interpreted on the basis that pretreatment of PGJ inhibited NFκB activation, AKT activity and expression of COX-2 in HT-29 cells [67].

It is not clear, if the antioxidants in dietary plants polyphenol can explain all of the protective effect against oxidative stress-related chronic diseases. Synergistic effect between the supplements PGJ & LAB - fermented sobya biopeptides may be acting in coordination to protect against oxidative stress events. In agreement with our finding, apricot cultivars grown in Spain showed low contents of bioactive compounds with mean polyphenol concentration of 179.8 mg GAE/100 g [68]. Interestingly, heat-processed apricots have excellent antioxidative properties due to the high melanoidins content. Derived melanoidin is responsible for the significant elevation of antioxidant capacity and protecting endothelial cells from hydrogen peroxide - induced oxidative mitochondrial damage and cell death [69]. Evidence obtained from the present trial is based on a healthy adult population group, may not be generalizable to individuals with a disease or specific risk factors. Inability to apply molecular markers or food-specific signatures such as metabolomic analysis is a further limitation due to protocol limitation.

Conclusion

The nutrition intervention with mixtures of PGJ and probiotic fermented sobya had synergistic positive effects. PGJ enhances the antioxidant status in humans by decreasing the oxidative damage in lipids by decreasing urinary TBARS and improving the antioxidant mechanisms; while probiotic fermented sobya stimulates erythrocytes GST activity. The present study demonstrated that designing effective preventive strategies aiming at reducing the risk of chronic diseases is a cost effective safe initiative in contrast to the action of drugs developed by the pharmaceutical industry. Quantification among individuals of biologically effective pomegranate dose, interacting with critical cellular targets for curing or preventing various illnesses warrants further investigations. Research concerning increased knowledge on the depth of the role of nutrients in the health promotion and.

Competing interests

The authors declare that they have no competing interests.

Authors' contribution

MG conceived the study and was responsible for the human trial and the collection of the biological fluids. He also did the laboratory investigation and performed the statistical analysis. AM participated in the design of the study and coordination. LH participated in the design of the study, the statistical analysis and wrote the manuscript. MH was responsible for the ANOVA test. All authors read and approved the final manuscript.

Acknowledgment

The authors are grateful to the volunteers participating in the trial for their patience and compliance.

Author details

[1]Department of Nutrition & Food Sc, National Research Center, Giza, Dokki, Egypt. [2]Department of Biochemistry, Faculty of Agriculture, Cairo University, Giza, Egypt. [3]Department of Agronomy, Faculty of Agric, Cairo University, Giza, Egypt.

References

1. Circu ML, Aw TY. Glutathione and modulation of cell apoptosis. Biochim Biophys Acta. 1823;2012:1767–77.
2. Sies H. Oxidative stress. Introductory remarks. In: Oxidative Stress (Sies, H., ed.), 1985;pp. 1-8. Academic Press, London, U.K.
3. Caillet P, Canoui-Poitrine F, Vouriot J, et al. Comprehensive geriatric assessment in the decision-making process in elderly patients with cancer: ELCAPA study. J Clin Oncol. 2011;29(27):3636–42.
4. Itoh Y, Shinya K, Kiso M, Watanabe T, Sakoda Y, Hatta M, Muramoto Y, Tamura D, Sakai-Tagawa Y, Noda T, et al. In vitro and in vivo characterization of new swine-origin H1N1 influenza viruses. Nature. 2009;460(7258):1021–5.
5. Paz-Elizur T, Sevilya Z, Leitner-Dagan Y, Elinger D, Roisman LC, Livneh Z. DNA repair of oxidative DNA damage in human carcinogenesis: potential application for cancer risk assessment and prevention. Cancer Lett. 2008;18;266(1):60-72.
6. Egypt Demographic and Health Survey. 2014;Pp 52. http://dhsprogram.com/pubs/pdf/PR54/PR54.pdf.
7. Bengmark, Lansky EP, Newman RA. Punica granatum (pomegranate) and its potential for prevention and treatment of inflammation and cancer. J Ethnopharmacol. 2007;109:177–206.
8. WHO. 2008-2013 action plan for the global strategy for the prevention and control of noncommunicable diseases. 2008. Pp 1-42. http://www.who.int/nmh/publications/ncd_action_plan_en.pdf.
9. Alomar MJ. Factors affecting the development of adverse drug reactions. Saudi Pharmac J. 2014;22:83–94.
10. Vertuani S, Angusti A, Manfredini A. The Antioxidants and Pro-Antioxidants Network: An Overview. Current Pharmaceutical Design. 2004;10:1677–94.
11. Fleg JL, Forman DE, Berra K. Secondary prevention of atherosclerotic cardiovascular disease in older adults. Circulation. 2013;128:2422–46.
12. Ministry of agriculture Egypt. Annual report- statistical data. 2014; Pp1-10. http://egypt.opendataforafrica.org/kddlloe/egypt-agriculture-sheet.
13. Kesarwani A, Chiang P, Chen S. Distribution of Phenolic compounds and antioxidative activities of rice kernel and their relationships with agronomic practice. Sci W J. 2014;14:1–6.
14. Seeram NP, Aviram M, Zhang Y, Henning SM, Feng L, Dreher M, Heber D. Comparison of antioxidant potency of commonly consumed polyphenol-rich beverages in the United States. J Agric Food Chem. 2008;56:1415–22.
15. Borges et al., 2010, Viuda-Martos M, Fernández-López J, Pérez-Álvarez JA. Pomegranate and its many functional components as related to human health: a review. Compr Rev Food Sci Food Saf. 2010; 9: 635–54.
16. Guo X, Tresserra-Rimbau A, Estruch R, Miguel A, Martínez-González M, Medina-Remón A. Effects of Polyphenol, measured by a biomarker of total polyphenols in urine, on cardiovascular risk factors after a long-term follow-up in the PREDIMED study. Oxidative Medicine and Cellular Longevity. 2016;16:1–11.
17. Shih A. Anthocyanins induce the activation of phase II enzymes through the antioxidant response element pathway against oxidative stress-induced apoptosis. J Agric Food Chem. 2007;55:9427–35.
18. Kullisaar T, Zilmer M, Mikelsaar T, Vihalemm H, Annuk C, et al. Two antioxidative lactobacilli strains as promising probiotics. Int J Food Microbiol. 2002;72:215–24.
19. Songisepp E, Kals J, Kullisaar T, Mända r R, Hütt P, Zilmer M, Mikelsaar M. Evaluation of the functional efficacy of an antioxidative probiotic in healthy volunteers. Nutr J. 2005;4:22.
20. Cagno R, Coda R, Angelis M, Gobbetti M. Exploitation of vegetables and fruits through lactic acid fermentation. Food Microbiology. 2013;33(1):1–10.
21. Alsayadi M et al. Evaluation of anti-Hyperglycemic and anti-hyperlipidemic activities of water kefir as probiotic on Streptozotocin- induced diabetic Wistar rats. J Diabetes Mellitus. 2014;4:85–95.
22. Zhang S, Liu L, Su Y, Li H, Sun Q, Liang X, et al. Antioxidative activity of lactic acid bacteria in yogurt. Afr J Microbiol Res. 2011;5:5194–201.
23. Fouad M, Moustafa A, Hussein L, Romeilah R, Gouda M. In-vitro antioxidant and antimicrobial activities of selected fruit and vegetable juices and fermented dairy products commonly consumed in Egypt. RJPBCS. 2015;6(2):541–50.
24. Melgarejo P, Calín-Sánchez A, Carbonell-Barrachina AA, Martínez-Nicolás JJ, Legua P, Martínez R, Hernández F. Antioxidant activity, volatile composition and sensory profile of four new very-early AP (Prunus armeniaca L.). J Sci Food Agric. 2013;30:20–8. doi:10.1002/jsfa.6201 [Epub ahead of print].
25. Martel F, Monteiro R, Calhau C. Effect of polyphenols on the intestinal and placental transport of some bioactive compounds. Nutr Res Revs. 2010;23: 47–64.
26. Hertog MGL, Sweetnam PM, Fehily AM, Elwood PC, Kromhout D. Antioxidant flavonols and ischaemic heart disease in a Welsh population of men. The Caerphilly study. Am J Clin Nutr. 1997;65:1489–94.
27. Singleton VL, Rossi JA. Colorimetry of total phenolics with phosphomolybdic-phosphotungstic acid reagents. Am J Enol Vitic. 1965;16:144–58.
28. Roura E, Lacueva CA, Estruch R, Lamuela-Ravento RM. Total polyphenol intake estimated by a modified Folin_Ciocalteu assay of urine. Clin Chem. 2006;52:749–52.
29. Hussein L, Medina A, Barrionnevo A, Lammuela-Raventos RM, Andres-Lacueva C. Normal distribution of urinary polyphenol excretion among Egyptian males 7_14 years old and changes following nutritional intervention with tomato juice (Lycopersicon esculentum). Intern J Food Sc Nutr. 2009;6:15–23.
30. Brand-Williams W, Cuvelier ME, Berset C. Use of free radical method to evaluate antioxidant activity. Lebensm Wiss Technology. 1995;28:25–30.
31. Shimada K, Fujikawa K, Yahara K, Nakamura T. Antioxidative properties of xanthone on the auto oxidation of soybean in cylcodextrin emulsion. J Agr Food Chem. 1992;40:945–8.
32. Ohkawa H, Ohishi N, Yagi K. Assay for lipid peroxides in animal tissues by thiobarbituric acid reaction. Anal Biochem. 1979;95:351–8.
33. Jaffe M. Uber den niederschlag, welchen pikrinsaure in normalen hrn erzeugt und uber eine neue reaction des kreatinins. Z Physiol Chem. 1886;10:391–400.
34. Beutler E, Duron M, Kelly BM O. Improved method for the determination of blood. Glutathione. J Lab Clin Med. 1963;61:882–8.
35. Habig WJ, Pabst MJ, Jacoby WB. Glutathione S-transferase, the first enzymatic step in mercapturic acid formation. J Biol Chem. 1974;249:7130–9.
36. Steel RD, Torri JH and Dickey DA. Principles and Procedures of Statistics: A Biometrical Approach, 3rd ed,. Mc Graw-Hill, New York. 1997;666p.
37. Freed RP, Einensmith S, Gutez D, Reicosky VW, Smail, Wolberg P. MSTAT-C analysis of agronomic research experiments. East Lansing, USA: Michigan Univ; 1989.
38. Jakesevic M, Aaby K, Borge GI, Jeppsson B, Ahrné S, Molin G. Antioxidative protection of dietary bilberry, chokeberry and Lactobacillus plantarum HEAL19 in mice subjected to intestinal oxidative stress by ischemia-reperfusion. BMC Complement Altern Med. 2011;11:8–15.
39. Halvorsen BL, Holte K, Myhrstad MCW, Barikmo I, Hvattum E, Remberg SF, Wold AB, et al. A systematic screening of total anti oxidants in dietary plants. J Nutr. 2002;132:461–71.
40. Gil MI, Tomás-Barberán FA, Hess-Pierce B, Holcroft DM, Kader AA. Antioxidant activity of pomegranate juice and its relationship with phenolic composition and processing. J Agric Food Chem. 2013;48:4581–9.
41. Cam M, Hisil Y, Durmaz G. Classification of 8 pgjs based on antioxidant capacity measured by four methods. Food Chemistry. 2009;112:721–6.

42. Holst B, Williamson G. A critical review of the bioavailability of glucosinolates and related compounds. Nat Prod Rep. 2004;21(3):425–47.
43. Lhoste EF, Ouriet V, Bruel S, Flinois JP, Bre' zillon C, Magdalou J, Che' ze, C, et al. The human colonic microflora influences the alterations of xenobiotic-metabolizing enzymes by catechins in male F344 rats. Food Chem Toxicol. 2003;41(5):695–702.
44. Mertens-Talcott SU, Jilma-Stohlawetz P, Rios J, Hingorani L, Derendorf H. Absorption, metabolism, and antioxidant effects of pomegranate (Punica granatum L.) Polyphenols after ingestion of a standardized extract in healthy human volunteers. J Agric Food Chem. 2006;54:8956–61.
45. Seeram NP, Lee R, Heber D. Bioavailability of ellagic acid in human plasma after consumption of ellagitannins from pomegranate (Punica granatum juice). Clin Chim Acta. 2004;348:63–8.
46. Pfeiffer P, Papp N, Abrankó L, Blázovics A, Pedryc A, Stefanovits-Bányai É. Accumulation of antioxidants in apricot fruit through ripening: Characterization of a genotype with enhanced functional properties. Biol Res. 2011;44:339–44.
47. Kemperman RA, Bolca S, Roger LC, Vaughan EE. Novel approaches for analysing gut microbes and dietary polyphenols: challenges and opportunities. Microbiology. 2010;156(11):3224–31.
48. Cerda B, Espin JC, Parra S, et al. The potent in vitro antioxidant ellagitannins from pomegranate juice are metabolised into bioavailable but poor antioxidant hydroxy-6H-dibenzopyran-6-one derivatives by the colonic microflora of healthy humans. Eur J Nutr. 2004;43:205–20.
49. Osawa R, Kuroiso K, Goto S, Shimizu A. Isolation of Tannin-Degrading Lactobacilli from Humans and Fermented Foods. Appl Environ Microbiol. 2000;66(7):3093–7.
50. Simmering R, Pforte H, Jacobasch G, Blaut M. The growth of the flavonoid-degrading intestinal bacterium, Eubacterium ramulus, is stimulated by dietary flavonoids in vivo. FEMS Microbiol Ecol. 2002;40:243–8.
51. Salinas AE, Wong MG. Glutathione S-Transferases – a review. Curr Med Chem. 1999;6:279–309.
52. Pool-Zobel BL, Selvaraju V, Sauer J, Kautenburger T, Kiefer J, Richter KK, Soom M, Wolfl S. Butyrate may enhance toxicological defence in primary, adenoma and tumor human colon cells by favourably modulating expression of glutathione- S-transferases genes, an approach in nutrigenomics. Carcinogenesis. 2005;26:1064–76.
53. Durgaprasad S, Ganesh PC, Vasanthkumar, Jose FA. A pilot study of the antioxidant effect of curcumin in tropical pancreatitis S. Indian J Med Res. 2005;122:315–8.
54. Boateng J, Verghese M, Shackelford L, Walker LT, Khatiwada J, Ogutu S, Williams DS, Jones J, Guyton M, Asiamah D, et al. Selected fruits reduce azoxymethane (AOM)-induced aberrant crypt foci (ACF) in Fisher 344 male rats. Food Chem Toxicol. 2007;45:725–32.
55. Munjal U, Scharlau D, Glei M. Gut fermentation products of inulin-type fructans modulate the expression of xenobiotic-metabolising enzymes in human colonic tumour cells. Anticancer Res. 2012;32(12):5379–86.
56. Ito H, Gonthier M-P, Manach C, Morand C, Mennen L, Remesy C, Scalbert A. Polyphenol levels in human urine after intake of six different polyphenol-rich beverages. Br J Nutr. 2006;94:500–9.
57. Edmands WM, Ferrari P, Rothwell JA, Rinaldi S, Slimani N, Barupal DK, Biessy C, Jenab M. Polyphenol metabolome in human urine and its association with intake of polyphenol-rich foods across European countries. Am J Clin Nutr. 2015;102:905–13.
58. Pe'rez-Jime'nez J, Hubert J, Hooper L, Cassidy A, Manach C, Williamson G, Scalbert A. Urinary metabolites as biomarkers of polyphenol intake in humans: a systematic review. Am J Clin Nutr. 2010;92:801–9.
59. Scalbert A, Zamora-Ros R. Bridging evidence from observational and intervention studies to identify flavonoids most protective for human health. Am J Clin Nutr. 2015;101(5):897–8. doi:10.3945/ajcn.115.110205.
60. Naylor S. Biomarkers: current perspectives and future prospects. Expert Rev Mol Diagn. 2003;3:525–9.
61. Jurenka JS. Therapeutic applications of pomegranate (Punica granatum L.): a review. Altern Med Rev. 2008;13:128–44.
62. Kris-Etherton PM, Lefevre M, Beecher GR, Gross MD, Keen CL, Etherton T. Bioactive compounds in ntrition and health-researchmethodologies for establishing biological function:the antioxidant and anti-inflammatory effects. Of flavonoids on atherosclerosis. Annu. Rev. Nutr. 2004;24:511–38.
63. Hussein L, Abdel-Rahim E, Afify A, Ezz El-Arab A, Labib E. Effectiveness of Apricots (Prunus armeniaca), Pomegranate (Punica granatum) Juice and Lactic Acid Fermented Sobya on Plasma Levels of Lipid Profile Parameters and Total Homocysteine among Egyptian dults. Food and Nutrition Sciences. 2014;5:2225–36.
64. Umner MD, Elliott-Eller M, Weidner G, Daubenmier JJ, Chew MH, Marlin R, et al. Effects of pomegranate juice consumption on myocardial perfusion in patients with coronary heart disease. Am J Cardiol 2005; 96: 810–14. Pubmed Abstract | Publisher Full Text
65. Basu A, Penugonda K. Pomegranate juice: a heart-healthy fruit juice. Nutr Reviews. 2009;67:49–56.
66. Kumar R, Goswami S, Singh K, Gyanendra K, Raj D. Modulation of redox signal transduction in plant system through induction of free radical / ROS scavenging redox - sensitive enzymes and metabolites. AJCS. 2013;7(11):1744–51.
67. Surh YJ. NF-kappa B, and Nrf2 as potential chemopreventive targets of some anti-inflammatory and antioxidative phytonutrients with anti-inflammatory and antioxidative activities. Asia Pac J Clin Nutr. 2008;1:269–72.
68. Brat P, George S, Annick B, Chaffaut L, Scalbert A, Mennen L, Arnault N, Amiot MJ. Daily polyphenol intake in France from fruit and vegetables. J Nutr. 2006;136:2368–73.
69. Cossu A, Posadino AM, Giordo R, Emanueli C, Sanguinetti AM, et al. Apricot melanoidins prevent oxidative endothelial cell death by counteracting mitochondrial oxidation and membrane depolarization. Plos one. 2012;7(11), e48817. doi:10.1371/journal.pone.0048817.

2

Effect of a high protein diet and/or resistance exercise on the preservation of fat free mass during weight loss in overweight and obese older adults

Amely M. Verreijen[1*], Mariëlle F. Engberink[1], Robert G. Memelink[1], Suzanne E. van der Plas[1], Marjolein Visser[2,3] and Peter J.M. Weijs[1,3]

Abstract

Background: Intentional weight loss in obese older adults is a risk factor for accelerated muscle mass loss. We investigated whether a high protein diet and/or resistance exercise preserves fat free mass (FFM) during weight loss in overweight and obese older adults.

Methods: We included 100 overweight and obese adults (55–80 year) in a randomized controlled trial (RCT) with a 2 × 2 factorial design and intention-to-treat analysis. During a 10-week weight loss program all subjects followed a hypocaloric diet. Subjects were randomly allocated to either a high protein (1.3 g/kg body weight) or normal protein diet (0.8 g/kg), with or without a resistance exercise program 3 times/week. FFM was assessed by air displacement plethysmography.

Results: At baseline, mean (±SD) BMI was 32 ± 4 kg/m^2. During intervention, protein intake was 1.13 ± 0.35 g/kg in the high protein groups vs. 0.98 ± 0.29 in the normal protein groups, which reflects a 16.3 ± 5.2 g/d higher protein intake in the high protein groups. Both high protein diet and exercise did not significantly affect change in body weight, FFM and fat mass (FM). No significant protein*exercise interaction effect was observed for FFM. However, within-group analysis showed that high protein in combination with exercise significantly increased FFM (+0.6 ± 1.3 kg, $p = 0.011$).

Conclusion: A high protein diet, though lower than targeted, did not significantly affect changes in FFM during modest weight loss in older overweight and obese adults. There was no significant interaction between the high protein diet and resistance exercise for change in FFM. However, only the group with the combined intervention of high protein diet and resistance exercise significantly increased in FFM.

Trial registration: Dutch Trial Register, number NTR4556, date 05-01-2014.

Keywords: Older adults, Obesity, Weight loss, Fat free mass, High protein diet, Resistance exercise

* Correspondence: a.verreijen@hva.nl
[1]Department of Nutrition and Dietetics, Faculty of Sports and Nutrition, Amsterdam University of Applied Sciences, Dr. Meurerlaan 8, 1067 SM Amsterdam, Netherlands
Full list of author information is available at the end of the article

Background

Older adults represent the fastest growing population in Europe, but also in the rest of the world [1]. The prevalence of obesity among this age group is 20–30% which has dramatically increased in the past decades [1]. Obesity in older adults is a serious health problem related with multiple chronic health conditions and plays an important role in non-fatal disability [2], which in turn may contribute to lower quality of life [2].

Weight loss leads to metabolic and functional benefits [3]. However, a potential drawback of weight loss in older adults is the accompanying loss of skeletal muscle mass [4], which in turn might accelerate the development of sarcopenia [5]. Strategies to reduce the loss of skeletal muscle mass during weight loss include resistance exercise and sufficient intake of high quality protein [6, 7]. Resistance exercise stimulates muscle protein synthesis, which in turn supports muscle mass preservation and muscle function [8]. In addition, high dietary protein intake has been shown to stimulate muscle protein synthesis in older adults [1, 9–11]. Several studies indicate that, in contrast to young adults, older adults might be resistant to anabolic stimuli from protein, which implies a blunted post prandial response [12, 13].

The number of weight loss trials in overweight or obese older adults is limited, and trials combining resistance exercise with a high protein diet are scarce [14]. We previously studied the effect of a high whey protein-, leucine- and vitamin D-enriched supplement on muscle mass preservation during a 13-week weight loss program including 3 times/week resistance exercise in obese older adults [15]. Subjects in the intervention group received a supplement containing 21 g whey protein (10 servings/wk), whereas the control group received an isocaloric control supplement. This study showed that the intervention group significantly preserved their muscle mass compared to the control group with an effect size of 0.95 kg (95% CI: 0.09;1.81).

Generally, dieticians give dietary advice regarding weight loss treatment based on regular foods, not including any specific supplements. Porter-Starr et al. [16] recently evaluated the effect of a high protein hypocaloric diet using meal-based protein foods in obese older adults over a 6-month period. They found a positive effect on physical performance, but no significant effect on fat free mass (FFM). No studies so far have evaluated the effects of a high protein diet using regular foods with or without resistance exercise on the preservation of FFM during weight loss in older overweight and obese subjects. In the present study we therefore evaluated the effects of a high protein diet and/or resistance training on preservation of FFM, fat mass (FM) loss, waist circumference loss and improvement of handgrip strength and physical performance during a 10-week weight loss trial in overweight and obese adults aged 55 years and over.

Methods

Subjects

Overweight and obese men and women (≥55 y) with BMI ≥ 28 kg/m^2, or BMI > 25 kg/m^2 with waist circumference > 88 cm (women) or > 102 cm (men), were recruited from the Amsterdam area through local flyers and advertisements. Potential subjects were excluded when they had participated in any weight loss program three months prior to screening; when participation in the resistance training program was considered unsafe according to a physiotherapist; or when they were not able to comply with the full study protocol. All women were postmenopausal and did not use hormone replacement therapy. A full description of the eligibility criteria is online available in the Dutch Trial Register (NTR4556, www.trialregister.nl). The study was approved by the Medical Ethics Committee Independent Review Board Nijmegen, Netherlands (NL43226.072.14) and written informed consent was obtained from all subjects. The study took place from May 2014 through December 2014 at the Amsterdam University of Applied Sciences in The Netherlands.

Design and randomization procedures

We performed a 10-week randomized controlled trial with a 2-by-2 factorial design combining the factors 'high protein diet' and 'resistance exercise'. Eligible subjects were randomly allocated to either the control group (C) receiving a hypocaloric normal protein dietary advice, the high protein diet group (Pr) receiving a hypocaloric high protein dietary advice, the exercise group (Ex) receiving a hypocaloric normal protein dietary advice with an exercise program, or to the high protein diet and exercise group (PrEx) receiving both a hypocaloric high protein dietary advice and an exercise program. Randomization envelopes with four different codes stratified by gender were generated using a random number generator by the study coordinator. Body composition, waist circumference, handgrip strength and physical performance were assessed at study baseline and after 5 and 10 weeks of intervention.

Hypocaloric diet and protein advice

All subjects followed a hypocaloric diet of 600 kcal below estimated energy needs [17]. Energy needs were estimated by multiplying measured resting energy expenditure using indirect calorimetry (Vmax Encore n29; Viasys Healthcare, Houten, the Netherlands) with the estimated physical activity level using a 3-day physical activity record. Prescribed dietary protein intake was 0.8 g/kg body weight (BW) for the normal protein dietary advice, and 1.3 g/kg for the high protein dietary advice (using current BW for BMI < 30 kg/m^2 or using BW at BMI 27.5 kg/m^2 for those with a BMI ≥ 30 kg/m^2) [18].

For each subject the amount of energy (kcal) and protein (g) was calculated and incorporated in the dietary advice, which was given at study baseline, together with a specific food variation list for either the high protein or the normal protein diet. Foods were not provided. During intervention, subjects of all groups received five dietary consultations; two times during a face-to-face visit at week 5 and 9, and three times by telephone in week 2, 4 and 7. Dietary intake was assessed by a 3-day food record at baseline, after 5 and 10 weeks of intervention. Intake after 5 and 10 weeks was used to evaluate compliance to the prescribed diet. Food records were checked for completeness during study visits and additional information about unclear items or amounts was obtained. Total energy and macronutrient intakes were calculated using a computerized Dutch Food Composition Table [19].

Exercise program

The exercise program involved resistance training 3 days a week for 1-h sessions. The training started with a 10-min warming up followed by two sets of 50 s of the following exercises: squats, lunges, chest press, shoulder press, biceps curls, triceps extensions, standing rows, step-ups and crunches. During the 10-week period the number of sets was gradually increased from 2 – 3 set for all exercises, the time to perform the exercises increased from 50 – 75 s, and resistance was increased by using dumbbells, elastic bands, medicine balls and a step bench. The training ended with 5-min cooling down. The exercise program was developed by certified trainers and a physiotherapist and training sessions were supervised by certified trainers. Attendance to the training sessions was recorded by the trainer.

Measurement of body composition, waist circumference, handgrip strength and physical performance

Body composition including FFM (primary outcome) and FM was determined using air displacement plethysmography (BODPOD, Life Measurement Inc., Concord, CA). BW was measured on the calibrated scale as part of the BODPOD system. Waist circumference was measured in a standing position halfway between the anterior superior iliac spine and the lower rib after normal expiration. Handgrip strength was measured with an isometric handgrip dynamometer (JAMAR 5030 J1, Sammons Preston Rolyan, Bollingbrook, CA) while the subject was seated with the elbow flexed at 90°. Three consecutive measures of handgrip strength (kg) at both hands were recorded to the nearest 0.1 kg and the sum of the maximum value of left and right hand was calculated. Physical performance was assessed with a 400-m gait speed test (m/s) [20], a 4-m gait speed test (fastest of 2 repetitions of usual gait speed, (m/s)), and a chair stand test (s) [21].

Statistical analysis

Double-data entry was performed and discrepancies were checked and adjusted. Statistical analyses were performed with FFM change as primary outcome. A sample size of $n = 21$ per study group, $n = 84$ in total, provided 80% power to detect an absolute difference of 0.5 kg FFM with SD 0.4 kg and $P < 0.05$ (2-sided) [22, 23].

Subject characteristics and dietary intake at baseline were compared between groups using an independent samples t-test or the Fisher Exact test. Intention-to-treat analysis was performed using last observations carried forward for subjects with missing week 5 and/or week 10 measurements. Between group differences on outcome variables were analysed using a mixed linear model including time, protein (high/normal), exercise (yes/no) as fixed factors, subject as random factor and sex and baseline value of the outcome variable as covariates. For all outcome variables the interaction for protein*exercise was tested. This interaction tested whether the effect in the exercise groups is dependent on whether the subjects received the high or the normal protein diet (and vice versa). Within group changes over 10 weeks were estimated using a paired t-test.

Statistical analyses were performed using SPSS software (version 22.0, IBM). Data in text and tables are expressed as means with SD, unless stated otherwise. Statistical significance was defined as a two-tailed $P < 0.05$.

Results

Subjects

We randomized 122 subjects into the four study groups. Before the baseline visits 22 subjects declined study participation for personal reasons. The number of subjects screened, excluded, randomized, and included in the analysis is shown in Fig. 1. Mean age of the study population was 62.4 ± 5.4 y, 36% was male, mean BMI was 32.2 ± 4.3 kg/m^2 and 66% was obese. There were no relevant differences in subject's characteristics between the study groups at study baseline (Table 1). Of the 100 subjects with a baseline visit, 32 subjects dropped out during the study because of adverse events not related to the study ($n = 7$), adverse events related to the study ($n = 1$, lash), personal reasons ($n = 14$), or unknown reasons ($n = 10$).

Dietary intake and adherence to exercise program

There were no differences between groups in self-reported mean dietary intake at baseline and the energy reduction during treatment (Table 2). Protein intake during the trial was 1.13 ± 0.35 g/kg/d in the high protein groups. Protein intake was on average 87% of the protein target of 1.3 g/kg/d, with 29% of the subjects reaching this target. In the normal protein groups the protein intake during the trial was 0.98 ± 0.29 g/kg/d, which was on average 123% of the

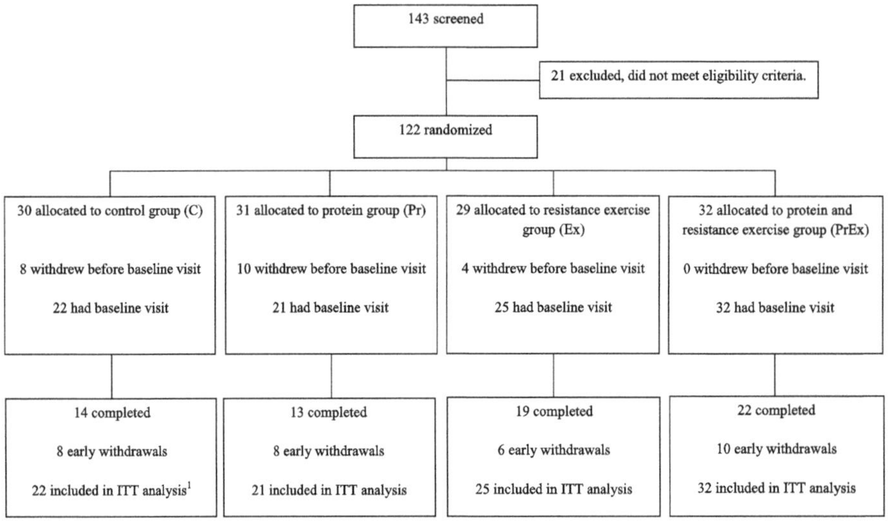

Fig. 1 Flow chart of number of subjects screened, randomized, completed intervention and included in the analysis. [1] For one subject no body composition data were available at baseline, therefore $n = 21$ subjects were included in the intention to treat (ITT) analysis for the primary outcome fat free mass

protein target, with 78% of the subjects reaching the protein target of 0.8 g/kg/d. The high protein groups had on average a 16.3 ± 5.2 g/d higher protein intake during intervention ($p = 0.002$) compared to the normal protein groups.

With respect to the exercise program, mean adherence was 2.8 ± 0.3 times/week.

Effects on body weight, waist circumference, FFM and FM

The 10-week weight loss trial resulted in a significantly decreased BW, waist circumference and FM in all groups. Overall loss in BW was -2.1 ± 2.6 kg, without significant effects of protein and exercise. Comparable results were observed for changes in waist circumference, where a mean decrease of −4 ± 4 cm was observed with no significant effects of protein and exercise (Table 3). Figure 2 shows that the intervention did not significantly affect change in FFM, with exception of the high protein-exercise group which showed a significant increase in FFM of 0.6 ± 1.3 kg ($p = 0.011$). There was no significant effect of high protein and exercise on change in FFM and FM, but exercise significantly decreased body fat percentage with 0.8% ($p = 0.048$).

Table 1 Baseline characteristics of 100 obese older subjects by treatment[a]

Characteristic	Control ($n = 22$)	Protein ($n = 21$)	Exercise ($n = 25$)	Protein + Exercise ($n = 32$)	p-value[b]
Sex, n (% male)	6 (27%)	8 (38%)	9 (36%)	13 (41%)	0.786
Origin, % Caucasian	82%	86%	68%	84%	0.418
Age, y	63.4 ± 4.3	61.9 ± 6.1	63.1 ± 6.0	61.5 ± 5.1	0.529
Body weight, kg	92.7 ± 5.1	93.0 ± 15.3	90.7 ± 14.7	93.5 ± 14.4	0.912
BMI, kg/m^2	33.2 ± 4.8	32.1 ± 4.6	32.2 ± 4.7	31.6 ± 3.4	0.584
BMI ≥ 30 kg/m^2, n (%)	16 (73%)	13 (62%)	16 (64%)	21 (66%)	0.886
Waist circumference, cm[c]	110 ± 13	110 ± 12	107 ± 13	107 ± 9	0.761
Fat mass, %[c]	45.3 ± 8.2	44.7 ± 8.5	43.2 ± 8.7	41.6 ± 7.8	0.383
Fat free mass, kg[d]	51.0 ± 13.1	51.2 ± 10.4	51.5 ± 11.5	54.8 ± 12.7	0.584
Handgrip strength, kg[e]	62.2 ± 22.0	65.2 ± 17.4	70.1 ± 21.8	73.9 ± 24.3	0.234
4-m gait speed, m/s[f]	1.17 ± 0.33	1.32 ± 0.28	1.28 ± 0.22	1.25 ± 0.18	0.284
400-m gait speed, m/s[f]	1.40 ± 0.17	1.42 ± 0.20	1.49 ± 0.21	1.51 ± 0.22	0.133
Time to complete 5 stands, s[f]	13.5 ± 3.2	12.6 ± 3.1	11.1 ± 3.0	11.7 ± 3.4	0.058

[a]Data are presented as means ± SD or as number (percentage); [b]Significance level (two-sided p-value) for comparison between groups using One-Way ANOVA or Chi-square test (sex, origin and BMI group); [c]n protein + exercise group = 31; [d]n control group = 21; [e]Sum of maximum of left and right hand; n protein group = 20; [f] n exercise group = 24

Table 2 Dietary intake in the study groups at baseline and during intervention[a]

		Control (*n* = 20)	Protein (*n* = 21)	Exercise (*n* = 25)	Protein + Exercise (*n* = 31)	*P* value[b]	Protein groups (*n* = 52)	Control groups (*n* = 45)	*P* value[c]
Energy, kcal/d	Baseline	1928 ± 849	1932 ± 539	1877 ± 522	2061 ± 621	0.730	2009 ± 587	1900 ± 678	0.397
	During intervention	1650 ± 531	1726 ± 449	1569 ± 463	1784 ± 579	0.452	1761 ± 526	1605 ± 490	0.137
Protein, g/day	Baseline	85.7 ± 31.0	82.6 ± 21.4	82.6 ± 23.4	93.2 ± 31.2	0.425	88.9 ± 27.9	83.9 ± 26.7	0.372
	During intervention	76.6 ± 21.1	89.3 ± 22.6	73.9 ± 22.4	92.8 ± 32.9	0.025	91.4 ± 29.0	75.1 ± 21.6	0.002
Protein, g/kg/day	Baseline	0.95 ± 0.36	0.92 ± 0.34	0.93 ± 0.30	1.00 ± 0.31	0.825	0.97 ± 0.32	0.94 ± 0.33	0.662
	During intervention	0.87 ± 0.29	1.02 ± 0.36	0.84 ± 0.23	1.02 ± 0.35	0.081	1.02 ± 0.35	0.86 ± 0.26	0.008
Protein, g/adj_kg/day[d]	Baseline	1.12 ± 0.45	1.04 ± 0.30	1.08 ± 0.36	1.14 ± 0.39	0.820	1.10 ± 0.35	1.10 ± 0.39	0.972
	During intervention	1.00 ± 0.27	1.13 ± 0.33	0.97 ± 0.32	1.13 ± 0.37	0.177	1.13 ± 0.35	0.98 ± 0.29	0.027
Protein, en%[e]	Baseline	18.5 ± 3.3	17.6 ± 3.4	17.9 ± 3.7	18.3 ± 3.6	0.838	18.0 ± 3.5	18.2 ± 3.5	0.814
	During intervention	18.9 ± 2.2	21.1 ± 3.5	18.9 ± 3.0	21.2 ± 4.6	0.033	21.1 ± 4.1	19.0 ± 2.6	0.002
Carbohydrate, en%	Baseline	44.2 ± 5.2	43.3 ± 6.5	45.3 ± 6.0	43.7 ± 8.6	0.760	43.5 ± 7.7	44.8 ± 5.7	0.343
	During intervention	46.2 ± 5.8	40.4 ± 6.1	47.1 ± 6.4	43.3 ± 6.2	0.002	42.2 ± 6.3	46.7 ± 6.1	0.001
Fat, en%	Baseline	33.1 ± 6.3	34.1 ± 5.6	32.3 ± 6.9	32.0 ± 7.7	0.832	33.3 ± 6.9	32.8 ± 6.6	0.825
	During intervention	30.9 ± 5.7	33.3 ± 5.7	29.2 ± 6.9	30.6 ± 7.1	0.214	31.7 ± 6.7	30.0 ± 6.4	0.204

[a]Data represent means ± SD using last observations carried forward; Intake during intervention is mean intake data at week 5 and 10; [b]Significance level of differences between four groups using One-Way ANOVA; [c]Significance level of differences between protein and non-protein groups using the t-test; [d]Protein in g/kg/day with adjusted weight using current weight for BMI < 30 kg/m^2 or using weight at BMI 27.5 kg/m^2 for BMI ≥ 30 kg/m^2, to make it comparable to the protein target; [e]en% stands for % of energy intake

Table 3 Change in outcome measures at 10 weeks of intervention with protein and exercise effects[a]

	Control (*n* = 22)	Protein (*n* = 21)	Exercise (*n* = 25)	Protein + Exercise (*n* = 32)	Protein effect Beta (95% CI)[b]	*P*[c]	Exercise effect Beta (95% CI)[b]	*P*[c]	Protein * Exercise interaction Beta (95% CI)[d]	*P*[e]
Body weight, kg	−1.7 ± 1.8*	−2.1 ± 3.6*	−2.6 ± 2.9*	−2.0 ± 2.2*	+0.1 (−0.7;1.0)	0.763	−0.3 (−1.1;0.5)	0.472	NS	
BMI, kg/m^2	−0.6 ± 0.6*	−0.8 ± 1.1*	−1.0 ± 1.0*	−0.9 ± 0.9*	−0.0 (−0.3;0.3)	0.924	−0.2 (−0.5;0.1)	0.213	NS	
Waist circumference, cm	−3 ± 4*	−3 ± 4*	−4 ± 4*	−3 ± 3*[f]	+0.3 (−0.9;1.4)	0.673	−0.4 (−1.6;0.8)	0.555	NS	
Fat mass, kg	−1.5 ± 2.5*[g]	−2.1 ± 3.4*	−2.8 ± 3.7*	−2.6 ± 2.4*	−0.0 (−1.0;0.9)	0.946	−0.8 (−1.7;0.2)	0.124	NS	
Fat percentage, %	−1.0 ± 2.1*[g]	−1.3 ± 2.2*	−1.9 ± 3.3*	−2.1 ± 2.0*	−0.1 (−0.9;0.6)	0.736	−0.8 (−1.6;−0.0)	0.048	NS	
Fat free mass, kg	−0.0 ± 1.4[g]	0.0 ± 1.5	+0.2 ± 2.3	+0.6 ± 1.3*	+0.1 (−0.4;0.7)	0.666	+0.3 (−0.2;0.9)	0.233	NS	
Handgrip strength, kg[h]	+1.8 ± 6.6	−1.7 ± 6.5	−1.8 ± 11.6	+2.0 ± 6.0	−2.2 (−6.4;2.1)	0.311	−1.9 (−6.0;2.1)	0.346	6.2 (0.6;11.8)	0.030
4-m gait speed, m/s	+0.13 ± 0.24*	+0.08 ± 0.26	+0.08 ± 0.13*[i]	+0.20 ± 0.24*	−0.04 (−0.15;0.06)	0.440	−0.04 (−0.14;0.06)	0.476	0.14 (0.00;0.28)	0.045
400-m gait speed, m/s	+0.04 ± 0.15	+0.07 ± 0.10*	+0.07 ± 0.07*[i]	+0.08 ± 0.15*	+0.02 (−0.03;0.06)	0.445	+0.01 (−0.03;0.06)	0.554	NS	
Repeated chair stands, s	−1.6 ± 2.1*	−1.6 ± 1.7*	−1.0 ± 2.7[i]	−1.4 ± 2.7*	−0.1 (−0.9;0.6)	0.703	−0.2 (−0.9;0.6)	0.643	NS	

[a]Data represent means ± SD using last observations carried forward; [b]Estimate of protein or exercise effect at week 10 using mixed linear model including time, sex, protein (high/normal), exercise (yes/no) and baseline value; [c]Significance level of estimate of protein or exercise effect at week 10 using mixed linear model; [d] Estimate of interaction effect of protein*exercise at week 10 using mixed linear model including time, sex, protein (high/normal), exercise (yes/no), protein*exercise and baseline value only presented when the interaction effect was significant ($P < 0.1$). The effect of the combined protein-exercise intervention can be calculated by summating the beta's of the protein effect, the exercise effect and the interaction protein*exercise effect; [e]Significance level of the interaction effect of protein*exercise at week 10 using mixed linear model; [f]$n = 31$; [g]$n = 21$; [h]Sum of maximum of left and right hand, n protein group = 20; [i]$n = 24$; [*] Significant mean change at week 10 within group using a paired t-test; NS not significant ($P \geq 0.1$)

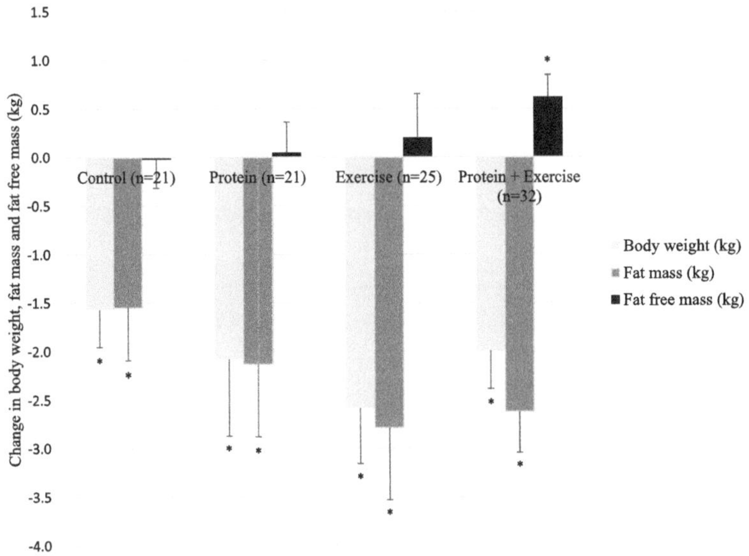

Fig. 2 Change in body weight, fat mass and fat free mass in the four study groups. Data represent mean changes over 10 weeks with SEM using last observations carried forward for subjects with missing week 5 and/or week 10 measurements. * indicates within group change using a paired t-test

There was no significant protein*exercise interaction for FM and FFM.

Effects on handgrip strength and physical performance

No significant change in handgrip strength was observed over time whereas all physical performance tests improved over time. However, no significant effects of protein and exercise on handgrip strength and physical performance tests were observed (Table 3). There was a significant interaction for protein*exercise for handgrip strength ($p = 0.030$) and 4-m gait speed ($p = 0.045$), indicating that combining a high protein diet with exercise had greater positive effects on handgrip strength and 4-m gait speed than high protein diet or exercise only (Table 3).

Discussion

In the present randomized controlled trial in overweight and obese older adults during weight loss, we observed no significant effect of the high protein diet (although at a lower level than targeted) and resistance exercise on FFM preservation and no statistically significant interaction between high protein and resistance exercise. However, only in the group with the combined intervention of high protein diet and resistance exercise program, FFM significantly increased.

The recommended dietary allowance (RDA) for protein is 0.8 g/kg/d and is age-independent [24]. However, the recent expert opinion on protein requirements of older adults is higher, and recommended protein intake ranges from 1.0 – 1.2 g/kg/d [25]. Specific recommendations for obese older adults during weight loss do not exist. Weijs et al. [26] showed that protein requirements under the challenged conditions of weight loss may be substantially higher than 0.8 g/kg/d, and are probably even higher than 1.2 g/kg/d in order to preserve muscle mass.

In this study we demonstrated that it is difficult to reach a 1.3 g/kg/d protein intake using a hypocaloric high protein diet based on regular food products (mean intake was 1.13 g/kg/d).

Although subjects in the high protein groups had a 16 g per day higher protein intake compared to the normal protein groups (mean intake was 0.98 g/kg/d), the difference in protein intake might have been too small in order to detect an effect on preservation in FFM. Previously, we studied the effect of a high-whey protein, leucine and vitamin D supplement during weight loss on muscle mass preservation in older obese adults [15]. In that study, the difference in protein intake was 28 g/d with an intake of 1.11 g/kg/d in the intervention group and 0.85 g/kg/d in the control group. This difference resulted in a muscle preserving effect of 0.95 kg. However, besides the difference in protein intake, also other components of the supplement, including leucine, vitamin D and other micronutrients might explain the effect on preservation of FFM in that study.

Two other possible explanations for the absence of a high-protein effect on FFM preservation in the present study should be considered. Firstly, older adults might require a minimum threshold of protein with one eating moment to raise muscle protein synthesis levels. Previous studies showed that a minimal amount of 20 g of high quality protein per meal is needed to stimulate protein synthesis above baseline levels [27]. In our former study, the protein supplement was, ten times per week, supplied as 21 g protein at once [15]. In the current study, only 39% of the subjects in the high protein groups had in total at least one eating moment with ≥ 20 g protein over the recorded days during intervention (week 5 and 10).

A second explanation for the absence of a high-protein effect on FFM preservation is the protein composition of the diet. Whey protein has been shown to be very effective in stimulating postprandial muscle protein accretion in older men [28, 29], which has been ascribed to its fast digestion and to the high leucine content. Since we did not focus on specific types of proteins during dietary counseling it is likely that the amount of leucine known to stimulate muscle protein synthesis (at least 2 g per meal [12]) for older adults was not reached for most subjects in our study.

We observed no overall exercise effect, except for relative fat mass (Table 3). However, when analysing the interaction between gender and exercise a significant interaction for FFM with beta +1.1 kg (95%–CI: –0,0;2,3) was shown, indicating that FFM in males responds stronger to the exercise program than FFM in females. This is in line with expectations based on literature [30].

We observed a significant improvement in physical performance during 10-weeks intervention in all groups. We did, however, not observe an additional improvement in physical performance as a results of higher protein intake or resistance training. A suggested explanation could be that the observed FM loss overruled the possible effects of improvements in physical functioning due to high protein and exercise [31].

Previous studies have shown that on average 25–30% of weight loss is lean mass in older obese adults [14]. In our study, all groups including the control group preserved their FFM. It could be speculated that subjects in the control group increased their level of physical activities and sports activities themselves to compensate for the fact that they were not allowed to participate in the exercise group training sessions. A slight increase in physical activity level during intervention was observed for all groups, and this was not different between the groups, which could partly explain the FFM preservation even in the control group. Another explanation could be the relatively high intake of protein in the control groups (average was 0.98 g/kg), which further reduced the protein intake contrast between groups and might have been beneficial for FFM preservation.

A limitation of this study is the unequally distributed number of subjects that withdrew from participation in the study groups before the baseline measurements. Group allocation could be a reason for declining further participation. Another limitation was the lower than expected magnitude of weight loss, which can be partly explained by the preservation of (C, Pr, Ex groups) or gain (PrEx group) in FFM. Furthermore, we advised a -600 kcal/d reduction in energy intake, which was not achieved based on the analyses of the 3-d food records. Most of previous successful weight loss trials in overweight older adults [14] had weekly group sessions with a dietitian. In our study, the subjects had a bi-weekly consultation, which may also have resulted in the limited weight loss observed. Since the amount of weight loss is modest, the change in FFM is also small. Additionally, the duration of the study might have been too short to achieve sufficient weight loss for group differences in FFM preservation due to protein intake to manifest. Finally, our study was designed and powered to find an effect of protein on FFM with a 0.5 g/kg/d difference between groups; however, only a 0.15 g/kg/d difference in protein intake was achieved, therefore making it difficult to draw firm conclusions regarding a higher versus control protein intake during weight loss with or without resistance exercise.

In conclusion, the lower than targeted protein intake of 1.13 g/kg/d obtained by consuming regular protein rich foods did not significantly affect FFM and FM change during modest weight loss in older overweight and obese subjects. There was no significant interaction between the high protein diet and resistance exercise for FFM. However, only the group with the combined intervention of the high protein diet and the resistance exercise program significantly increased in FFM. This suggests that combining protein with resistance exercise is beneficial for FFM preservation during weight loss in older adults, which should be confirmed by future studies using a larger protein contrast.

Abbreviations

BW: Body weight; C: Control group; Ex: Exercise group; FFM: Fat free mass; FM: Fat mass; ITT: Intention-to-treat; Pr: High protein diet group; PrEx: High protein diet and exercise group

Acknowledgments

We gratefully acknowledge the expert assistance of Minse de Bos-Kuil, Martinet Streppel, Michael Davidson, Suzan Bakker, Yalcin Batur, Darshan Brassinga, Sandra Brug, Roukaya Eter, Inge Evers, Daan van Geebergen, Merel Godyla, Jordy de Groot, Madelief Jambroes, Lois Kaersenhout, Jonathan Klaassen, Roos Klaver, Hetty Korsten, Nikki Kremer, Sofie Krop, Bram Kurk, Yasmine Lhassani, Aline Meijlink, Anna Mickiewicz, Qudsia Mirza, Elise Plat, Mariëtte van Rijmenam, Sadia Rodjan, Anna Rootjes, Eva Sayers, Kim Schut, Esther Sjouwerman, Emiel van der Steen, Alicia Toby, Maarten Troost, Tirza Wennekes, Linda Zevenhek.

Funding

This research did not receive any specific grant from funding agencies in the public, commercial, or not-for-profit sectors.

Availability of data and materials

The datasets used and/or analysed during the current study available from the corresponding author on reasonable request.

Authors' contributions

The authors' contributions were as follows: PJMW and AMV: designed the research (project conception, development of overall research plan, and study oversight); SEvdP, AMV, RGM: conducted the research (hands-on conduct of the experiments and data collection); AMV, MFE, PJMW analyzed the data or performed the statistical analysis; AMV, MFE, RGM, MV, and PJMW wrote the manuscript; and PJMW: had primary responsibility for the final content. AMV, MFE, RGM, SEvdP, MV and PJMW had no conflict of interest. All authors read and approved the final manuscript.

Competing interests

The authors declare that they have no competing interests.

Consent for publication
Not applicable.

Ethics approval and consent to participate
The study was approved by the Medical Ethics Committee Independent Review Board Nijmegen, Netherlands (NL43226.072.14) and written informed consent was obtained from all subjects.

Author details
[1]Department of Nutrition and Dietetics, Faculty of Sports and Nutrition, Amsterdam University of Applied Sciences, Dr. Meurerlaan 8, 1067 SM Amsterdam, Netherlands. [2]Department of Health Sciences, Faculty of Earth and Life Sciences, VU University Amsterdam, De Boelenlaan 1085, 1081 HV Amsterdam, Netherlands. [3]Department of Nutrition and Dietetics, Internal Medicine, VU University Medical Center, De Boelenlaan 1117, 1081 HV Amsterdam, Netherlands.

References
1. Mathus-Vliegen EM. Obesity management task force of the european association for the study of obesity. Prevalence, pathophysiology, health consequences and treatment options of obesity in the elderly: a guideline. Obes Facts. 2012;5:460–83.
2. Groessl EJ, Kaplan RM, Barrett-Connor E, Ganiats TG. Body mass index and quality of well-being in a community of older adults. Am J Prev Med. 2004; 26(2):126–9.
3. Bales CW, Buhr G. Is obesity bad for older persons? a systematic review of the pros and cons of weight reduction in later life. J Am Med Dir Assoc. 2008;9(5):302–12.
4. Houston DK, Nicklas BJ, Zizza CA. Weighty concerns: the growing prevalence of obesity among older adults. J Am Diet Assoc. 2009;109(11):1886–95.
5. Miller SL, Wolfe RR. The danger of weight loss in the elderly. J Nutr Health Aging. 2008;12(7):487–91. Review.
6. Kim JE, O'Connor LE, Sands LP, Slebodnik MB, Campbell WW. Effects of dietary protein intake on body composition changes after weight loss in older adults: a systematic review and meta-analysis. Nutr Rev. 2016;74(3):210–24.
7. Weinheimer EM, Sands LP, Campbell WW. A systematic review of the separate and combined effects of energy restriction and exercise on fat-free mass in middle-aged and older adults: implications for sarcopenic obesity. Nutr Rev. 2010;68(7):375–88.
8. Frimel TN, Sinacore DR, Villareal DT. Exercise attenuates the weight-loss-induced reduction in muscle mass in frail obese older adults. Med Sci Sports Exerc. 2008;40:1213–9.
9. Wolfe RR, Miller SL, Miller KB. Optimal protein intake in the elderly. Clin Nutr. 2008;27:675–84.
10. Bosse JD, Dixon BM. Dietary protein in weight management: a review proposing protein spread and change theories. Nutr Metab (Lond). 2012;9:81.
11. Bauer J, Biolo G, Cederholm T, Cesari M, Cruz-Jentoft AJ, Morley JE, et al. Evidence-based recommendations for optimal dietary protein intake in older people: a position paper from the PROT-AGE study group. J Am Med Dir Assoc. 2013;14(8):542–59.
12. Breen L, Phillips SM. Skeletal muscle protein metabolism in the elderly: Interventions to counteract the 'anabolic resistance' of ageing. Nutr Metab (Lond). 2011;8:68.
13. Burd NA, Yang Y, Moore DR, Tang JE, Tarnopolsky MA, Phillips SM. Greater stimulation of myofibrillar protein synthesis with ingestion of whey protein isolate v. micellar casein at rest and after resistance exercise in elderly men. Br J Nutr. 2012;108:958–62.
14. Waters DL, Ward AL, Villareal DT. Weight loss in obese adults 65 years and older: a review of the controversy. Exp Gerontol. 2013;48(10):1054–61.
15. Verreijen AM, Verlaan S, Engberink MF, Swinkels S, de Vogel-van den Bosch J, Weijs PJ. A high whey protein-, leucine-, and vitamin D-enriched supplement preserves muscle mass during intentional weight loss in obese older adults: a double-blind randomized controlled trial. Am J Clin Nutr. 2015;101(2):279–86.
16. Porter Starr KN, Pieper CF, Orenduff MC, McDonald SR, McClure LB, Zhou R, et al. Improved function with enhanced protein intake per meal: a pilot study of weight reduction in frail, obese older adults. J Gerontol A Biol Sci Med Sci. 2016;71(10):1369–75.
17. Dutch Institute for Health Improvement CBO. Guideline diagnostics and treatment of obesity in adults and children. Utrecht: Van Zuiden Communications; 2008.
18. Weijs PJ, Sauerwein HP, Kondrup J. Protein recommendations in the ICU: g protein/kg body weight - which body weight for underweight and obese patients? Clin Nutr. 2012;31(5):774–5.
19. RIVM/Voedingscentrum. Dutch Food Composition Database (NEVO). The Hague; 2011.
20. Sayers SP, Guralnik JM, Newman AB, Brach JS, Fielding RA. Concordance and discordance between two measures of lower extremity function: 400 meter self-paced walk and SPPB. Aging Clin Exp Res. 2006;18(2):100–6.
21. Guralnik JM, Simonsick EM, Ferrucci L, Glynn RJ, Berkman LF, Blazer DG, et al. A short physical performance battery assessing lower extremity function: association with self-reported disability and prediction of mortality and nursing home admission. J Gerontol. 1994;49:M85–94.
22. Noakes M, Keogh JB, Foster PR, Clifton PM. Effect of an energy-restricted, high-protein, low-fat diet relative to a conventional high-carbohydrate, low-fat diet on weight loss, body composition, nutritional status, and markers of cardiovascular health in obese women. Am J Clin Nutr. 2005;81(6):1298–306.
23. Leidy HJ, Carnell NS, Mattes RD, Campbell WW. Higher protein intake preserves lean mass and satiety with weight loss in pre-obese and obese women. Obesity (Silver Spring). 2007;15(2):421–9.
24. EFSA Panel on Dietetic Products, Nutrition and Allergies (NDA). Scientific opinion on dietary reference values for protein. EFSA J. 2012;10:2557.
25. Deutz NE, Bauer JM, Barazzoni R, Biolo G, Boirie Y, Bosy-Westphal A, et al. Protein intake and exercise for optimal muscle function with aging: recommendations from the ESPEN Expert Group. Clin Nutr. 2014;33(6):929–36.
26. Weijs PJ, Wolfe RR. Exploration of the protein requirement during weight loss in obese older adults. Clin Nutr. 2016;35(2):394–8.
27. Moore DR, Churchward-Venne TA, Witard O, Breen L, Burd NA, Tipton KD, et al. Protein ingestion to stimulate myofibrillar protein synthesis requires greater relative protein intakes in healthy older versus younger men. J Gerontol A Biol Sci Med Sci. 2015;70(1):57–62.
28. Pennings B, Boirie Y, Senden JM, Gijsen AP, Kuipers H, van Loon LJ. Whey protein stimulates postprandial muscle protein accretion more effectively than do casein and casein hydrolysate in older men. Am J Clin Nutr. 2011; 93:997–1005.
29. Hector AJ, Marcotte GR, Churchward-Venne TA, Murphy CH, Breen L, von Allmen M, et al. Whey protein supplementation preserves postprandial myofibrillar protein synthesis during short-term energy restriction in overweight and obese adults. J Nutr. 2015;145(2):246–52.
30. Sanal E, Ardic F, Kirac S. Effects of aerobic or combined aerobic resistance exercise on body composition in overweight and obese adults: gender differences. A randomized intervention study. Eur J Phys Rehabil Med. 2013; 49(1):1–11.
31. Davison KK, Ford ES, Cogswell ME, Dietz WH. Percentage of body fat and body mass index are associated with mobility limitations in people aged 70 and older from NHANES III. J Am Geriatr Soc. 2002;50(11):1802–9.

3

Association between energy drink intake, sleep, stress, and suicidality in Korean adolescents: energy drink use in isolation or in combination with junk food consumption

Subin Park[1], Yeeun Lee[2] and Junghyun H. Lee[3*]

Abstract

Background: A considerable amount of research suggests that the frequent use of caffeinated energy drinks may be associated with undesirable effects, particularly so in children and adolescents. This study aimed to investigate the associations between energy drink intake and mental health problems, in isolation or in combination with junk food consumption, in a nationally representative sample of Korean adolescents.

Methods: Data from the 2015 Korean Youth Risk Behavior Web-Based Survey, collected from 68,043 adolescents aged 12–18 years (mean age 15.09 ± 1.72 years), were analyzed. Questionnaires were administered to collect information related to dietary behavior including energy drink intake and junk food consumption. Single item measures of sleep dissatisfaction, stress, depression, suicidal ideation, suicide plan, and suicide attempt were also administered. Associations between energy drink intake and sleep dissatisfaction, perceived severe stress, persistent depressive mood, and suicidality were investigated, and a multivariate approach was taken so that additional variance from demographic and lifestyle factors could be controlled for statistically.

Results: Energy drink intake was significantly associated with sleep dissatisfaction (adjusted odd ratios [AORs] = 1.64 and 1.25), severe stress (AORs = 2.23 and 1.38), depressive mood (AOR = 2.59 and 1.51), suicidal ideation (AORs = 3.14 and 1.43), suicide plan (AORs = 4.65 and 1.78), and suicide attempt (AORs = 6.79 and 1.91), with a higher risk for more frequent use of energy drinks (≥5 times/wk) than for less frequent use (1–4 times/wk). The detrimental effect of energy drinks on mental health was particularly prominent in frequent junk food consumers.

Conclusions: Our data suggest that energy drink intake had detrimental effects related to stress, sleep dissatisfaction, mood, and suicidality, in isolation or in combination with junk food consumption, in Korean adolescents. However, the cross-sectional study design prevents our ability to assess causal relationships.

Keywords: Energy drinks, Junk food, Mood, Suicide, Adolescents

* Correspondence: leejunghyun1@gmail.com
[3]Department of Psychiatry, National Center for Mental Health, 127, Yongmasan-ro, Gwangjin-gu, Seoul 04933, South Korea
Full list of author information is available at the end of the article

Energy drinks are highly caffeinated soft drinks that are marketed as providing mental and physical stimulation and improving energy, athletic performance, and concentration [1]. Concern has been raised because such products sometimes bypass legislation regarding caffeine content [2, 3], and therefore have the potential to put users at risk of intoxication [4, 5]. Energy drinks did not become widely available in South Korea until 2010. Energy drinks boasted an explosive total volume growth of 665 % from introduction in 2010 to 2012, when consumption totaled around 19.9 m liters [6]. Particularly, among teenagers who are overburdened with studying and examinations, the consumption rates are increasing because of its concentration enhancement and awakening and fatigue-relieving effects [5, 7]. Students in South Korea study longer hours and sleep shorter hours than students in other Organization for Economic Cooperation & Development (OECD) countries. In 2009, Korean students studied an average of 7 h 50 min per day, compared to 5 h 21 min in Japan, 5 h 04 min in the US, 3 h 49 min in England, and 6 h 6 min in Finland, and slept an average of 7 h 30 min per day, compared to 8 h 47 min in the US, 8 h 36 min in England, and 8 h 31 min in Finland [8].

Caffeine and sugar content are the main ingredients in energy drinks [9, 10]. Caffeine is most widely known as central nervous system stimulant, which activates noradrenaline and serotonin neurons [11]. Caffeinated energy drinks may also cause activation of methylxanthine [12, 13] which may related to psychological condition including memory, anxiety, or sleep [11], even though these effects seem to vary according to individual sensitivity to the methylxanthine [11, 13]. Excess sugar is also likely to linked to low level of serotonin and brain function [14]. Caffeine use does appear to have important implications in the school environment. Its high consumption has been associated with difficulty sleeping and tiredness in the mornings [15], falling asleep at school [16], behavioral problems [17], violence and conduct disorder [18], and low academic achievement [19].

The frequency and amount of consumption of many food and drink products is known to be highly intercorrelated [20]. For instance, fast food consumption is positively associated with energy drink intake and soft drink consumption, and negatively associated with fruit, vegetable, and milk intake in adolescents [21]. The effects of energy drinks may be best understood in combination with other aspects of diet. With increasing consumption of high-caffeinated energy drinks, an increase in the intake of junk food (processed and snack foods, which are high in fat and/or sugar) is of particular concern in Korean children and adolescents [22]. Previous studies found a relationship between a junk food diet and hyperactive behaviors, depressed mood, and lethargy in children and adolescents [20, 23, 24]. Thus, both energy drink and junk food consumption may adversely affect adolescents' mood and behavior.

The current study aimed to examine the associations between energy drink intake and self-reported sleep dissatisfaction, stress, depression, and suicidality in a nationally representative sample of Korean adolescents. The combined effects of energy drink intake and junk food consumption were also investigated. It was hypothesized that 1) energy drink intake is related to mental health problems such as sleep dissatisfaction, depression, and suicidality and 2) frequent energy drink intake in combination with frequent junk food consumption would be the strongest predictor of such undesirable outcomes.

Methods

Participants and procedures

Data from the 2015 Korean Youth Risk Behavior Web-Based Survey (KYRBS) were used. The KYRBS is an anonymous self-reported online survey conducted annually since 2005 by the Korea Centers for Disease Control and Prevention to identify teenagers' health behaviors with the subjects ranging from middle school freshmen to high school seniors. Using stratified cluster sampling, the middle and high school student samples that represent the teenager population were extracted. After given the instructions of the survey, the students who agreed to participate did the survey during class. Personal data including the respondents' names, schools, phone numbers, addresses, and resident registration numbers were not collected. In 2015, the survey included a total of 800 schools, i.e. 400 middle schools and 400 high schools each, and a total of 70,632 respondents participated. Regarding gender, 35,204 male students and 32,839 female students participated, reaching 96.7 % of participation rate. The average age of the respondents was 15.09 ± 1.72, ranging from 12 to 18. As it can be searched from other sources easily [25], the description of sampling method and survey process will not be discussed in detail further. The KYRBS was reviewed and approved by the institutional review board of Korea Centers for Disease Control and Prevention (2014-06EXP-02-P-A). The KYRBS data used for the present study is openly available [26].

Measurements

Predictor variables

Frequency of energy drink intake during the previous week was assessed on a seven-point scale where 1 = *never*, 2 = *once or twice a week*, 3 = *three or four times a week*, 4 = *five or six times a week*, 5 = *once a day*, 6 = *twice a day*, and 7 = *three times or more a day*. Participants were classified into three groups: highly frequent energy drink intake (≥5 times/week), moderately frequent energy drink intake (1–4 times/week), and infrequent energy drink intake (<1 time/week).

Covariates

Sociodemographic variables included gender, age, school type (middle school, high school), place of residence (name of city), and residential type (residence with family, with relatives, with friends, alone, dormitory, or residence in a facility). Places of residence were dichotomized as rural vs. urban area, and residential type was dichotomized as residence with vs. without family. Perceived academic achievement was assessed using a 5-point Likert scale (high, high-middle, middle, low, low-middle, and low) and further dichotomized as high achievement vs. others.

The frequency of intense-level physical activities was evaluated asking the following. "In recent 7 days, how many days did you engage in physical activities (such as, riding bikes at a rapid speed, lifting up heavy loads, swimming fast and so on) for more than 20 minutes that made you sweat or pant heavily?" The scales were given from 1(none) to 6(more than 5 days a week). Those who engaged in moderate level physical activities for more than five times a week or those who engaged in intense level physical activities for more than three times a week were categorized as 'physically active' group [10, 27].

Frequency of junk food consumption during a previous week was assessed on a seven-point scale where 1 = *never,* 2 = *once or twice a week,* 3 = *three or four times a week,* 4 = *five or six times a week,* 5 = *once a day,* 6 = *twice a day,* and 7 = *three times or more a day.* Junk food consumption was dichotomized as infrequent consumption (≤2 times/week) vs. frequent consumption (≥3 times/week). Lifetime alcohol use was assessed with the following question: "Have you ever used alcohol?" The response options were "yes" or "no."

Outcome variables

The degree of sleep dissatisfaction was measured with the following question: "In the last week, how satisfactory was your sleep in terms of relieving your fatigue?" The response options were very satisfactory (1), satisfactory (2), average (3), unsatisfactory (4), and very unsatisfactory (5). On the basis of the responses, participants were classified into the following two groups for multivariate logistic regression analyses: ≥ average satisfaction with sleep (1–3) and (ii) < average satisfaction with sleep (4–5) [27].

The degree of perceived stress was measured as following: "Usually, to what degree are you stressed? The answers ranged from 1) not at all 2) not so much 3) a little bit 4) quite much 5) very much [26].

The depressed feeling experience in the recent 12 months was measured as following: "Have you experienced sadness or despair to the degree that stopped your daily routine for two weeks?" [26].

Suicidal ideation was evaluated with the following question: "In recent 12 months, have you ever thought of committing a suicide?" Suicide plan was evaluated with the following question: "In recent 12 months, have you planned a suicide in detail?" Suicide attempt was evaluated with the following question: "In recent 12 months, have you ever attempted a suicide?" [26].

Statistical analyses

Univariate logistic regression tests were performed to compare sociodemographic and lifestyle factors between groups (high energy drink use vs. non-use; moderate energy drink use vs. non-use). Odds ratios (ORs) and 95 % confidence intervals (CIs) were calculated using energy drink intake (highly or moderately frequent intake) as the predictor and each sociodemographic and lifestyle factor as the main outcome variables.

Next, to analyze the associations between the adolescents' energy drink intake and mental health variables, multivariate logistic regression tests were performed using energy drink intake as the principal predictor and each mental health variable as the main outcome variables, after controlling for age, gender, school type, area of residence, residential type, level of academic achievement, level of physical activity, and junk food and alcohol consumption.

Next, in order to further examine the nature of the relationships observed, the variables for frequency of energy drink and junk food consumption were combined so that all four possible groupings of frequent/infrequent intake could be investigated in relation to the dichotomous mental health outcomes, using binary logistic regression analysis. Because consuming energy drinks less than once a week and junk food less than three times a week were considered to be the healthiest dietary practices, the infrequent junk food/energy drink condition was chosen as the comparison group. If the confidence intervals were found not to overlap, then the difference between groups was considered to be significant.

All analyses took into account the sampling design parameters, weighting, clustering, and stratification factor. The proportion of general subject characteristics was weighted according to the respondent's probability of being selected for the sex-, grade-, and school type-specific distributions for the region [25, 26]. SPSS (version 21.0; SPSS Inc., Chicago, IL) was used to perform all statistical analyses, and a p-value less than 0.05 was considered to be significant.

Results

The estimated prevalence of highly frequent energy drink intake (≥5 times a week) was 1.4 %, and prevalence of moderately frequent energy drink intake (1–4 times/week) was 10.5 %. Compared to those who had energy drinks less than once a week, those who had energy drinks 5 times or more per week were more likely to be male (OR = 1.79), attend high school (OR = 1.21), live in a rural area (OR = 1.19), achieve higher academic performance (OR = 1.35), eat junk food (OR = 5.70), drink alcohol (OR = 1.35), be physically active (OR = 1.43), and not to live with their family (OR = 3.73). Those whose energy drink intake frequency was between 1–4 times per week showed similar sociodemographic and lifestyle characteristics as those whose energy drink intake was 5 times or more per week, except that they were less likely to achieve higher academic performance compared to those whose energy drink intake was less than once per week (OR = 0.87) (Table 1).

After adjusting for age, gender, school type, area of residence, residential type, academic achievement, junk food and alcohol consumption, and physical activity, participants who used energy drinks frequently were more likely to experience sleep dissatisfaction (adjusted odd ratios [AORs] = 1.64 and 1.25), severe stress (AORs = 2.23 and 1.38), depressive mood (AOR = 2.59 and 1.51), suicidal ideation (AORs = 3.14 and 1.43), suicide plan (AORs = 4.65 and 1.78), and suicide attempt (AORs = 6.79 and 1.91), compared to participants who used energy drinks infrequently or did not use energy drinks, with higher AORs for highly frequent use of energy drinks than for moderately frequent use of energy drinks (Table 2).

In order to further examine the nature of the relationships observed, the frequency of energy drink intake and junk food consumption variables were combined, and the prevalence of mental health problems across the four groups according to frequent/infrequent intake were compared. Compared to the infrequent energy drinks and infrequent junk food group, the frequent energy drinks and/or frequent junk food group were more likely to experience sleep dissatisfaction (AORs = 1.58, 1.32, and 1.30), severe stress (AORs = 1.78, 1.47, and 1.24), depressed mood (AORs = 2.48, 1.55, and 1.39), suicidal ideation (AORs = 2.55, 1.47, and 1.30), suicide plan (AORs = 3.94, 2.96, and 1.65), and suicide attempt (AORs = 5.01, 2.11, and 1.58), with the highest AORs for the frequent energy drinks and frequent junk food group followed by the frequent energy drinks and infrequent junk food group and the infrequent energy drinks and frequent junk food group (Table 3). In particular, the frequent energy drinks and frequent junk food group showed significantly higher risk for depressive mood, suicidal ideation, suicide plan, and suicide attempt compared to the other three groups.

Discussion

Our findings indicate that energy drink consumption is associated with multiple mental health problems in adolescents. Our findings also reveal this deleterious effect was most significant in combination with junk food consumption.

In the present study, approximately 12 % of adolescents consumed energy drinks at least once every week. The adolescents with frequent energy drink intake were more likely to be male and physically active, which is

Table 1 Sociodemographic and lifestyle characteristics of adolescents with frequent energy drink and infrequent energy drink consumption

	Highly frequent energy drinks (≥5/wks) (*N* = 945)	Moderately frequent energy drinks (1-4/wks) (*N* = 7262)	Infrequent energy drinks (*N* = 59836)	Highly frequent energy drinks vs. infrequent energy drinks	Moderately frequent energy drinks vs. infrequent energy drinks
	%	%	%	OR (95 % CI)	OR (95 % CI)
Sex, males	65.0	59.8	51.0	1.79 (1.75-1.82)	1.43 (1.42-1.44)
High school	57.5	54.0	52.8	1.21 (1.18-1.23)	1.05 (1.04-1.06)
Rural residence	7.2	8.1	6.1	1.19 (1.14-1.23)	1.36 (1.35-1.38)
Non-residence with family	13.5	5.5	4.0	3.73 (3.63-3.83)	1.40 (1.38-1.43)
High academic achievement	16.4	11.2	12.7	1.35 (1.32-1.38)	0.87 (0.86-0.87)
Junk food consumption (≥3 times /wk)	46.5	23.8	13.2	5.70 (5.59-5.80)	2.05 (2.03-2.07)
Lifetime alcohol use	54.6	49.0	39.6	1.35 (1.34-1.37)	1.46 (1.45-1.48)
Physically active	47.4	42.5	38.7	1.43 (1.40-1.45)	1.17 (1.16-1.18)
	Mean (SD)	Mean (SD)	Mean (SD)	Mean difference (95 % CI)	Mean difference (95 % CI)
Age, yrs	15.44 (1.78)	15.13 (1.76)	15.07 (1.72)	0.37 (0.35-0.39)	0.06 (0.05-0.07)

Table 2 Association between energy drink intake and mental health problems in Korean adolescents

	Highly frequent energy drinks (≥5/wks) (*N* = 945)	Moderately frequent energy drinks (1-4/wks) (*N* = 7262)	Infrequent energy drinks (*N* = 59836)	Highly frequent energy drinks vs. infrequent energy drinks	Moderately frequent energy drinks vs. infrequent energy drinks
	%	%	%	AOR (95 % CI)	AOR (95 % CI)
Sleep dissatisfaction	52.0	43.2	37.8	1.64 (1.61-1.67)	1.25 (1.25-1.26)
Perceived stress	53.1	41.7	34.3	2.23 (2.19-2.27)	1.38 (1.37-1.39)
Persistent depressive mood	46.0	31.0	22.3	2.59 (2.54-2.65)	1.51 (1.49-1.52)
Suicidal ideation	29.9	15.5	10.9	3.14 (3.07-3.21)	1.43 (1.42-1.45)
Suicide plan	18.2	6.4	3.3	4.65 (4.53-4.78)	1.78 (1.75-1.81)
Suicide attempt	15.1	4.2	2.0	6.79 (6.59-7.00)	1.91 (1.87-1.95)

AOR: odd ratios adjusted for age, gender, school type, residential area, residence type, academic achievement, alcohol and junk food consumption, and physical activity

consistent with previous findings [28, 29]. Masculinity and sports-related identity may be associated with male adolescents' frequent energy drink consumption [29]. The adolescents with frequent energy drink intake, in particular those who consumed energy drinks 5 or more days per week, also tended to reside in a rural area where access to healthy food are limited [30]. It is possible that being separated from family may affect their unregulated dietary habits [31, 32]. In addition they were inclined to consume junk food, which suggests that energy drink and junk food consumption habits tend to co-occur. Our results are compatible with previous findings indicating that junk food consumption is accompanied by other unhealthy eating behaviors [21, 33]. It is notable that highly frequent energy drink consumption, but not moderately frequent consumption, was positively related to high academic achievement in our study. This finding was somewhat inconsistent with previous studies that reported the association between energy drink intake and lower academic performance [28, 34]. Considering the tendency to increase study hours at the cost of sleeping hours among Korean students [8], students whose grades are in the upper ranks may habitually use highly caffeinated drinks with high frequency for its wakening effect. Although some students may have benefited from the instant physiological effects to enhance cognitive performances [35], further research is needed to clarify the effect of energy drink intake on students' academic performance in the long term.

Frequent energy drink intake was significantly associated with a wide range of mental health problems, including sleep dissatisfaction, stress, depressive mood, and suicidality, irrespective of sociodemographic factors, physical activity, alcohol use, and junk food consumption. Particularly, adolescents who consumed energy drinks for 5 days or more every week were at the greatest risk of the aforementioned mental health problems. These findings are consistent with previous studies on the adverse health effects of energy drink consumption [5, 34, 36–38]. In particular, considering a relatively high prevalence of suicidal behavior (i.e., suicidal ideation rates 19.1 % and suicide attempt rates 4.9 %) in Korean adolescents [39, 40], it should be noted that suicide attempt in adolescents who consumed energy drinks five

Table 3 Comparisons of mental health problems according to energy drink and junk food consumption

	Frequent energy drinks/frequent junk food (A) (*N* = 2123)	Frequent energy drinks/infrequent junk food (B) (*N* = 6084)	Infrequent energy drinks/frequent junk food (C) (*N* = 7746)	Infrequent energy drinks/infrequent junk food (D) (*N* = 52090)	C versus D	B versus D	A versus D
	%	%	%	%	AOR (95 % CI)	AOR (95 % CI)	AOR (95 % CI)
Sleep dissatisfaction	47.9	43.0	43.7	36.9	1.30 (1.29-1.31)	1.32 (1.31-1.33)	1.58 (1.56-1. 60)
Perceived stress	45.6	42.2	38.8	33.7	1.24 (1.23-1.25)	1.47 (1.46-1.48)	1.78 (1.76-1.80)
Persistent depressive mood	41.7	29.6	28.2	21.4	1.39 (1.38-1.40)	1.55 (1.54-1.56)	2.48 (2.45-2.51)
Suicidal ideation	24.0	14.7	13.7	10.5	1.30 (1.29-1.32)	1.47 (1.45-1.49)	2.55 (2.51-2.59)
Suicide plan	13.2	5.9	5.1	3.0	1.65 (1.62-1.68)	1.96 (1.93-1.99)	3.94 (3.86-4.03)
Suicide attempt	10.0	3.9	3.1	1.9	1.58 (1.54-1.61)	2.11 (2.07-2.16)	5.01 (4.89-5.14)

AOR: odd ratios adjusted for age, gender, school type, area of residence, residential type, level of academic achievement, level of physical activity, and alcohol use

times or more per week was 7 times as high as those adolescents who consumed energy drinks less than once per week.

Caffeine, the main active ingredient in energy drinks, reduces both sleep duration and sleep quality, manifested by increased wake time after sleep onset and decreased proportion of deep sleep [15, 41, 42]. This may lead to subsequent consumption in reaction to feeling tired on the following day, which can create a vicious cycle of energy drink consumption and poor sleep quality. Also, caffeine overdose can induce nervousness and irritable mood [4], and abstinence of caffeine is highly associated with dysphoric mood states for habitual consumers, which implies caffeine withdrawal [43, 44]. The mood fluctuations and irritability caused by caffeine overdose or withdrawal may account for high levels of perceived stress, depressive mood symptoms, and suicidal behavior in the adolescents who frequently consumed energy drinks.

Taken together, although energy drink consumption may have temporary psychoactive effects such as mood enhancement or reduced fatigue [45, 46], the current study sheds more light on its potential detrimental effects. There is an argument that the removal of the negative consequences of caffeine withdrawal, such as drowsiness or dysphoric mood, may account for the seemingly positive effects of caffeine [47–49]. Accordingly, adolescents who consume energy drinks may frequently experience decreased alertness and depressive mood as withdrawal symptoms of caffeine, which may cause dependence on the caffeinated beverages in order to maintain the normal level of activation, rather than benefitting from its positive effects.

As hypothesized, energy drink intake combined with frequent junk food consumption showed the highest risk for mental health problems in general. Food additives, sugar intake, a low micro-nutrient intake, and polyunsaturated fatty acid (PUFA) deficiency associated with frequent junk food consumption predisposes children to behavioral symptoms, such as hyperactivity, delinquency, and aggressive behaviors [50–53]. In prior studies, chronic high fat food consumption led to hypo-affective states with increased hypothalamic-pituitary-adrenocortical axis reactivity [54], and changed brain reward circuitry into depressive behaviors with an increased brain-derived neurotrophic factor (BDNF) and cAMP response element binding protein (CREB) activity [55]. In addition, consumption of sweetened desserts was reported to lead to peaks and troughs in blood sugar, along with associated periods of hyperactivity and lethargy [20, 52]. Thus, frequent junk food consumption can aggravate the mood effects of caffeine contained in energy drinks. Considering the aforementioned association between junk food consumption and energy drink intake, the danger of adolescents' associated dietary habits demands special attention.

This study has several limitations that deserve discussion. First, due to the cross-sectional design of this study, causal relationships between energy drink intake and mental health problems cannot be determined. Given that energy drink consumption did not predict psychiatric problems at 6-month follow up [38], the association may be bi-directional and reverse causality should also be considered. For example, adolescents who are under stress may be more likely to consume energy drinks for an instant mood elevation effect [56]. Second, sleep dissatisfaction, perceived stress, depressive mood, and suicidality were measured using one item each, rather than with standardized multi-item measures. This may limit the validity of measurements of these variables [26]. Third, information on the constituents of energy drinks and the type of junk food subjects were lacking. Energy drinks contain various ingredients such as caffeine, sugar, guarana, taurine, ginseng, and bitter orange [10]. There are several evidences supporting the differential effects of these ingredients on cognitive performance and mood [35, 57, 58], although only a few studies investigated the interactive cognitive effects of caffeine, taurine and sugar [35, 57]. Further researches are needed to clarify the interactive effects of various ingredients of energy drinks on mood and behaviors. Fourth, data about the number of years the subjects were consuming the drink or the total amount of energy drink intake were also lacking. Finally, energy drink intake and suicide attempts may have been underreported because of concerns over disclosing suicide attempts and frequent use of energy drinks. Therefore, future studies are needed to further clarify the causal relationships among energy drink intake, emotional problems, and other associated food consumption. However, the strength of the present study is its inclusion of data from 68,043 adolescents from a nationally representative sample in South Korea, which improves the external validity of the study results.

Conclusions

In conclusion, study findings indicate that adolescents who consume energy drinks regularly are at great risk of mental health problems, particularly when in combination with junk food consumption. Furthermore, the risk of mental health problems was significantly different between highly frequent and moderately frequent consumers. Therefore, the amount of energy drink intake should be carefully monitored, and an educational intervention on the negative effects of energy drinks is needed for adolescents who consume energy drinks regularly.

Abbreviations
BDNF: Brain-derived neurotrophic factor; CIs: Confidence intervals; CREB: cAMP response element binding protein; KYRBS: Korean Youth Risk Behavior Web-Based Survey; OECD: Organization for Economic Cooperation & Development; ORs: Odds ratios; PUFA: Polyunsaturated fatty acid

Acknowledgements
We thank Ms. Yuji Jung for clerical assistance.

Funding
This work was supported by a clinical research grant (No. 2016-03) from the National Center for Mental Health, Republic of Korea.

Availability of data and materials
The dataset supporting the conclusions of this article is available in the Korea Youth Risk Behavior Web-based Survey website [http://yhs.cdc.go.kr/new/index.asp].

Authors' contributions
JHL, SP contributed in the conception and design of the study. SP, JHL, YL participated in data interpretation, manuscript drafting and revisions. All authors read and approved the final version of the manuscript.

Competing interests
The authors declare that they have no competing interests.

Consent for publication
Not applicable.

Ethics approval and consent to participate
The KYRBS was reviewed and approved by the institutional review board of Korea Centers for Disease Control and Prevention (2014-06EXP-02-P-A). The KYRBS data used for the present study is openly available.

Author details
[1]Department of Research Planning, Mental Health Research Institute, National Center for Mental Health, Seoul, South Korea. [2]Department of psychology, Korea University, Seoul, South Korea. [3]Department of Psychiatry, National Center for Mental Health, 127, Yongmasan ro, Gwangjin-gu, Seoul 04933, South Korea.

References

1. Meadows-Oliver M, Ryan-Krause P. Powering up with sports and energy drinks. J Pediatr Health Care. 2007;21(6):413–6.
2. McCusker RR, Goldberger BA, Cone EJ. Caffeine content of energy drinks, carbonated sodas, and other beverages. J Anal Toxicol. 2006;30(2):112–4.
3. Pomeranz JL. Advanced policy options to regulate sugar-sweetened beverages to support public health. J Public Health Policy. 2012;33(1):75–88.
4. Reissig CJ, Strain EC, Griffiths RR. Caffeinated energy drinks–a growing problem. Drug Alcohol Depend. 2009;99(1-3):1–10.
5. Seifert SM, Schaechter JL, Hershorin ER, Lipshultz SE. Health effects of energy drinks on children, adolescents, and young adults. Pediatrics. 2011; 127(3):511–28.
6. Euromonitor. Energy drinks in South Korea. London: Euromonitor International; 2016.
7. Heckman MA, Sherry K, de Mejia EG. Energy Drinks: an assessment of their market size, consumer demographics, ingredient profile, functionality, and regulations in the United States. Compr Rev Food Sci Food Saf. 2010;9(3): 303–17.
8. Ministry for Health WaFA. State of children and adolescents. Seoul: Ministry for Health, Welfare and Family Affairs; 2010.
9. McLellan TM, Lieberman HR. Do energy drinks contain active components other than caffeine? Nutr Rev. 2012;70(12):730–44.
10. Rath M. Energy drinks: what is all the hype? The dangers of energy drink consumption. J Am Acad Nurse Pract. 2012;24(2):70–6.
11. Nehlig A, Daval JL, Debry G. Caffeine and the central nervous system: mechanisms of action, biochemical, metabolic and psychostimulant effects. Brain Res Brain Res Rev. 1992;17(2):139–70.
12. Daly JW, Butts-Lamb P, Padgett W. Subclasses of adenosine receptors in the central nervous system: interaction with caffeine and related methylxanthines. Cell Mol Neurobiol. 1983;3(1):69–80.
13. Bruce M, Scott N, Lader M, Marks V. The psychopharmacological and electrophysiological effects of single doses of caffeine in healthy human subjects. Br J Clin Pharmacol. 1986;22(1):81–7.
14. Moller SE. Serotonin, carbohydrates, and atypical depression. Pharmacol Toxicol. 1992;71 Suppl 1:61–71.
15. Orbeta RL, Overpeck MD, Ramcharran D, Kogan MD, Ledsky R. High caffeine intake in adolescents: associations with difficulty sleeping and feeling tired in the morning. J Adolesc Health. 2006;38(4):451–3.
16. Calamaro CJ, Mason TB, Ratcliffe SJ. Adolescents living the 24/7 lifestyle: effects of caffeine and technology on sleep duration and daytime functioning. Pediatrics. 2009;123(6):e1005–1010.
17. Jackson DA, Cotter BV, Merchant RC, Babu KM, Baird JR, Nirenberg T, Linakis JG. Behavioral and physiologic adverse effects in adolescent and young adult emergency department patients reporting use of energy drinks and caffeine. Clin Toxicol. 2013;51(7):557–65.
18. Kristjansson AL, Sigfusdottir ID, Frost SS, James JE. Adolescent caffeine consumption and self-reported violence and conduct disorder. J Youth Adolesc. 2013;42(7):1053–62.
19. James JE, Kristjansson AL, Sigfusdottir ID. Adolescent substance use, sleep, and academic achievement: evidence of harm due to caffeine. J Adolesc. 2011;34(4):665–73.
20. Wiles NJ, Northstone K, Emmett P, Lewis G. 'Junk food' diet and childhood behavioural problems: results from the ALSPAC cohort. Eur J Clin Nutr. 2009; 63(4):491–8.
21. French SA, Story M, Neumark-Sztainer D, Fulkerson JA, Hannan P. Fast food restaurant use among adolescents: associations with nutrient intake, food choices and behavioral and psychosocial variables. Int J Obes Relat Metab Disord. 2001;25(12):1823–33.
22. Song Y, Joung H, Engelhardt K, Yoo SY, Paik HY. Traditional v. modified dietary patterns and their influence on adolescents' nutritional profile. Br J Nutr. 2005;93(6):943–9.
23. Zahedi H, Kelishadi R, Heshmat R, Motlagh ME, Ranjbar SH, Ardalan G, Payab M, Chinian M, Asayesh H, Larijani B, et al. Association between junk food consumption and mental health in a national sample of Iranian children and adolescents: the CASPIAN-IV study. Nutrition. 2014;30(11-12):1391–7.
24. Park S, Cho SC, Hong YC, Oh SY, Kim JW, Shin MS, Kim BN, Yoo HJ, Cho IH, Bhang SY. Association between dietary behaviors and attention-deficit/hyperactivity disorder and learning disabilities in school-aged children. Psychiatry Res. 2012;198(3):468–76.
25. Korea Centers for Disease Control and Prevention. Korea youth risk behavior web-based survey: survey summaries. Cheongwon: Korea Centers for Disease Control and Prevention; 2014.
26. Park S, Kim Y. Prevalence, correlates, and associated psychological problems of substance use in Korean adolescents. BMC Public Health. 2016;16:79.
27. Park S. Associations of physical activity with sleep satisfaction, perceived stress, and problematic Internet use in Korean adolescents. BMC Public Health. 2014;14:1143.
28. Pettit ML, DeBarr KA. Perceived stress, energy drink consumption, and academic performance among college students. J Am Coll Heal. 2011;59(5):335–41.
29. Miller KE. Wired: energy drinks, jock identity, masculine norms, and risk taking. J Am Coll Heal. 2008;56(5):481–90.
30. Lutfiyya MN, Lipsky MS, Wisdom-Behounek J, Inpanbutr-Martinkus M. Is rural residency a risk factor for overweight and obesity for US children? Obesity. 2007;15(9):2348–56.
31. Papadaki A, Hondros G, Scott JA, Kapsokefalou M. Eating habits of university students living at, or away from home in Greece. Appetite. 2007;49(1):169–76.
32. Umberson D. Family status and health behaviors: Social control as a dimension of social integration. J Health Soc Behav. 1987;28(3):306–319.
33. Paeratakul S, Ferdinand DP, Champagne CM, Ryan DH, Bray GA. Fast-food consumption among US adults and children: dietary and nutrient intake profile. J Am Diet Assoc. 2003;103(10):1332–8.
34. Jin M-J, Yoon C-H, Ko H-J, Kim H-M, Kim A, Moon H-N, Jung S-P. The relationship of caffeine intake with depression, anxiety, stress, and sleep in Korean adolescents. Korean J Fam Med. 2016;37(2):111–6.
35. Scholey AB, Kennedy DO. Cognitive and physiological effects of an "energy drink": an evaluation of the whole drink and of glucose, caffeine and herbal flavouring fractions. Psychopharmacology. 2004; 176(3-4):320–30.

36. Sawah MA, Ruffin N, Rimawi M, Concerto C, Aguglia E, Chusid E, Infortuna C, Battaglia F. Perceived stress and coffee and energy drink consumption predict poor sleep quality in podiatric medical students: a cross-sectional study. J Am Podiatr Med Assoc. 2015;105(5):429–34.
37. Mash HBH, Fullerton CS, Ramsawh HJ, Ng THH, Wang L, Kessler RC, Stein MB, Ursano RJ. Risk for suicidal behaviors associated with alcohol and energy drink use in the US Army. Soc Psychiatry Psychiatr Epidemiol. 2014; 49(9):1379–87.
38. Richards G, Smith AP: Breakfast and Energy Drink Consumption in Secondary School Children: Breakfast Omission, in Isolation or in Combination with Frequent Energy Drink Use, is Associated with Stress, Anxiety, and Depression Cross-Sectionally, but not at 6-Month Follow-Up. Front Psychol. 2016;9(7):106.
39. Juon HS, Nam JJ, Ensminger ME. Epidemiology of suicidal behavior among Korean adolescents. J Child Psychol Psychiatry. 1994;35(4):663–76.
40. Kang E-H, Hyun MK, Choi SM, Kim J-M, Kim G-M, Woo J-M. Twelve-month prevalence and predictors of self-reported suicidal ideation and suicide attempt among Korean adolescents in a web-based nationwide survey. Aust N Z J Psychiatry. 2015;49(1):47–53.
41. Roehrs T, Roth T. Caffeine: sleep and daytime sleepiness. Sleep Med Rev. 2008;12(2):153–62.
42. Pollak CP, Bright D. Caffeine consumption and weekly sleep patterns in US seventh-, eighth-, and ninth-graders. Pediatrics. 2003;111(1):42–6.
43. Richardson NJ, Rogers PJ, Elliman NA, O'Dell RJ. Mood and performance effects of caffeine in relation to acute and chronic caffeine deprivation. Pharmacol Biochem Behav. 1995;52(2):313–20.
44. Goldstein A, Wallace ME. Caffeine dependence in schoolchildren? Exp Clin Psychopharmacol. 1997;5(4):388.
45. Haskell CF, Kennedy DO, Wesnes KA, Scholey AB. Cognitive and mood improvements of caffeine in habitual consumers and habitual non-consumers of caffeine. Psychopharmacology. 2005;179(4):813–25.
46. Smith A. Effects of caffeine on human behavior. Food Chem Toxicol. 2002; 40(9):1243–55.
47. James JE, Rogers PJ. Effects of caffeine on performance and mood: withdrawal reversal is the most plausible explanation. Psychopharmacology. 2005;182(1):1–8.
48. Rogers PJ, Richardson NJ. Why do we like drinks that contain caffeine? Trends Food Sci Technol. 1993;4(4):108–11.
49. James JE. Does caffeine enhance or merely restore degraded psychomotor performance? Neuropsychobiology. 1994;30(2-3):124–5.
50. Bellisle F. Effects of diet on behaviour and cognition in children. Br J Nutr. 2004;92 Suppl 2:S227–232.
51. Benton D. The impact of diet on anti-social, violent and criminal behaviour. Neurosci Biobehav Rev. 2007;31(5):752–74.
52. Benton D. Sucrose and behavioral problems. Crit Rev Food Sci Nutr. 2008; 48(5):385–401.
53. Sinn N, Bryan J, Wilson C. Cognitive effects of polyunsaturated fatty acids in children with attention deficit hyperactivity disorder symptoms: a randomised controlled trial. Prostaglandins Leukot Essent Fat Acids. 2008; 78(4-5):311–26.
54. Sharma S, Fernandes M, Fulton S. Adaptations in brain reward circuitry underlie palatable food cravings and anxiety induced by high-fat diet withdrawal. Int J Obes. 2013;37(9):1183–91.
55. Sharma S, Fulton S. Diet-induced obesity promotes depressive-like behaviour that is associated with neural adaptations in brain reward circuitry. Int J Obes. 2013;37(3):382–9.
56. Smit H, Cotton J, Hughes S, Rogers P. Mood and cognitive performance effects of "energy" drink constituents: caffeine, glucose and carbonation. Nutr Neurosci. 2004;7(3):127–39.
57. Giles GE, Mahoney CR, Brunye TT, Gardony AL, Taylor HA, Kanarek RB. Differential cognitive effects of energy drink ingredients: caffeine, taurine, and glucose. Pharmacol Biochem Behav. 2012;102(4):569–77.
58. Seidl R, Peyrl A, Nicham R, Hauser E. A taurine and caffeine-containing drink stimulates cognitive performance and well-being. Amino Acids. 2000;19(3-4):635–42.

4

Development of a standardized measure to assess food quality: a proof of concept

L. H. Jomaa[1], N. C. Hwalla[2] and J. M. Zidek[3*]

Abstract

Background: Food-based dietary guidelines are promoted to improve diet quality. In applying dietary recommendations, such as the MyPlate, the number of servings in a food group is the unit of measure used to make food selections. However, within each food group, different foods can vary greatly in their nutritional quality despite often having similar energy (caloric) values. This study aimed to develop a novel unit of measure that accounts for both the quantity of energy and the quality of nutrients, as defined by caloric and micronutrient density, respectively, in foods and to demonstrate its usability in identifying high quality foods within a food group.

Methods: A standardized unit of measure reflecting the quality of kilocalories for nutrition (qCaln) was developed through a mathematical function dependent on the energy content (kilocalories per 100 g) and micronutrient density of foods items within a food group. Nutrition composition of 1806 food items was extracted from the USDA nutrient database. For each food item analyzed, qCaln ratios were calculated to compare qCaln to its caloric content. Finally, a case example was developed comparing two plates adapted from the MyPlate.

Results: Examples of food items with highest and lowest qCaln ratios were displayed for five food groups: vegetables, fruits/fruit juices, milk/dairy products, meats/meat alternatives, and breads/cereals. Additionally, the applicability of the qCaln was presented through comparing two plates, adopted from the USDA MyPlate, to show differences in food quality.

Conclusions: The newly developed qCaln measure can be used to rank foods in terms of their nutrient density while accounting for their energy content. The proposed metric can provide consumers, public health professionals, researchers, and policy makers with an easy-to-understand measure of food quality and a practical tool to assess diet quality among individuals and population groups.

Keywords: Novel measure, Food quality, Nutrient density, Nutrient profiling, qCaln

Background

Identifying best methods to measure food and diet quality is an ongoing scientific and policy-level challenge facing public health professionals, researchers, and decision-makers. Over the years, several approaches and methods have been proposed to assess food and diet quality, including diet quality indices and various nutrient profiling methods.

Diet quality indices were developed to measure conformance of individuals and population groups to international and national dietary guidelines and recommendations, such as the U.S. dietary guidelines (MyPlate) [1]. The Healthy Eating Index (HEI) 2005 and the alternative HEI (AHEI 2010) are examples of diet quality indices that have been extensively used by public health professionals and researchers in a variety of settings and age groups. The HEI 2005 and the more accurate and up-to-date AHEI 2010 are based on the Dietary Guidelines for Americans whereby researchers assess the frequency of consuming food items and the nutrient intake within and among food groups, respectively, compared to these dietary guidelines [2]. Both indices were successful in finding associations between diet and health outcomes, such as obesity and chronic diseases including diabetes, cardiovascular diseases, and cancer [3]. However, limitations exist with these diet quality indices. A major shortcoming is the difficulty of determining which foods within a food group

* Correspondence: jeremyzidek@gmail.com
[3]Jeremy Zidek, Futura Food, 113 Creekside Drive, State College, PA 16801, USA
Full list of author information is available at the end of the article

score better than others. When making food selections, it is also not immediately obvious to a consumer that a food will score high or low on the HEI. Furthermore, consumers may not be able to discern which foods within a food group are of high nutritional quality or nutrient density, and which foods are of lower quality, especially for foods that lack nutrition facts labels like fresh fruits and vegetables.

The nutrient profiling method, defined as the science of ranking foods based on nutrient composition [4, 5], represents an alternative approach proposed by researchers to improve assessment of food and diet quality. Numerous methods have been proposed and used by researchers, regulatory agencies, and food industry to develop, test, and validate nutrient profile models [4], however, these approaches still have their limitations. Some nutrient profiling approaches were developed with the aim of increasing healthy micronutrient consumption. Others focused on less desirable nutrients that need to be limited, such as saturated fat, added sugars, and sodium, or a combination of both beneficial and less desirable nutrients that need to be limited [5]. Although various nutrient profiling models have been validated against established indicators of diet quality and can aid in the value-based selection of quality foods [6, 7], a singular based score of quality that can account both for the macro- and micro-nutrient content of foods has yet to be achieved.

Challenges are faced when interpreting currently used diet quality indices and nutrient profiling measures, particularly in non-research settings, when consumers are requested to meet food-based dietary guidelines (FBDGs) and nutrition recommendations. For example, in applying dietary recommendations, such as the US MyPlate [8], the number of servings in a food group is the unit of measure used to make food selections. However, within each food group, different foods can vary greatly in their nutritional quality despite often having similar energy (caloric) values. The complexity of diet quality indices and nutrient profiling approaches hinder consumers' ability to make healthier dietary choices. This is particularly challenging in the midst of a complex food environment that has a wide array of food products with contradictory health and nutrition claims and, at best, confusing food-labeling systems (front-of-package labels and nutrition facts labels). These environmental conditions coupled with difficult-to-understand diet quality measures add to the confusion of average consumers and may lead to poor dietary choices [9, 10].

In order to address this problem, the present study aimed to create a novel unit of measure that accounts for both the quantity of energy (kilocalories per 100 g) and the quality of nutrients, as defined by micronutrient density, in foods and to demonstrate the usability of this novel measure to facilitate the assessment of food quality. Specific objectives of the study included 1) developing a standardized unit of measure reflecting the quality of kilocalories for nutrition (qCaln) that can account for the caloric and nutrient density per food item, 2) comparing food items per food groups based on the newly developed qCaln measure, and 3) testing the applicability of qCaln measure through demonstrating different food plates with various qCaln ratio scores.

Findings from this study can provide a new measure that allows for merging multiple nutritional parameters into one simple, standardized unit. In addition, this newly proposed measure could provide researchers and public health professionals with a relatively easier tool to assess the diet quality of individuals and population groups in comparison to other nutrient profiling tools and diet quality indices.

Methods

Development of qCaln measure

Generally, food energy has been measured in kilocalories (kcal, or Cal), which accounts for the energy in the macronutrients (carbohydrates, fats, and proteins) included in the sum total of ingredients in any food item. The quality of the food, however, is more often than not, determined by the amount and distribution of key micronutrients in food. Energy, macronutrient and micronutrient content of all food items within the Nutritionist Pro software (version 5.1.0, 2014, SR 24, First Data Bank, Nutritionist Pro, Axxya Systems, San Bruno, CA) were included in the computations. The food composition database in this software was based on the United States Department of Agriculture (USDA) National Nutrient Database for Standard Reference, release 27 [11]. In addition, a small number of local foods and beverages commonly consumed among Lebanese and Middle Eastern populations were considered in the calculations and were denoted as (AUB) in the figures, where applicable. Local foods and beverages were compared to culturally-specific food composition tables [12].

The qCaln is a function of the caloric content (per 100 g) from macronutrients and the amount and distribution of micronutrients (per 100 g) in a particular food such that:

$$qCaln = Cal + Cal * \left\{\sum_{i=1}^{n} w_i * S_i\right\} \quad (1)$$

where "Cal" is the amount of kilocalories per 100 g in the food ingredient, w_i is the weighting for each micronutrient I, "S_i" is the micronutrient score for each micronutrient "I", and n is the amount of micronutrients included in the calculation. The value w_i is the relative weighting for importance to each of the micronutrients.

Equation 1 allows for as many micronutrients as necessary to describe the nutrient density, and the authors recognize that some populations may require different types and distributions of micronutrients. For the purpose of this paper, a total of 10 micronutrients were selected for inclusion in the qCaln formula. The 10 micronutrients that were considered for this paper and their units are: vitamin A (RE), vitamin D (μg), vitamin C (μg), calcium (mg), iron (mg), zinc (mg), dietary fiber (g), saturated fat (g), total sugar (g), and sodium (mg). Total sugar was used instead of added sugar given that data on the latter is currently less readily available, and previous research has shown that using total sugar as a nutrient to limit is a reasonable option [6]. The selection of these nutrients were based on a number of factors: 1) the high prevalence of micronutrient deficiencies at a global level and their serious adverse health effects due, in part, to inadequate dietary intake of certain nutrients, including vitamin A, iron and zinc [13–17]; 2) the strong associations observed between diet-related chronic diseases and the high consumption of saturated fat, sugars, and sodium [18–21]; (3) recommended nutrients or nutrients that are restricted with upper limits according to international food agencies such as the Food and Drug Administration (FDA) in the US [22, 23] and the French Food Standard Agency (AFSSA) [24, 25]; and 4) comparable choice of nutrients reported in previous nutrient profiling indices such as the naturally nutrient rich (NNR) score [26] nutritional quality index (NQI) [27] and ratio of recommended to restricted food components (RRR) [28]. Equal weights for all micronutrients were considered in this study when calculating the qCaln measure. The equal weightings among micronutrients was based on the same assumption as that of the dietary reference intakes (DRIs) developed for healthy people, whereby the same relative importance is assumed among micronutrients [29]. Although some population groups may have additional physiological needs, such as during infancy or pregnancy, and individuals residing in developing nations may be at higher risk of certain micronutrient deficiencies, including iron and zinc deficiencies, the qCaln was developed to address the food quality regardless of the health and physiological status of consumers.

Thus, each micronutrient was assigned an equal weighting w_i of 0.10 as the weighting scores indicate that each micronutrient is equally important in a diet. For the purposes of this study, weightings for the selected micronutrients were considered identical, and weightings for micronutrients that were not included in the calculation were assumed to be "0". Saturated fat, total sugar, and sodium were negatively weighted in the qCaln calculation, indicating that these micronutrients need to be limited to prevent cardio-metabolic risk factors, including elevated blood sugar, cholesterol, or blood pressure levels [30–33].

Equation 1 can then be expanded such that,

$$\begin{aligned} \text{qCaln} = {} & \text{Cal} + \text{Cal} * \{w_i * (S_{VA} + S_{VD} \\ & + S_{VC} + S_{Ca} + S_{Fe} + S_{Zn} \\ & + S_{DF} - S_{satfat} - S_{Sugar} - S_{Na})\}\,. \end{aligned} \tag{2}$$

For each food item, and for each micronutrient "i", a micronutrient score "S_i" was calculated. The calculation is based on the amount of the selected micronutrient in the food item relative to other food items in the same food group to ensure proper comparison. The distribution of each selected micronutrient among all foods within each food group was tested for normality and were found to be close to a normal distribution. Given a normal distribution, the value of S_i will depend on the standard score (otherwise known as z-score or z-value) of the micronutrient. The equation for the standard score of a micronutrient amount relative to the rest of the food group is given by:

$$z = \frac{x - \mu}{\sigma} \tag{3}$$

where 'x' is the amount of a selected micronutrient (for example, "mg per serving size"), μ is the sample mean of the same micronutrient with all food items in that food group, and σ is the sample standard deviation of that micronutrient within the same foods included in the food group. Once the z-score was calculated, the critical value, or percentile score of the value z by integrating for the probability of our test value z being less than Z as $Z \to \infty$, was calculated. This value gives the probability that any statistic is less than the calculated z-score in Eq. 3 and is given by integrating the probability density function,

$$P(a \le x \le b) = \int_a^b f(x)\,dx \tag{4}$$

where

$$f(x) = \frac{1}{\sqrt{2\pi\sigma^2}}\, e^{\frac{-(x-\mu)^2}{2\sigma^2}}. \tag{5}$$

Equation 4 represents the area under a continuous curve f (x), and Eq. 5 represents the density function. Equation 5 cannot be integrated in terms of functions that can be expressed as exponentials, polynomials, trigonometric, logarithmic, and rational functions. Therefore, the probability P_i of a micronutrient i was estimated based on z-score tables such that $(0 \le P_i \le 1)$. Then, for each micronutrient i,

$$S_i = 2P_i - 1. \tag{6}$$

Once S_i was calculated for each micronutrient i, Eq. 2 was used to calculate the qCaln value for each food item taking into consideration all the selected micronutrients in the sample of food items within that food group. Thus, it follows that foods with critical z scores above the 50th percentile ($0.5 < P_i \leq 1.0$) will have a greater qCaln value than the listed value of Cal indicating higher quality food, and foods with lower than the 50th percentile ($0.0 \leq P_i < 0.5$) have qCaln values less than the listed Cal, indicating less quality. Also, it follows from Eqs. 2 and 6 that the minimum qCaln value would approach 0.0 and the maximum value would approach a value twice the amount of Cal ($qCaln_{max} = 2 * Cal$).

Calculation of qCaln ratio

After calculating S_i for each micronutrient, a qCaln value per 100 g was calculated for 1806 different food items from five different food groups. These 5 main food groups were: 1.) breads and cereals, 2.) dairy products, 3.) fruits and juices, 4.) vegetables, 5.) and meat and meat alternatives. Using the weightings from Eq. 1 and the data from the USDA National Nutrient Database [11], the qCaln ratio, was calculated to compare qCaln to Cal for each food item analyzed. A complete example showing qCaln results for each food within the vegetables food group is shown in an Additional file 1 [see "qCaln-Vegetables.csv"]. Ratios of qCaln that are greater than 1.0 can be interpreted as higher quality food per calorie, whereas qCaln ratios that are less than 1.0 represent lower micronutrient content per food item compared to its caloric content.

$$qCaln\ Ratio = \frac{qCaln}{Cal}. \tag{7}$$

Comparison of food plates

To show the applicability of the qCaln ratio, two separate plates were compared. Each plate was based on FBDG recommendations from USDA MyPlate [8] and consisted of at least one serving of food from fruits and fruit juices, vegetables, meat and meat alternatives, milk and dairy products, and breads and cereals. Figure 6 shows the two plates selected for comparison. Table 1 lists the contents for each plate compared. Each food item listed was assumed to be one portion size of food. The qCaln ratio was then calculated for each food item and averaged for the entire plate of food items.

Results

Comparison of qCaln of food items within same food groups

Of the 1806 total food items analyzed, 534 had qCaln ratio values > 1.0 when compared to kilocalorie (Cal) content, and 1272 had ratios < 1.0. Ratios that are > 1.0 can be interpreted as higher quality food per calorie, whereas qCaln ratios < 1.0 represent lower micronutrient content per food item compared to its caloric content. Figures 1, 2, 3, 4 and 5 show the highest and lowest qCaln ratios (qCaln ratio = qCaln / kcal) for the vegetables, fruits and fruit juices, milk and dairy products, meats and meats alternatives, and breads and cereals food groups, respectively.

Figure 1 shows some of the highest 10 qCaln ratios and some of the lowest 10 qCaln ratios in the Vegetables food group (196 vegetables were analyzed for qCaln values). A table including the calculations of the qCaln ratio for each food item in the vegetables food group considered in this manuscript is included as Additional file 1.

Figure 2 shows some of the highest 10 qCaln ratios and some of the lowest 10 qCaln ratios in the Fruits and Juices food group (320 fruits and juices were analyzed for qCaln values).

Figure 3 shows some of the highest 10 qCaln ratios and some of the lowest 10 qCaln ratios in the Dairy food group (160 dairy products were analyzed for qCaln values).

Figure 4 shows some of the highest 10 qCaln ratios and some of the lowest 10 qCaln ratios in the meat and meat Alternatives food group (770 meat and meat alternative foods were analyzed for qCaln values).

Figure 5 shows some of the highest 10 qCaln ratios and some of the lowest 10 qCaln ratios in the Breads and Cereals food group (360 breads and cereals were analyzed for qCaln values).

In the case of vegetables, the highest 10 qCaln ratios included spinach, leeks, green peppers, collards, and turnip (greens), whereas those of the lowest qCaln ratios, reflecting lower micronutrient content to caloric

Table 1 Contents of each USDA MyPlate example for comparison

Food group	Plate 1	Plate 2
Fruits and fruit juices	Apple, cherry, orange, pineapple	Grapes, kiwi, banana
Vegetables	Carrot, green pepper, tomato	Tomato, onion
Breads and cereals	Oat bran muffin, white toasted bread, and wheat (white wheat) bread	White pita bread, spaghetti pasta
Meat and meat alternatives	Egg, pork sausage, bacon	Meatless meatballs (meat alternative), hot dog
Milk and dairy products	Whole milk	Fruit-flavored yogurt

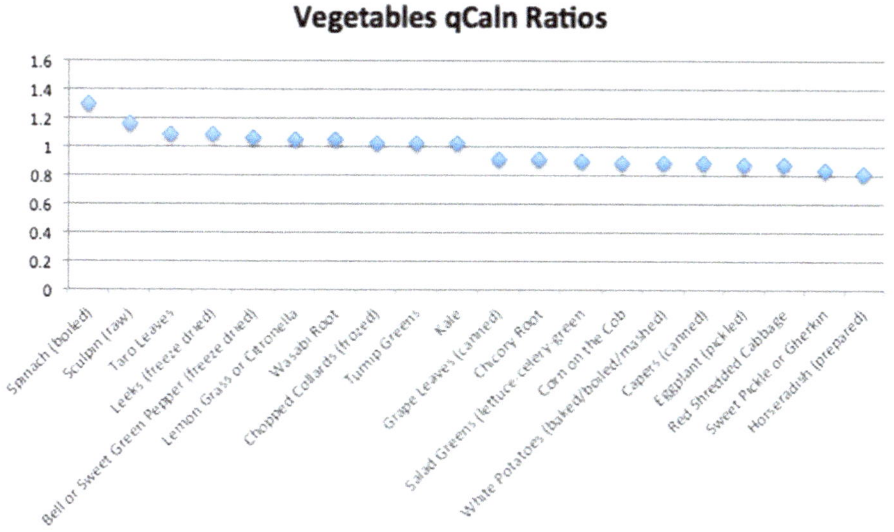

Fig. 1 Spectrum of qCaln ratios for selected vegetables

content, were sweet pickles, pickled eggplants, canned capers, and red cabbage. For fruits, food items with the highest qCaln ratios were dried mixed fruits (prune, apricot, and pear), dry cranberry beans, wild raspberries, cherries, and blackberries, and those of the lower qCaln ratios were canned juices and fruits canned in syrup such as papaya, plums, and loquats. These results are in line with dietary recommendations that highlight the high nutrient yet low energy density of green leafy vegetables and other fresh fruits and vegetables that are not preserved in salt or sugar. It is worth noting that the sugar content of canned fruits and fruit juices was a major contributor to lower qCaln ratios for fruit items. When analyzing the dairy products, food items with the highest quality were low-fat, non-fat, and low sodium varieties of milk and cheese as these items score lower in terms of fat and thus caloric content and have lower sodium levels, which is found in abundance within dairy products and could contribute to elevated sodium intake levels.

Figure 6 displays a comparison of two meals superimposed on the USDA MyPlate along with each food item's qCaln ratio. Where applicable, foods are assumed to be fresh. The bread in the right image is assumed to be white pita bread. The meatballs in the right plate are assumed to be meatless meatballs.

Finally, two separate meals were compared that would be considered good diet choices for each plate according

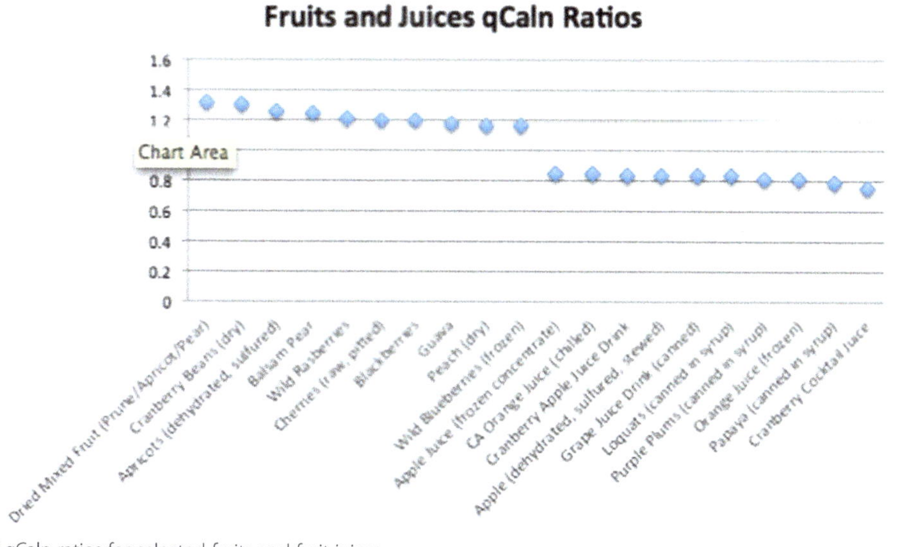

Fig. 2 Spectrum of qCaln ratios for selected fruits and fruit juices

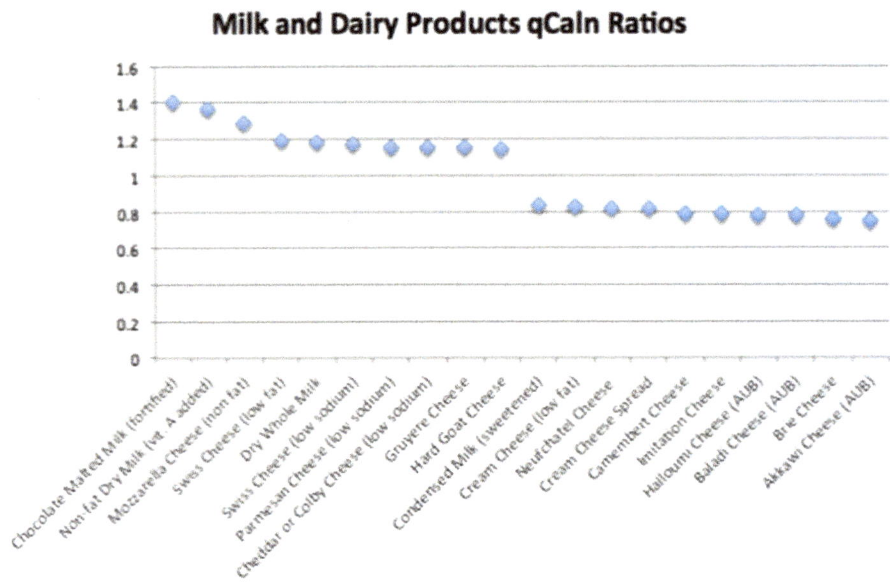

Fig. 3 Spectrum of qCaln ratios for foods in the milk and dairy group

to the MyPlate guidelines [8]. Note the generally higher values of qCaln ratios in Plate 1 compared to Plate 2. The average qCaln ratio for Plate 1 is 0.969, while the average qCaln ratio for Plate 2 is 0.927. Oranges and cherries have higher qCaln ratios (1.04 and 1.20, respectively) than grapes and bananas (0.86 and 0.94, respectively). For the meat and meat alternatives food group, eggs would be considered a better selection than meatless meatballs (1.00 to 0.98, respectively), but the hot dog on Plate 2 is a better choice than either the cooked sausage pork or bacon on Plate 1. However, as shown in the figure above, if the eggs on Plate 1 are made from egg whites only, then the qCaln ratio value drops from 1.00 to 0.82. Therefore, what is gained by reducing saturated fat (egg whites relative to eggs with yolks) is outweighed by the loss of various micronutrients contained in the egg yolk. The selection of whole milk in Plate 1 would also be a better selection than a yogurt cup (full fat variety) in Plate 2 with fruit flavoring (0.92 to 0.85, respectively).

Discussion

This study aimed to develop a new unit of measure that accounts for both the caloric and micronutrient density of foods and to demonstrate the usability of this novel measure in assessing food quality. The qCaln was the

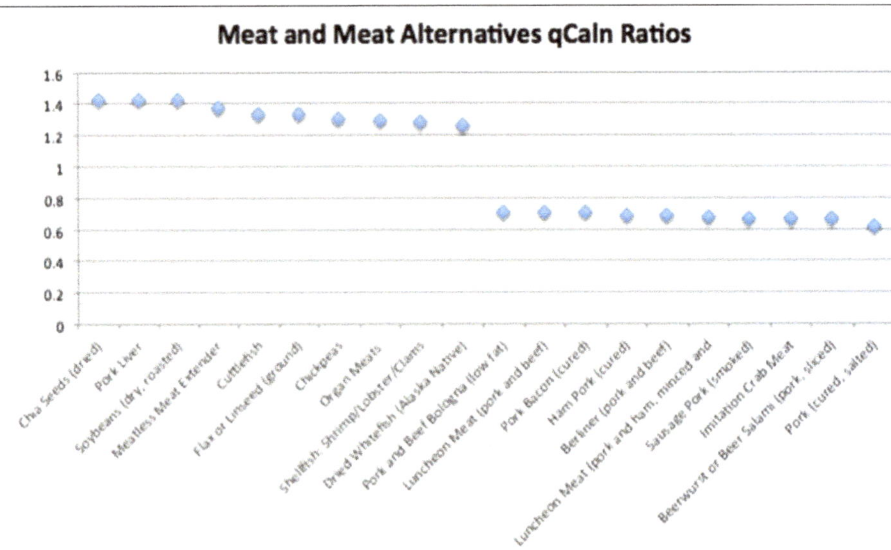

Fig. 4 Spectrum of qCaln ratios for foods in the meat and meat alternatives food group

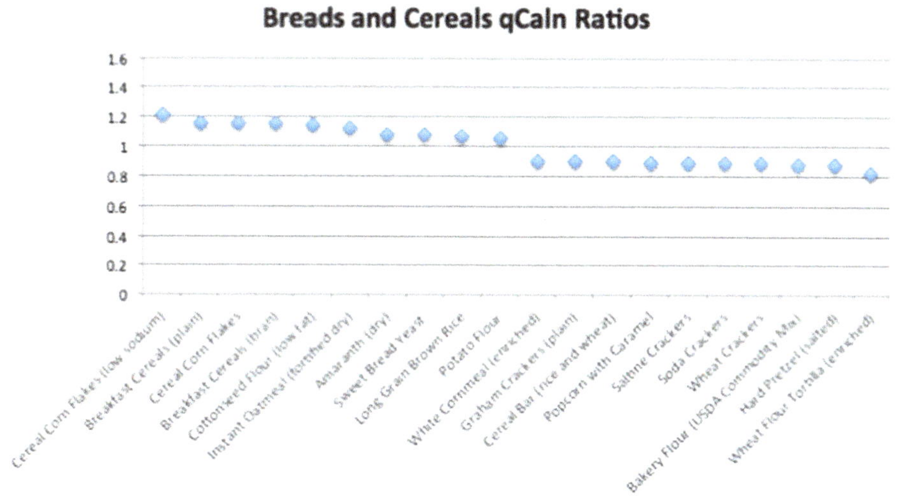

Fig. 5 Spectrum of qCaln ratios for foods in the breads and cereals food group

standardized unit developed based on the caloric density and the amount and distribution of micronutrients per 100 g in a particular food. Results showed that food items in any food group can be analyzed based on their qCaln values. In addition, through calculating a qCaln ratio for each food item, the caloric and micronutrient contents of a food were compared with the food's energy density (caloric value) in one single measure. Using the qCaln ratio, higher quality foods could be differentiated easily from lower quality foods. More specifically, the qCaln ratios of food items within each of the food groups, including vegetables, fruits/fruit juices, milk/dairy products, breads/cereals, and meats/meat alternatives, were compared to each other in this paper.

The advantages of the proposed approach over other existing food quality measures and nutrient profiling approaches lies in simplifying complex nutrient composition data into a singular based score that reflects both nutrient and energy density. The definition of nutrient dense foods have expanded over the years due to numerous attempts by researchers, regulatory agencies, and food companies to identify adequate criteria for ranking foods based on their nutrient composition. Some of the models highlighted the importance of limiting certain nutrients, such as total fat, saturated fat, sugar, or sodium, that were associated with adverse health outcomes, when defining nutrient-density [34, 35]. Other approaches emphasized recommended or desirable nutrients that may not be adequately consumed by population groups yet have favorable health benefits, including vitamins, minerals, and fiber [36], or included a combination of both, nutrients to be promoted and others that need to be limited [4, 6]. Despite the importance of these attempts in advancing the field of nutrient profiling, the majority of the approaches fell short of identifying a single measure to encompass the complexity of food and its nutritional value.

The selection of the 10 micronutrients that were included in the calculation of the qCaln accounted for two groups of nutrients: those that are not consumed in sufficient amounts and contribute, in part, to micronutrient deficiencies across various population groups [13–17] and less desirable nutrients that are consumed in abundance worldwide such as saturated fat, sugar, and

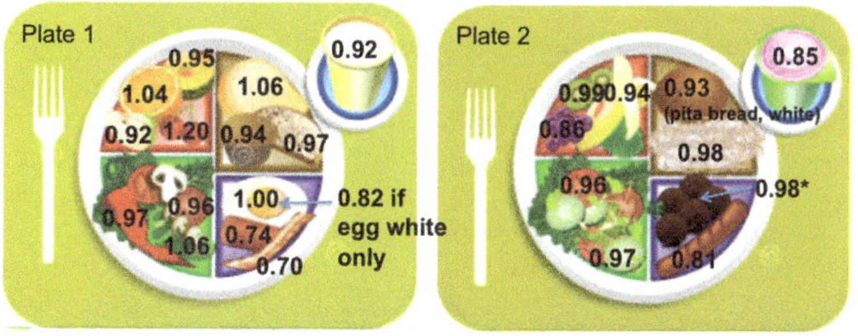

Fig. 6 Comparison of two meals superimposed on the USDA MyPlate with qCaln ratios

sodium [18–21]. In addition, the number and choice of micronutrients considered in the qCaln calculation were similar, albeit not identical, to other nutrient profiling methods such as the NNR score, [26, 28], the NQI) [27] the RRRr food scores [22] and nutritional adequacy score of individual foods and limited nutrient score (SAIN/LIM system). Furthermore, the choice of the micronutrients in the present study was not dependent on nutrients that are consumed in low or high amounts in a specific country or context, but rather included a more comprehensive and global approach. This is in line with the recommendations from Drewnowski and Fulgoni, 2008 [4], who urged that the choice of nutrients included in nutrient profiling methods should be based on diets from different countries rather than focusing on a specific country or context, such as the United States. In fact, the formula for calculating qCaln presented in this study can be easily expanded or reduced based on objective research designed to identify the optimum number of micronutrients in nutrient profiling techniques.

It is worth noting that the percent daily value (%DV) of each micronutrient was not included in the calculation for qCaln within the present study for a number of reasons. First, Eqs. 3, 4, 5 and 6 described in the methodology ensure that the amount of a given micronutrient in a given food is compared to the normal distribution of that micronutrient relative to all foods within its food group. Therefore, dividing these contents by the %DV would lead to the same distribution and "S-score" (Eq. 6) used in the qCaln calculation. Second, the use of %DV relative to qCaln values of a particular food when compared to a food group would be better used for overall meal and diet construction, allowing for comparisons of foods between food groups. By accounting for the %DV in future calculations of the qCaln, this measure could be used for meal construction to educate consumers on making healthier dietary choices in an attempt to meet their daily dietary needs.

Applications of the qCaln measure: nutrition education and dietary counseling

The proposed qCaln allows for a better interpretation of the food quality not only by researchers but also consumers. The qCaln can be linked to food-based dietary guidelines depicted visually through the MyPlate, MyPyramid, and the Mediterranean Diet Pyramid among other education models used by health care professionals to educate consumers about healthy dietary choices. For example, promoting the consumption of low-fat and low-sodium dairy products that have higher qCaln ratios (i.e. higher nutrient density with lower fat and sodium content as well as higher calcium and vitamin D), can assist consumers in meeting their beneficial nutrient requirements while avoiding less desirable nutrients. Similarly, promoting the consumption of fresh fruits like oranges rather than orange juice from frozen concentrate or sweetened fruit juices can help in making smarter food choices.

Training consumers to select foods with higher qCaln values, where appropriate, can help improve diet quality and meet dietary recommendations. Currently, dietary guidelines are presented to the public as recommendations in terms of serving sizes of food groups that are promoted to be consumed, such as whole grains, low fat dairy products, and foods to avoid including those high in sugar and fat. These recommendations are usually based on studies highlighting the daily optimal intakes of energy, and macro- as well as micro-nutrients among humans (acceptable macronutrient distribution ranges and DRIs, respectively). Despite the extensive efforts exerted by nutrition professionals to relay dietary guidelines in simple and interactive manners, consumers still face challenges in interpreting these recommendations. Difficulties arise when consumers are asked to make healthy dietary choices from a wide array of food products available on the market and with various nutrition facts labeling systems. In addition, deciphering the labeling systems, which include the amount of calories, macronutrient, and micronutrient content of foods, requires health and nutrition literacy at the consumer end, which may be lacking by various population groups and in numerous contexts. This is further complicated with the diversity of units, serving sizes, and nutrients listed on nutrition facts labels in differing countries, in addition to front-of-package labels along with other competing marketing slogans and techniques. Furthermore, fresh produce and certain types of meats and dairy products lack nutrition labels and the choice among the myriad of produce on the market leaves consumers confused as to which of the food items within each of the food groups are the most nutritious. The qCaln measure can merge the multiple nutritional measures including, caloric content of food, and the macro- and micronutrient content of food into one simple, standardized unit. In addition, the qCaln can be linked to optimal daily nutrient intakes of individuals and allows for daily meal construction. This linkage will allow consumers to make food purchases with conscious dietary knowledge rather than just preference, taste, convenience, and cost. The qCaln, if deemed valid in various contexts, could be used in addition to food labeling either on the front or the side of products, and on menus at various points of purchase with the potential for expanding nutrition education and supporting nutrition labeling systems that are already in place. Future research should evaluate the experiences of consumers towards the use of the qCaln and their success in attempting to make healthier dietary choices at different points of sales (supermarkets, restaurants, work-site cafeterias, schools, etc.).

Using the qCaln, as a composite score that takes into consideration energy and nutrient density, is not only valuable for consumers but also researchers and health professionals who seek to assess the diet quality of individuals and population groups. The proposed measure can provide a simple method to assess nutrient profiles of individual food items within the same food category while also providing investigators with a relatively simple tool to assess the overall nutrient profiles of individuals (for example, the average qCaln ratios of consumers over a specific period of time such as week or month). The latter measure can be then linked to other global measures of diet quality, such as the HEI and diet diversity scores.

Applications of the qCaln measure: linking nutrition to agriculture

One of the main benefits and applications of the qCaln is to help individuals make better food item choices and improve their overall dietary intake. In fact, nutrition programs that attempt to increase awareness and proper consumption of micronutrients achieve some of the highest benefit-cost ratios, even in the short term [37]. However, improving dietary intake is not dependent only on the knowledge of the consumers regarding quality of foods through targeted nutrition awareness programs but also on the quantity and quality of agricultural produce available in the market and accessible to consumers. Nevertheless, the link between the evidence provided by these nutrition programs and agricultural practices is, at best, limited. In addition, there is a dearth in robust monitoring and evaluation tools to assess the impact of agriculture on nutrition outcomes [38]. Thus, it is important to generate easy-to-understand measures that can be compatible for both fields to best inform how to grow healthy food in a sustainable manner while respecting individuals and populations' food choices, preferences, and traditions [39]. Researchers, public health professionals, farmers, and consumers can be trained to interpret the qCaln measure, as a relatively easier tool to use compared to other more complex agricultural and nutrition indicators. The qCaln could then be used to bridge the gap between nutrition and agriculture by tracking quality energy produced to quality energy consumed through the qCaln. However, the applicability of qCaln in linking agricultural management practices aimed at sustainable crop production with nutritional outcomes is worth more thorough explorations in future studies.

Limitations

Findings from this paper need to be interpreted in light of a number of limitations. First, equal weights were assumed for all included micronutrients in the calculation for the qCaln. Although the use of equal-weighted scores has been used extensively by other researchers when developing nutrient profiling methods [4], targeted differential weightings for micronutrients have been suggested for context-specific cases such as biological quality of nutrients in food, bioavailability, and distribution of nutrients in the food supply [4]. Also, researchers have been showing the importance of altering the relative weightings of micronutrients in profiling to fit populations [40]. Thus, the formula for the qCaln can be further improved through reflecting different dietary needs and increasing or limiting intakes of specific nutrients for various segments of the population, such as increasing folate and vitamin B12 for pregnant women or limiting sodium and saturated fats for individuals at risk of hypertension or cardiovascular diseases.

Another limitation of the qCaln calculations in the present study is the lack of inclusion of bioavailability data and the effect of food preparation on micronutrient content of foods. For example, animal-based protein sources are more readily digested and absorbed allowing for higher bioavailability of essential micronutrients compared to plant-based sources, and cooked vegetables that are prepared through steaming have different micronutrient contents compared to boiled or baked vegetables [41]. To address these limitations, bioavailability and food preparation factors could be added to the proposed qCaln equation in future studies to allow for a better depiction of the quality of the foods and diets consumed by individuals. Additionally, the validity of this measure needs to be tested against other diet quality indices, including the HEI and diet diversity scores, and a number of nutrient profiling methods, such as the Nutrient-Rich Food Index (NRF) [6], and the SAIN/LIM scoring system [24]. The measure could also be tested against other objective health outcomes and biomarkers such as obesity, hypertension, and diabetes; and using more sophisticated validation techniques including 'goodness of fit' models (Drewnowski and Fulgoni 2008). Finally, further attention is needed to consider other attributes of food. For example, the qCaln could be compared to the Nutrient Rich Foods Index [7] to compare foods of varying food quality relative to cost. The qCaln, as a single number unit of measure, would allow for easy comparison of food quality to cost.

Conclusion

The proposed unit of measure reflects a novel nutrient profiling approach that accounts for both the quantity of energy (caloric density) and the quality of nutrients in foods into one standardized metric and demonstrates the usability of this new measure to facilitate the assessment of food quality. Results show that the qCaln can be used to rank foods in terms of their nutrient and energy content simultaneously, making food selections within a food group easier to understand. This easy-to-use tool can be applied by public health professionals, regulatory agencies, and the food industry to promote the selection of healthier nutrient-dense yet low in energy content foods and assist consumers in meeting dietary guidelines and nutrition recommendations. In addition, this novel metric could be further validated by researchers in comparison to other nutrient profiling and diet quality measures to test its usability in assessing diet quality of individuals and population groups. This metric can have other applications and can be further expanded beyond the nutrition research serving as the impetus for nutrition-sensitive agriculture through tracking of food quality from production to consumption.

Additional files

Additional file 1: Calculated qCaln ratios for each food item in the vegetables food group. (CSV 13 kb)

Abbreviations
%DV: Percent daily value; AHEI: Alternative healthy eating index; DRIs: Dietary reference intakes; FBDG: Food-based dietary guidelines; HEI: Healthy eating index; NNR: Naturally nutrient rich score; qCaln: Quality of kilocalories for nutrition; SAIN/LIM: Nutritional adequacy scores of individual foods and limited nutrient score; USDA: United States department of agriculture

Acknowledgements
The authors would like to acknowledge the assistance of Ms. Ruba Cheaib in compiling the food and nutrient composition data from the USDA nutrient database.

Funding
University Research Board at the American University of Beirut.

Availability of data and materials
The datasets generated and/or analyzed during the current study are available from the corresponding author on reasonable request.

Authors' contributions
LJ and JZ equally contributed to developing the methodology for the qCaln and preparing this manuscript. NH provided guidance and direction on qCaln comparison techniques, particularly with MyPlate, and contributed to the writing of the manuscript. All authors read and approved the final manuscript.

Competing interests
The authors declare that they have no competing interests.

Consent for publication
Not applicable.

Ethics approval and consent to participate
Not applicable.

Author details
[1]Lamis Jomaa, Faculty of Agricultural and Food Sciences, American University of Beirut, Beirut, Lebanon. [2]Nahla Hwalla, Faculty of Agricultural and Food Sciences, American University of Beirut, Beirut, Lebanon. [3]Jeremy Zidek, Futura Food, 113 Creekside Drive, State College, PA 16801, USA.

References
1. Choose MyPlate.gov. USDA Food and Nutrition Services; 2016.
2. Guenther PM, Casavale KO, Reedy J, Kirkpatrick SI, Hiza HA, Kuczynski KJ, Kahle LL, Krebs-Smith SM. Update of the healthy eating index: HEI-2010. J Acad Nutr Diet. 2013;113:569–80.
3. Chiuve SE, Fung TT, Rimm EB, Hu FB, McCullough ML, Wang M, Stampfer MJ, Willett WC. Alternative dietary indices both strongly predict risk of chronic disease. The J Nutr. 2012;142:1009–18. jn. 111.157222.
4. Drewnowski A, Fulgoni V. Nutrient profiling of foods: creating a nutrient-rich food index. Nutr Rev. 2008;66:23–39.
5. Drewnowski A, Fulgoni VL. Nutrient density: principles and evaluation tools. Am J Clin Nutr. 2014;99:1223S–8S.
6. Fulgoni VL, Keast DR, Drewnowski A. Development and validation of the nutrient-rich foods index: a tool to measure nutritional quality of foods. J Nutr. 2009;139:1549–54.
7. Drewnowski A. The nutrient rich foods index helps to identify healthy, affordable foods. Am J Clin Nutr. 2010;91:1095S–101S.
8. Choose MyPlate.gov [http://www.choosemyplate.gov/]. Accessed 30 June 2016.
9. Drewnowski A, Specter S. Poverty and obesity: the role of energy density and energy costs. Am J Clin Nutr. 2004;79:6–16.
10. Drewnowski A. Obesity and the food environment: dietary energy density and diet costs. Am J Prev Med. 2004;27:154–62.
11. U.S. Department of Agriculture ARS. USDA national nutrient database for standard reference. 2014.
12. Pellet P, Shadarevian S. Food composition. Tables for use in the Middle East. Beirut: American University of Beirut; 1970.
13. Diaz JR, de las Cagigas A, Rodriguez R. Micronutrient deficiencies in developing and affluent countries. Eur J Clin Nutr. 2003;57 Suppl 1:S70–2.
14. Ahmed T, Hossain M, Sanin KI. Global burden of maternal and child undernutrition and micronutrient deficiencies. Ann Nutr Metab. 2012;61 Suppl 1:8–17.
15. Bailey RL, West Jr KP, Black RE. The epidemiology of global micronutrient deficiencies. Ann Nutr Metab. 2015;66 Suppl 2:22–33.
16. Micronutrient deficiencies. Vitamin A deficiency [http://www.who.int/nutrition/topics/vad/en/]. Accessed 30 June 2016.
17. Micronutrient Deficiencies. Iron deficiency anaemia [http://www.who.int/nutrition/topics/ida/en/]. Accessed 30 June 2016.
18. Flock MR, Kris-Etherton PM. Dietary guidelines for Americans 2010: implications for cardiovascular disease. Curr Atheroscler Rep. 2011;13:499–507.
19. Huth PJ, Fulgoni VL, Keast DR, Park K, Auestad N. Major food sources of calories, added sugars, and saturated fat and their contribution to essential nutrient intakes in the US diet: data from the national health and nutrition examination survey (2003–2006). Nutr J. 2013;12:1.
20. Nishida C, Uauy R, Kumanyika S, Shetty P. The joint WHO/FAO expert consultation on diet, nutrition and the prevention of chronic diseases: process, product and policy implications. Public Health Nutr. 2004;7:245–50.
21. Musaiger AO. Diet and prevention of coronary heart disease in the Arab Middle East countries. Med Princ Pract. 2002;11:9–16.
22. Scheidt DM, Daniel E. Composite index for aggregating nutrient density using food labels: ratio of recommended to restricted food components. J Nutr Educ Behav. 2004;36:35–9.
23. Food Labeling Guide. Guidance for Industry: A Food Labeling Guide [http://www.fda.gov/Food/GuidanceRegulation/GuidanceDocumentsRegulatoryInformation/LabelingNutrition/ucm2006828.htm]. Accessed 30 June 2016.
24. Darmon N, Vieux F, Maillot M, Volatier JL, Martin A. Nutrient profiles discriminate between foods according to their contribution to nutritionally adequate diets: a validation study using linear programming and the SAIN, LIM system. Am J Clin Nutr. 2009;89:1227–36.
25. AFSSA: Définition de profils nutritionnels pour l'accès aux allégations nutritionnelles et de santé: propositions et arguments. [Setting of nutrient profiles for accessing nutrition and health claims: proposals and arguments.] 2008.
26. Drewnowski A. Concept of a nutritious food: toward a nutrient density score. Am J Clin Nutr. 2005;82:721–32.
27. Hansen RGWB, Sorenson AW. Nutrition quality index of food. Westport: AVI Publishing Co; 1979.

28. Zelman K, Kennedy E. Naturally nutrient rich… putting more power on Americans' plates. Nutr Today. 2005;40:60–8.
29. Otten JJ, Hellwig JP, Meyers LD. Dietary reference intakes: the essential guide to nutrient requirements. Washington: National Academies Press; 2006.
30. Micha R, Mozaffarian D. Saturated fat and cardiometabolic risk factors, coronary heart disease, stroke, and diabetes: a fresh look at the evidence. Lipids. 2010;45:893–905.
31. Michas G, Micha R, Zampelas A. Dietary fats and cardiovascular disease: putting together the pieces of a complicated puzzle. Atherosclerosis. 2014;234:320–8.
32. Graudal NA, Hubeck-Graudal T, Jürgens G. Effects of low-sodium diet vs. High-sodium diet on blood pressure, renin, aldosterone, catecholamines, cholesterol, and triglyceride (Cochrane review). Am J Hypertens. 2012;25:1–15.
33. Basu S, Yoffe P, Hills N, Lustig RH. The relationship of sugar to population-level diabetes prevalence: an econometric analysis of repeated cross-sectional data. PLoS One. 2013;8:e57873.
34. Nijman C, Zijp I, Sierksma A, Roodenburg A, Leenen R, Van den Kerkhoff C, Weststrate J, Meijer G. A method to improve the nutritional quality of foods and beverages based on dietary recommendations. Eur J Clin Nutr. 2007;61:461–71.
35. Scarborough P, Rayner M, Stockley L. Developing nutrient profile models: a systematic approach. Public Health Nutr. 2007;10:330–6.
36. Maillot M, Darmon N, Darmon M, Lafay L, Drewnowski A. Nutrient-dense food groups have high energy costs: an econometric approach to nutrient profiling. J Nutr. 2007;137:1815–20.
37. Behrman JR, Alderman H, Hoddinott J. Malnutrition and hunger. In: Global crises, golobal solutions. Cambridge: United Kingdom Cambridge University Press; 2004. p. 363–420.
38. Fanzo J, Lachat C, Sparling T, Olds T. The nutrition sensitivity of agriculture and food policies: a summary of eight country case studies, About SCN news. 2013.
39. Meerman J, Garrett J, Wüstefeld M. Development partners and country programming in nutrition and agriculture: preview of findings from a landscape review, SCN news. 2013. p. 10–8.
40. Arsenault JE, Fulgoni VL, Hersey JC, Muth MK. A novel approach to selecting and weighting nutrients for nutrient profiling of foods and diets. J Acad Nutr Diet. 2012;112:1968–75.
41. USDA Table of Nutrient Retention Factors [https://www.ars.usda.gov/ARSUserFiles/80400525/Data/retn/retn06.pdf]. Accessed 30 June 2016.

Vitamin D status among the elderly Chinese population: a cross-sectional analysis of the 2010–2013 China national nutrition and health survey (CNNHS)

Jing Chen[1†], Chunfeng Yun[2†], Yuna He[3], Jianhua Piao[1], Lichen Yang[1] and Xiaoguang Yang[1*]

Abstract

Background: Vitamin D inadequacy is common among the elderly, especially within the Asian population. The vitamin D status among healthy adults in the elderly Chinese population was evaluated.

Methods: A total of 6014 healthy adults aged 60 years or older (2948 men, 3066 women) participated in this descriptive cross-sectional analysis. Possible predictors of vitamin D inadequacy were evaluated via multiple logistic regression analyses.

Results: The median serum 25-hydroxyvitamin D (25(OH)D) levels were 61.0 nmol/l (interquartile range (IQR) 44.3–80.6, range 5.1–154.5) for men and 53.7 nmol/l (IQR 38.8–71.0, range 6.0–190.0) for women, with 34.1% (95% confidence interval (CI) 32.4–35.8) of men and 44.0% (95% CI 42.2–45.8) of women presenting vitamin D inadequacy (25(OH)D <50 nmol/l). According to the multivariate logistic regression analyses, vitamin D inadequacy was positively correlated with female gender (P <0.0001), underweight (P = 0.0259), the spring season (P <0.0001), low ambient UVB levels (P <0.0001) and living in large cities (P = 0.0026). For men, vitamin D inadequacy was positively correlated with the spring season (P = 0.0015), low ambient UVB levels (P <0.0001) and living in large cities (P = 0.0022); for women, vitamin D inadequacy was positively correlated with the spring season (P = 0.0005) and low ambient UVB levels (P <.0001).

Conclusions: Vitamin D inadequacy is prevalent among the elderly population in China. Because residing in regions with low ambient UVB levels increases the risk of vitamin D inadequacy both for men and women, vitamin D supplementation and sensible sun exposure should be encouraged, especially during the cooler seasons. Further studies are required to determine the optimal vitamin D intake and sun exposure levels to maintain sufficient vitamin D levels in the elderly Chinese population.

Keywords: Vitamin D, Elderly population, China, Risk factors, Environment

Background

Vitamin D status is related to many types of health outcomes among the elderly population and can contribute to musculoskeletal complications (including proximal myopathy, bone and muscle pain, secondary hyperparathyroidism, osteoporosis, and osteomalacia) [1], chronic diseases (cancer and cardiovascular diseases) [2], autoimmune diseases (systemic lupus erythematosus, multiple sclerosis, scleroderma or systemic sclerosis, autoimmune thyroid diseases, rheumatoid arthritis and primary biliary cirrhosis) [3, 4], and psychotic disorders (depression, self-neglect and cognitive impairment) [5–7]. All these diseases can cause disability among the elderly. Compared to individuals with sufficient vitamin D levels, older women with vitamin D deficiency were significantly older, heavier, and less physically active; furthermore, these

* Correspondence: xgyangcdc@vip.sina.com
[†]Equal contributors
[1]Department of Trace Element Nutrition, National Institute of Nutrition and Health, Chinese Center for Disease Control and Prevention, Room 103, Nanwei Road No. 29, Xicheng District, Beijing 100050, People's Republic of China
Full list of author information is available at the end of the article

women presented with more comorbidities [8]. A healthy vitamin D status in an elderly individual is important to avoid disability. Because the percentage of people in China aged 60 years and older is expected to reach 36.5% by 2050 and 39.6% by 2100 [9], the health of the elderly Chinese population is receiving increasing levels of attention.

The primary source of vitamin D for most human populations is sunlight exposure between approximately 9:00 and 15:00 h (local solar time) during the spring, summer and autumn seasons [10]. At more extreme latitudes, the solar elevation angles and ambient UVB levels are always low; thus, the UVB exposure periods required to produce an ideal quantity of vitamin D are sometimes impractical, especially during the cooler seasons. Vitamin D requirements are thought to vary with age, yet all age groups have been shown to exhibit a high prevalence of 25-hydroxyvitamin D (25(OH)D) insufficiency and secondary hyperparathyroidism [11]. The elderly population requires more vitamin D to produce the increased 25(OH)D concentrations necessary to overcome the hyperparathyroidism associated with their diminishing renal function [11]. Currently, vitamin D deficiency among the elderly population constitutes a widespread and urgent public health issue that must be remedied.

In the present study, the prevalence of vitamin D deficiency and insufficiency in a nationally representative sample of the Chinese population over 60 years old was evaluated. The primary risk factors of inadequate vitamin D levels among the elderly Chinese population was predicted based on age, gender, BMI, ambient UVB levels in the residential regions, vitamin D supplementation levels and hypertension. National vitamin D data are instrumental to the development of appropriate health monitoring of the elderly Chinese population, and the Chinese Center for Disease Control and Prevention could use these data to identify at-risk groups and provide advice regarding the use of vitamin D supplements.

Methods

Study design

Data for the present analysis were extracted from the China National Nutrition and Health Survey (CNNHS), 2010–2013. This survey was a nationally representative cross-sectional study conducted by the Chinese Center for Disease Control and Prevention to assess the health and nutrition of Chinese civilians. The survey randomly selected 150 districts (urban) or counties (rural) within all thirty-one provinces, autonomous regions and municipalities directly under the central Chinese government (except Taiwan, Hong Kong and Macao). The country was divided into four strata according to socioeconomic characteristics: large cities, small to medium cities, general rural areas and poor rural areas.

Participants and setting

This study used a stratified multistage probability sampling design and aimed to randomly survey approximately 40 people (20 men, 20 women) aged 60 years or older in each district or county. Participants who did not have adequate serum samples for 25(OH)D measurement and individuals with a history of either kidney disease or chronic liver disease were excluded. Finally, 2948 men and 3066 women were enrolled in the study. Serum samples were collected from the participants between June 2013 and March 2014, and the body mass index (BMI) was calculated as the weight (in kg) divided by the height (in m) squared. According to the Chinese definitions, underweight, overweight and obesity were defined using the BMI cut-off points of 18.5, 24 and 28 kg/m^2, respectively [12].

Data collection

Demographic data (age, ethnicity) and data on vitamin D supplement use and educational level were collected based on self-reports. After 5 min of rest in a seated position, blood pressure levels were measured twice from the right arm of each participant; the mean of the two measurements was used for analysis. Hypertension was defined as two separate blood pressure measurements >140/90 mmHg at least 6 h apart [13]. On the day after the participants provided written informed consent, blood samples were collected in the morning after a fasting period of 10–12 h and centrifuged within 0.5–1 h following collection. Serum samples were then aliquoted and stored at —80 °C until further analysis.

Measurement of serum 25-hydroxyvitamin D

Serum 25(OH)D levels were quantified by using 25-Hydroxyvitamin D radioimmunoassay kits (DiaSorin-RIA; DiaSorin Inc., Stillwater, MN) on a GC-2016 gamma counter (ANHUI UCTC ZONKIA SCIENTIFIC INSTRUMENTS CO. LTD, Anhui, China). The interassay coefficients of variation (CVs) were 3.8 and 3.5% at 24.8 and 57.5 nmol/l, respectively. The DiaSorin-RIA method used in this study was in acceptable agreement with an LC-MS/MS method that has been accepted by the College of American Pathologists (CAP) as a proficient test to assess vitamin D deficiency and insufficiency [14]. In our study, participants with a serum 25(OH)D concentration lower than 30 nmol/l were stratified as vitamin D deficient; those with a concentration between 30 and 50 nmol/l as vitamin D insufficient; and those with a concentration above 50 nmol/l as vitamin D sufficient [15]. Both vitamin D deficiency and vitamin D insufficiency were grouped together as vitamin D inadequacy (25(OH)D less than 50 nmol/l).

Ambient UVB measurements

The ambient UV radiation exposure levels for each participant was estimated using the Chinese administrative division codes of each participant's current residential address. Latitudinal and longitudinal coordinates were obtained for each code and matched against available UVB data available from a 1° latitude × 1° longitude grid of readings of a total ozone mapping spectrometer (TOMS) mounted on the Nimbus-7 satellite; the UVB data were obtained from an archived database at the NASA Goddard Space Flight Center. This database was used to estimate the average erythemally weighted UVB dose (J/m^2) reaching the Earth at each location between June 2013 and March 2014. The HDFtool in MATLAB 7.11.0 (R2010b) was utilized to extract relevant information from the database, and the annual average ambient UVB levels for the entire cohort were classified into tertiles.

Statistical analysis

The participants were divided into sub-classes according to a number of hypothesized predictors for vitamin D status: regional stratum, ambient UVB level at the place of residence, season (spring, March to May; summer, June to August; autumn, September to November; and winter, December to February), age, BMI, vitamin D supplement usage, and hypertension. The Kolmogorov-Smirnov test was used to analyse the normality of each sub-class, and the results indicated that most sub-classes did not follow a normal distribution. Therefore, a Kruskal-Wallis test followed by a Mann-Whitney *U* test was conducted to examine the relationships between vitamin D levels and the hypothesized predictors. To investigate the relationship between vitamin D inadequacy and several possible predictors (e.g., age, BMI, ambient UVB level at area of residence, vitamin D supplement use, hypertension), a multinomial logistic regression analysis was performed. The statistical software package SAS version 9.2 was used for data analysis. The primary analysis was descriptive and includes the 95% confidence interval (CI). Using two-sided tests, the significance level was set at $P < 0.05$.

Results

As a part of the CNNHS in 2010–2013, the serum 25(OH)D levels of 6014 healthy individuals over 60 years old (man 2948, women 3066) were analysed. The median ages were 67.5 years (interquartile range (IQR) 63.2–73.2, range 60.0–100.2) for men and 66.8 years (IQR 63.0–72.5, range 60.0–98.2) for women. Among elderly men, the median BMI level was 23.2 kg/m^2 (IQR 20.3–25.8, range 12.3–44.8) with 14.0% of the participants underweight (BMI <18.5 kg/m^2), 29.5% overweight (BMI = 24–28 kg/m^2) and 12.3% obese (BMI> 28 kg/m^2). Among elderly women, the median BMI level was 23.3 kg/m^2 (IQR 20.5–25.9, range 11.4–38.9) with 13.5% of the participants underweight (BMI <18.5 kg/m^2), 32.5% overweight (BMI = 24–28 kg/m^2) and 11.8% obese (BMI> 28 kg/m^2). In addition, 29.4% of the elderly men and 29.9% of the elderly women were classified as hypertensive. In total, only 0.3% of the elderly men and 0.3% of the elderly women reported using vitamin D supplements. The baseline characteristics and 25(OH)D values of all the participants are presented in Table 1.

Among elderly men, the median serum 25(OH)D levels were 61.0 nmol/l (IQR 44.3–80.6, range 5.1–154.5), with an estimated 7.8% (95% CI 6.9–8.8) presenting vitamin D deficiency (25(OH)D <30 nmol/l) and 26.3% (95% CI 24.7–27.9) showing signs of vitamin D insufficiency (30 nmol/l ≤25(OH)D <50 nmol/l). Among elderly women, the median serum 25(OH)D levels were 53.7 nmol/l (IQR 38.8–71.0, range 6.0–190.0), with an estimated 12.0% (95% CI 10.8–13.2) presenting vitamin D deficiency (25(OH)D <30 nmol/l) and 32.0% (95% CI 30.4–33.7) showing signs of vitamin D insufficiency (30 nmol/l ≤25(OH)D <50 nmol/l). (Table 1)

In the logistic regression analysis for all the participants (Table 2), the following factors were associated with vitamin D inadequacy (OR; 95% CI): gender (women: 1.544; 1.388–1.717; P <0.0001 relative to men), BMI (underweight: 1.238; 1.049–1.462; P = 0.0259 relative to normal weight); season (spring: 2.487; 1.849–3.346, P <0.0001 relative to summer); ambient UVB levels in region of residence (low: 2.233; 1.952–2.553; P <0 · 0001 relative to high) and regional strata (large cities: 1.287: 1.109–1.494; P = 0.0026 relative to general rural areas). According to a logistic regression analysis of men (Table 2), vitamin D inadequacy was associated with season (spring: 2.137; 1.398–3.268; P = 0.0015 relative to summer) ambient UVB levels at region of residence (low: 2.119; 1.743–2.575; P <0 · 0001 relative to high) and regional strata (large cities: 1.466; 1.179–1.823; P = 0.0022 relative to general rural areas). According to a logistic regression analysis of women (Table 2), vitamin D inadequacy was associated with season (spring: 2.858; 1.887–4.327; P = 0.0005 relative to summer) and ambient UVB levels at region of residence (low: 2.352; 1.954–2.832; P <.0001 relative to high).

Discussion

More than one-third of the elderly Chinese participants in the present study had vitamin D inadequacies (25(OH)D <50 nmol/l), even during the summer and autumn seasons. The prevalence of vitamin D deficiency peaked at approximately 40 and 50% for men and women, respectively, during the spring season. The prevalence of vitamin D levels <50 nmol/l among Chinese adults is 34.3%, which is similar to that of the

Table 1 Demographic characteristics of the elderly Chinese study participants

	Men							Women						
	n	25(OH)D (nmol/l)		Percentage with 25(OH)D levels			*P* value	n	25(OH)D (nmol/l)		Percentage with 25(OH)D levels			*P* value
		mean	SD	<30 nmol/l	30–50 nmol/l	>50 nmol/l			mean	SD	<30 nmol/l	30–50 nmol/l	>50 nmol/l	
Total	2948	63.3	25.1	7.8	26.3	65.9		3066	56.1	22.9	12	32	56	
Age group							0.7021							0.2938
60–69	1818	63.9	25.1	7.5	25.5	67		1987	56.4	23.1	11.2	32.7	56.1	
70–79	951	62.5	25	8.2	27.7	64.1		878	55.4	22.4	13.7	30.2	56.2	
80+	179	61.9	24.6	8.4	27.9	63.7		201	56	22.9	11.9	33.8	54.2	
BMI (kg/m2)							0.7826							0.3829
<18.5	414	62.7	25.9	6.8	30	63.3		398	56.1	24.5	12.6	33.4	54	
18.5–24.0	1303	63.9	24.9	7.7	25	67.3		1363	56.9	23.1	11.4	31.4	57.2	
24.0–28.0	870	63.2	25	8.2	25.4	66.4		957	55.3	22.1	13	31.5	55.6	
>28.0	361	62.2	24.9	8.6	29.1	62.3		348	55	21.8	10.9	34.5	54.6	
Ethnicity							0.006							0.2212
Han nationality	2719	63.7	25	7.3	26.2	66.5		2810	56.4	23	11.8	31.6	56.6	
Hui nationality	11	71.9	24.6	9.1	0	90.9		20	53.5	17.4	5	50	45	
Other nationality	218	57.8	25	13.8	28.9	57.3		236	52.2	20.7	14.4	36	49.6	
Regional strata							<0.0001							0.0005
Large cities	701	58.2	23	9.8	30.7	59.5		724	55.3	22.1	10.1	37.6	52.3	
Small to medium cities	875	65.6	26.5	6.6	25.9	67.4		885	55.8	23.5	12.2	33.7	54.1	
General rural areas	859	65.6	25.4	7.9	21.5	70.5		924	57.2	23.6	14.2	26.8	59	
Poor rural areas	513	62.4	23.8	6.8	29	64.1		533	55.6	21.3	10.3	30.8	58.9	
Vitamin D supplementation							0.8237							0.4676
No	2940	63.3	25.1	7.8	26.3	65.9		3057	56.1	22.9	12	32	56	
Yes	8	68.4	24.3	0	25	75		9	51.9	14	11.1	33.3	55.6	
Ambient UVB levels (J/m2)							<0.0001							<0.0001
Low	953	60.1	25.2	8.1	34	57.9		964	51.7	21.6	13.8	39.6	46.6	
Medium	953	62.9	25.3	8.6	26.9	64.5		1045	55.7	23.1	13.4	31.5	55.1	
High	1042	66.6	24.3	6.8	18.8	74.4		1057	60.5	22.9	8.9	25.6	65.5	
Hypertension							0.5523							0.6414
No	2081	63.9	25	7.5	25.9	66.6		2150	55.9	22.8	12.5	31.9	55.6	
Yes	867	61.9	25.2	8.5	27.3	64.1		916	56.6	22.9	10.7	32.3	57	
Education level							0.8044							0.0779
Illiteracy	248	61.2	24.9	9.3	27	63.7		254	55	25.9	15.8	30.3	53.9	
Literate	2700	63.5	25.1	7.7	26.3	66.1		2812	56.2	22.6	11.6	32.2	56.2	
Season							0.1786							<0.0001
Spring	125	56.1	25.1	13.6	32.8	53.6		132	49.1	18.9	16.7	40.2	43.2	
Summer	382	64.1	23.9	6.3	24.9	68.8		383	59	21.8	7.3	28.2	64.5	
Autumn	1943	63.8	25.5	7.5	26.4	66.1		2042	56.6	23.3	11.5	32.2	56.3	
Winter	498	62.6	24.2	8.6	25.5	65.9		509	53.7	22.4	16.1	32.2	51.7	

Mann-Whitney *U* test was used for comparisons of different sub-groups

Table 2 Associations of various lifestyle factors with vitamin D inadequacy among the elderly Chinese population

	Total (*n*=6014)		Men (*n*=2948)		Women (*n*=3066)	
	OR (95% CI)	*P* value	OR (95% CI)	*P* value	OR (95% CI)	*P* value
Gender						
Men	ref					
Women	1.544 (1.388–1.717)	<0.0001				
Age group						
60–69	ref		ref		ref	
70–79	1.066 (0.948–1.199)	0.9405	1.126 (0.952–1.332)	0.6001	1.01 (0.858–1.19)	0.5367
80+	1.149 (0.923–1.432)	0.3334	1.132 (0.816–1.572)	0.6947	1.159 (0.86–1.56)	0.3447
BMI (kg/m2)						
18.5–24.0	ref		ref		ref	
<18.5	1.238 (1.049–1.462)	0.0259	1.261 (0.994–1.6)	0.0857	1.225 (0.971–1.546)	0.1284
24.0–28.0	1.005 (0.885–1.141)	0.1451	0.974 (0.806–1.177)	0.1329	1.031 (0.868–1.226)	0.5529
>28.0	1.079 (0.904–1.289)	0.9713	1.11 (0.86–1.433)	0.7736	1.044 (0.815–1.336)	0.7716
Season						
Summer	ref		ref		ref	
Spring	2.487 (1.849–3.346)	<0.0001	2.137 (1.398–3.268)	0.0015	2.858 (1.887–4.327)	0.0005
Autumn	1.462 (1.235–1.731)	0.2201	1.269 (0.996–1.618)	0.3442	1.66 (1.313–2.098)	0.4294
Winter	1.591 (1.301–1.947)	0.6809	1.245 (0.929–1.667)	0.3491	1.977 (1.496–2.614)	0.1581
Ambient UVB (J/m2)						
High	ref		ref		ref	
Low	2.233 (1.952–2.553)	<0.0001	2.119 (1.743–2.575)	<0.0001	2.352 (1.954–2.832)	<0.0001
Medium	1.646 (1.442–1.877)	0.0939	1.665 (1.37–2.025)	0.1111	1.625 (1.358–1.944)	0.4636
Education level						
Illiteracy	ref		ref		ref	
Literate	0.854 (0.704–1.036)	0.1085	0.875 (0.661–1.158)	0.3515	0.837 (0.641–1.094)	0.1928
Region strata						
General rural areas	ref		ref		ref	
Large cities	1.287 (1.109–1.494)	0.0026	1.466 (1.179–1.823)	0.0022	1.147 (0.935–1.408)	0.2101
Small to medium cities	1.136 (0.987–1.307)	0.664	1.093 (0.887–1.346)	0.2145	1.18 (0.974–1.429)	0.0716
Poor rural areas	1.052 (0.894–1.238)	0.2912	1.234 (0.974–1.565)	0.6048	0.916 (0.732–1.145)	0.0573
Hypertension						
No	ref		ref		ref	
Yes	1.012 (0.894–1.145)	0.8529	0.911 (0.76–1.093)	0.3181	1.099 (0.928–1.301)	0.2751

Canadian population (36.8%) [16], slightly lower than that of the European population(40.4%) [17] and higher than that of the US population (24%) [18]. In this study, the median 25(OH)D level in Chinese adults was 61.0 nmol/l, which was similar with the studies in the US [18] (median 25(OH)D_3: 63.6 nmol/l) and Canadian populations (median 25(OH)D: 63.8 nmol/l) [16].

Seasonal variations were observed in the serum 25(OH)D concentrations among the participants, with the lowest serum 25(OH)D concentrations reported during the spring months. The 2007–2010 National Health and Nutrition Examination Survey (NHANES) provided the nationally representative serum 25(OH)D concentrations in the US, and seasonal differences in vitamin D status were also observed [18]. In addition, our result was similar to a previous study, which noted that the vitamin D status was poorest during the spring among the elderly population in northern China [19].

In this study, a significant gender difference regarding the risk of vitamin D deficiency was identified. Compared to older men, older women had a 1.544-fold increased risk of vitamin D deficiency; this result is similar with a previous study focused in Jinan (Shandong province, China), which reported that the men had a better vitamin D status than women [20]. Another study in Caucasian adults indicated that plasma 25(OH)D levels were lower in women overall, especially among older subjects [21]. The different hormone levels and lifestyles may be possible contributors to different vitamin D levels between men and women. Women are more likely to use sunglasses, sunscreen or other sun protection equipment than men [22], especially among the Chinese population [23]. In addition, multivariate linear regression analysis showed that lower vitamin D levels were strongly associated with sunscreen use [24].

Elderly individuals who were underweight had a higher risk of vitamin D deficiency than those at a normal weight. There has been extensive discussion regarding the relationship between vitamin D deficiency and body weight, with many studies reporting an inverse association between vitamin D deficiency and obesity [25–28]. The long-standing concept that fat tissue is a storage site for vitamin D has led many researchers to believe that the association between vitamin D deficiency and obesity may due to increased metabolic clearance of vitamin D through enhanced uptake in fat tissue [29] and/or decreased bioavailability of vitamin D once it is deposited in fat tissue [30]. However, identify an association between increased body weight and vitamin D deficiency was not identified in the present study. Furthermore, the low percentage of participants with a high BMI might have impaired the ability to detect this association. Blum et al. [31] reported that fat tissue and serum vitamin D concentrations were positively correlated, which indicated that we need to rediscover the cause responsible for the association between vitamin D deficiency and body weight. In our study, underweight individuals were at higher risk for vitamin D deficiency, an observation that was similar to those of previous reports [21, 32]. Although underweight people are more likely to be malnourished, which could result in vitamin D deficiency [32], the real cause is still unknown.

Men living in large cities are at increased risk for vitamin D deficiency than those living in rural areas. Air pollution in the cities can decrease the ambient UVB level and affected the vitamin D health of the urban population [33]; this may be an explanation why, in our study, older people living in big cities presented a poorer vitamin D status than rural residents. However, the differences between rural and urban citizens could not be observed among older women, who were more likely to be vitamin D deficient than men in this study. Almost half of the elderly women in China were categorized with vitamin D inadequacy; therefore, the different vitamin D statuses between the urban and rural populations were not as significant among older Chinese women.

Based on our logistic regression, the elderly population (men and women) living in regions with low ambient UVB levels are at higher risk of vitamin D inadequacy than individuals living in areas with high or medium ambient UVB levels. As skin exposure to UVB rays serves is a primary source of vitamin D for most people, the exposure period required to achieve an equivalent oral dose of approximately 1000 IU vitamin D increases with increasing latitude [10]; therefore, ambient UVB levels were an expected predictor of vitamin D inadequacy in our study. However, vitamin D deficiency is also common in regions with plentiful sunlight [34, 35]. In China, there was an increasing trend in the risk of vitamin D deficiency among pregnant women exposed to low ambient UVB levels [36].

The study presents some limitations. Several studies have shown that sun exposure is an important determinant of serum 25(OH)D levels [37, 38]; however, we were unable to determine the duration and region of sun exposure for each participant. Instead, we used the ambient UVB levels to estimate the sun exposure levels for the participants and found that these ambient UVB levels affect the serum 25(OH)D levels among the elderly Chinese population. Dietary calcium intake is another crucial factor that affects vitamin D status, and some experimental studies have shown that dietary calcium deficiency can lead to secondary vitamin D deficiency [39]. Unfortunately, we did not estimate the dietary calcium intake levels for each participant.

The study was a descriptive cross-sectional analysis. These results can only inform us of associations between potential predictive factors and vitamin D deficiency levels, but we cannot assess the root causes of the increased incidence of vitamin D deficiency and insufficiency among the elderly Chinese population, which may be another limitation of our study. Although the study was cross-sectional in nature, the findings suggest that exposure to elevated UVB levels may prevent vitamin D deficiency and insufficiency.

Conclusions

Vitamin D deficiency and insufficiency were common among the elderly Chinese population, with almost one-third of the participants classified as having vitamin D deficiency or insufficiency. These conditions are common among older women, individuals residing in regions with low ambient UVB levels and older men living in large cities. During the spring season, vitamin D deficiency and insufficiency are more pronounced than during any other season. Further studies must identify optimal durations of outdoor activity and the necessary vitamin D intake levels to maintain sufficient vitamin D levels (25(OH)D >50 nmol/l) among the elderly population in China.

Acknowledgements
The authors would like to thank all the study participants as well as the staff who worked on the 2010–2013 CNNHS.

Funding
The study was supported by the 2012 Chinese Nutrition Society (CNS) Nutrition Research Foundation—DSM Research Fund (grant number 2013-021) and a special fund for health-scientific research in the public interest (grant number 20120212) from the National Health and Family Planning Commission of the People's Republic of China. Without these funds, we could not complete this research.

Availability of data and material
The data that support the findings of this study are available from the National Institute for Nutrition and Health at the Chinese Center for Disease Control and Prevention. However, there are restrictions regarding the availability of these data, which were obtained under license for the current study and are thus not publicly available. However, data are from the corresponding author upon reasonable request and with permission from the National Institute for Nutrition and Health at the Chinese Center for Disease Control and Prevention.

Authors' contributions
JC and CY measured the participants' serum 25(OH)D levels, performed the statistical analyses and wrote the paper. YH was responsible for data management and analysis as well as manuscript revisions. JP participated in project management and interpretation of the results. LY participated in project coordination and revised the manuscripts. XY conceived of the study and participated in its design and coordination. All authors read and approved the final manuscript.

Competing interests
The authors declare that they have no competing interests.

Consent for publication
Not applicable.

Ethics approval and consent to participate
The study was conducted according to the guidelines set by the Declaration of Helsinki, and all procedures involving human subjects were approved by the Ethics Committee of the National Institute for Nutrition and Health at the Chinese Center for Disease Control and Prevention. All participants in this survey provided written informed consent.

Author details
[1]Department of Trace Element Nutrition, National Institute of Nutrition and Health, Chinese Center for Disease Control and Prevention, Room 103, Nanwei Road No. 29, Xicheng District, Beijing 100050, People's Republic of China. [2]Institute of Population Research, Peking University, Beijing 100871, People's Republic of China. [3]Department of Nutrition Surveillance, National Institute of Nutrition and Health, Chinese Center for Disease Control and Prevention, Beijing 100050, People's Republic of China.

References

1. Lips P. Vitamin D, deficiency and secondary hyperparathyroidism in the elderly: consequences for bone loss and fractures and therapeutic implications. Endocr Rev. 2001;22:477–501.
2. Michaelsson K, Baron JA, Snellman G, Gedeborg R, Byberg L, Sundstrom J, et al. Plasma vitamin D and mortality in older men: a community-based prospective cohort study. Am J Clin Nutr. 2010;92:841–8.
3. Abaza NM, El-Mallah RM, Shaaban A, Mobasher SA, Al-Hassanein KF, Abdel Zaher AA, et al. Vitamin D deficiency in Egyptian systemic lupus erythematosus patients: how prevalent and does it impact disease activity? Integr Med Insights. 2016;11:27–33.
4. Rosen Y, Daich J, Soliman I, Brathwaite E, Shoenfeld Y. Vitamin D and autoimmunity. Scand J Rheumatol. 2016;45:439–47.
5. Aung K, Burnett J, Smith SM, Dyer CB. Vitamin D deficiency associated with self-neglect in the elderly. J Elder Abuse Negl. 2006;18:63–78.
6. Barnard K, Colon-Emeric C. Extraskeletal effects of vitamin D in older adults: cardiovascular disease, mortality, mood, and cognition. Am J Geriatr Pharmacother. 2010;8:4–33.
7. Chei CL, Raman P, Yin ZX, Shi XM, Zeng Y, Matchar DB. Vitamin D levels and cognition in elderly adults in China. J Am Geriatr Soc. 2014;62:2125–9.
8. Bolland MJ, Bacon CJ, Horne AM, Mason BH, Ames RW, Wang TK, et al. Vitamin D insufficiency and health outcomes over 5 y in older women. Am J Clin Nutr. 2010;91:82–9.
9. United Nations Department of Economic and Social Affairs, Population Division. World population prospects: the 2015 revision, key findings and advance tables. In: Working paper No. ESA/P/WP.241. 2015.
10. Webb AR, Engelsen O. Calculated ultraviolet exposure levels for a healthy vitamin D status. Photochem Photobiol. 2006;82:1697–703.
11. Vieth R, Ladak Y, Walfish PG. Age-related changes in the 25-hydroxyvitamin D versus parathyroid hormone relationship suggest a different reason why older adults require more vitamin D. J Clin Endocrinol Metab. 2003;88:185–91.
12. National Health and Family Planning Commission of the People's Republic of China. People's republic of China health industry standards: criteria of weight for adults. 2013. WS/T 428–2013.
13. National High Blood Pressure Education Program Working Group. National high blood pressure education program working group report on hypertension in the elderly. Hypertension. 1994;23:275–85.
14. Yun C, Chen J, Yang C, Li Y, Piao J, Yang X. Comparison of two 25-hydroxyvitamin D immunoassays to liquid chromatography-tandem mass spectrometry in assessing samples from the Chinese population. Clin Chim Acta. 2015;448:22–6.
15. Francis R, Aspray T, Fraser W, Gittoes N, Javaid K, MacDonald H. Vitamin D and bone health: a practical clinical guideline for patient management. Scotland: National Osteoporosis Society; 2013.
16. Sarafin K, Durazo-Arvizu R, Tian L, Phinney KW, Tai S, Camara JE, et al. Standardizing 25-hydroxyvitamin D values from the Canadian health measures survey. Am J Clin Nutr. 2015;102:1044–50.
17. Cashman KD, Dowling KG, Skrabakova Z, Gonzalez-Gross M, Valtuena J, De Henauw S, et al. Vitamin D deficiency in Europe: pandemic? Am J Clin Nutr. 2016;103:1033–44.
18. Schleicher RL, Sternberg MR, Looker AC, Yetley EA, Lacher DA, Sempos CT, et al. national estimates of serum total 25-hydroxyvitamin D and metabolite concentrations measured by liquid chromatography-tandem mass spectrometry in the US population during 2007–2010. J Nutr. 2016;146:1051–61.
19. Yan L, Prentice A, Zhang H, Wang X, Stirling DM, Golden MM. Vitamin D status and parathyroid hormone concentrations in Chinese women and men from north-east of the People's Republic of China. Eur J Clin Nutr. 2000;54:68–72.
20. Feng X, Guo T, Wang Y, Kang D, Che X, Zhang H, et al. The vitamin D status and its effects on life quality among the elderly in Jinan, China. Arch Gerontol Geriatr. 2016;62:26–9.
21. Touvier M, Deschasaux M, Montourcy M, Sutton A, Charnaux N, Kesse-Guyot E, et al. Determinants of vitamin D status in Caucasian adults: influence of sun exposure, dietary intake, sociodemographic, lifestyle, anthropometric, and genetic factors. J Invest Dermatol. 2015;135:378–88.
22. Holman DM, Berkowitz Z, Guy Jr GP, Hawkins NA, Saraiya M, Watson M. Patterns of sunscreen use on the face and other exposed skin among US adults. J Am Acad Dermatol. 2015;73:83–92. e1.
23. Cheng S, Lian S, Hao Y, Kang N, Li S, Nie Y, et al. Sun-exposure knowledge and protection behavior in a North Chinese population: a questionnaire-based study. Photodermatol Photoimmunol Photomed. 2010;26:177–81.
24. Golan-Cohen A, Merzon E, Alhin O, Kitai E, Fogelman Y. Blood levels of vitamin D and health-functional status in asymptomatic individuals: a cross sectional study. J Eval Clin Pract. 2016;22(6):950–55.
25. Holick MF, Chen TC. Vitamin D deficiency: a worldwide problem with health consequences. Am J Clin Nutr. 2008;87:1080s–6s.
26. Gilbert-Diamond D, Baylin A, Mora-Plazas M, Marin C, Arsenault JE, Hughes MD, et al. Vitamin D deficiency and anthropometric indicators of adiposity in school-age children: a prospective study. Am J Clin Nutr. 2010;92:1446–51.
27. Tran B, Armstrong BK, McGeechan K, Ebeling PR, English DR, Kimlin MG, et al. Predicting vitamin D deficiency in older Australian adults. Clin Endocrinol (Oxf). 2013;79:631–40.

28. Souberbielle JC, Massart C, Brailly-Tabard S, Cavalier E, Chanson P. Prevalence and determinants of vitamin D deficiency in healthy French adults: the VARIETE study. Endocrine. 2016;1–8. https://www.ncbi.nlm.nih.gov/pubmed/?term=Prevalence+and+determinants+of+vitamin+D+deficiency+in+healthy+French+adults%3A+the+VARIETE+study.
29. Liel Y, Ulmer E, Shary J, Hollis BW, Bell NH. Low circulating vitamin D in obesity. Calcif Tissue Int. 1988;43:199–201.
30. Wortsman J, Matsuoka LY, Chen TC, Lu Z, Holick MF. Decreased bioavailability of vitamin D in obesity. Am J Clin Nutr. 2000;72:690–3.
31. Blum M, Dolnikowski G, Seyoum E, Harris SS, Booth SL, Peterson J, et al. Vitamin D(3) in fat tissue. Endocrine. 2008;33:90–4.
32. Kim KJ, Kim YJ, Kim SH, An JH, Yoo HJ, Kim HY, et al. Vitamin D status and associated metabolic risk factors among North Korean refugees in South Korea: a cross-sectional study. BMJ Open. 2015;5:e009140.
33. Agarwal KS, Mughal MZ, Upadhyay P, Berry JL, Mawer EB, Puliyel JM. The impact of atmospheric pollution on vitamin D status of infants and toddlers in Delhi. India Arch Dis Child. 2002;87:111–3.
34. Trilok Kumar G, Chugh R, Eggersdorfer M. Poor vitamin D status in healthy populations in India: a review of current evidence. Int J Vitam Nutr Res. 2015;85:185–201.
35. Smith G, Wimalawansa SJ, Laillou A, Sophonneary P, Un S, Hong R, et al. High prevalence of vitamin D deficiency in Cambodian women: a common deficiency in a sunny country. Nutrients. 2016;8:290.
36. Yun C, Chen J, He Y, Mao D, Wang R, Zhang Y, et al. Vitamin D deficiency prevalence and risk factors among pregnant Chinese women. Public Health Nutr. 2015;1–9. https://www.ncbi.nlm.nih.gov/pubmed/26585546.
37. Brot C, Vestergaard P, Kolthoff N, Gram J, Hermann AP, Sorensen OH. Vitamin D status and its adequacy in healthy Danish perimenopausal women: relationships to dietary intake, sun exposure and serum parathyroid hormone. Br J Nutr. 2001;86 Suppl 1:S97–103.
38. Maeda SS, Kunii IS, Hayashi L, Lazaretti-Castro M. The effect of sun exposure on 25-hydroxyvitamin D concentrations in young healthy subjects living in the city of Sao Paulo, Brazil. Braz J Med Biol Res. 2007;40:1653–9.
39. Clements MR, Johnson L, Fraser DR. A new mechanism for induced vitamin D deficiency in calcium deprivation. Nature. 1987;325:62–5.

6

The 2014 FDA assessment of commercial fish: practical considerations for improved dietary guidance

Jennifer McGuire[1*], Jason Kaplan[2], John Lapolla[2] and Rima Kleiner[1]

Abstract

The U.S. Food and Drug Administration (FDA) recently released its report: *A Quantitative Assessment of the Net Effects on Fetal Neurodevelopment from Eating Commercial Fish (As Measured by IQ and also by Early Age Verbal Development in Children)*. By evaluating the benefits and potential concerns of eating fish during pregnancy and breastfeeding, the analysis suggests that pregnant women consuming two seafood meals (8–12 oz) per week could provide their child with an additional 3.3 IQ points by age 9. Recent insights from behavioral economics research indicate that other factors, such as concerns about price and methylmercury (MeHg) exposure, appear to reduce fish consumption in many individuals.

To assess the net effects of eating commercial fish during pregnancy, we compared the consumption of select fish species necessary to achieve IQ benefits with the amount necessary to have adverse developmental effects due to MeHg exposure. For the species or market types evaluated, the number of servings necessary to reach MeHg exposure to observe an adverse effect was at least twice that the amount estimated to achieve peak developmental benefit.

We then reported average costs of fresh and canned or pouched fish, and calculated the cost per week for pregnant women to achieve maximum IQ benefits for their gestating child. Canned light tuna was the least expensive option at $1.83 per week to achieve maximum IQ benefit.

Due to their relatively low cost, canned and pouched fish products eaten with enough regularity are likely to provide peak cognitive benefits. Because of its popularity, canned and pouched tuna could provide some of the largest cognitive benefits from fish consumption in the U.S. Future FDA consumer advice and related educational initiatives could benefit from a broader perspective that highlights the importance of affordable and accessible fish choices. These observations underscore the importance of clear public health messaging that address both health benefits and such real-world considerations as cost and convenience.

Keywords: Fish, Pregnancy, Diet, Mercury, Development, Cognitive

Introduction

In May 2014, the FDA released *A Quantitative Assessment of the Net Effects on Fetal Neurodevelopment from Eating Commercial Fish (As Measured by IQ and also by Early Age Verbal Development in Children)*. The revised 2014 report builds on current data assessing fish consumption during pregnancy and provides a scientific basis for updated dietary advice. While the 2014 report addresses a specific subset of consumers, its findings are of general interest, especially since fetal development contributes to broad public health outcomes. Many fish species are a rich source of essential nutrients, such as protein, vitamin D, selenium, various minerals, and omega-3 fatty acids [1–4]; the nutritional benefits of fish, including the benefits for fetal cognitive development, are well established [4–6].

Despite evidence of nutritional benefit, American consumers have received seemingly contradictory advice about the nutritional value and methylmercury (MeHg) content of many fish species [7–10]. Furthermore, dietary decisions are also affected by a highly diverse market for fish with significant variability in price and geographic access [11–16].

* Correspondence: jmcguire@nfi.org
[1]National Fisheries Institute, 7918 Jones Branch Dr #700, McLean, VA 22102, USA
Full list of author information is available at the end of the article

To address the specific concerns, the FDA's 2014 report dedicated separate analyses to the positive developmental effects of eating various fish and to the independent developmental effects of MeHg exposure, using both analyses to predict net cognitive outcomes for different patterns of fish consumptionInclusive of MeHg exposure, a consistent association was observed between maternal fish consumption and improvements in neurodevelopmental functioning in U.S. children through 9 years of age [17]. Subsequent modeling yielded estimates of the likely change in a child's IQ due to the amount of a specific fish consumed during gestation. The curves tended to show a steep increase in predicted IQ, from slightly below average to moderately above average, when moving from low to recommended levels of fish consumption. Net cognitive benefits were consistently observed when consumption during pregnancy was more than 12 oz per week. Peak benefits varied for each type of fish but generally peaked at 1 to 3 meals per week, diminishing slightly at higher frequencies of consumption but maintaining overall cognitive benefit [17].

These data suggest that, for most fish species consumed in the US, recommended dietary levels do not cause significant MeHg exposure [17]. No adverse cognitive effects from MeHg are expected for most fish species when consumed at a level of 1 to 3 meals per week. Moreover, even at significantly higher levels of consumption than recommended, the negative effects of MeHg are predicted to be far smaller than the adverse effects of eating too little fish [17]. For example, about 120 light tuna sandwiches would need to be consumed each week before reaching the minimum MeHg exposure for adverse cognitive effects to be expected [17]. Lastly, there is a considerable difference between the recommended rate of fish consumption for maximum benefits during pregnancy (12 oz of various fish per week) reported in the current FDA advisory and the 2010 Dietary Guidelines for Americans and the amount currently eaten by pregnant women in the U.S. (1.89 oz per week) [17, 18].

Ideally, consuming the amount of seafood that offers peak benefit rates would lead to better cognitive development and health for many Americans. However, recent analyses on economic incentives and consumer attitudes have outlined challenges to adherence of dietary guidance, mainly attributed to concerns over cost and safety [11, 13, 20]. Consumers appear to overestimate risks of contaminant exposure and underestimate the risks of nutrient deficiency, an outcome with a greater likelihood of occurring [4, 21, 22]. Consumers of commercial fish have historically misinterpreted fish MeHg advisories and reduced their consumption of all fish as a "precaution" [4, 21, 23, 24]. This tendency has been vividly demonstrated in surveys and focus groups. Consumers surveyed in Belgium, for example, tended to have a higher awareness of contaminants in fish than of nutrients, and pregnant women in Boston showed a similar ignorance of nutritional benefits, while citing mercury contamination as a reason for avoiding fish altogether [3, 9].

Economic considerations also appear to limit fish intake. For instance, in opinion polling, fish consumption is influenced by the perception that fish are too expensive for routine consumption (Fig. 1) [25]. Though it is inaccurate for many fish species, this perception attests to the real economic forces that drive consumers toward inexpensive fish options.

FDA communications calibrated to emphasize nutritional benefits, appropriately present risk of MeHg exposure, and highlight the affordability of some fish products could have a major social impact and lead to improved

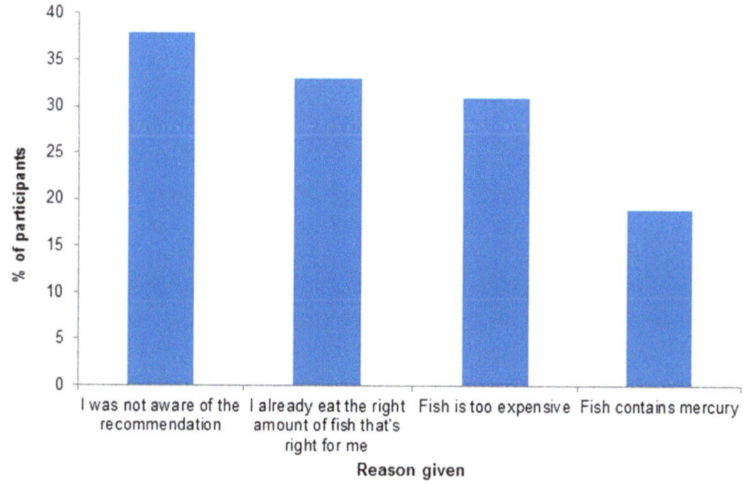

Fig. 1 Reasons for not eating the recommended amount of fish (aided), general population survey [25]. Survey participants were asked to check all that apply from four reasons provided to best describe why they do not eat the recommended amount of fish (at least 2 or 3 servings of any variety of fish or seafood each week)

dietary practices [4, 21, 26]. To that end, this review will supplement the FDA's findings with econometric analyses, providing insight into the real-world determinants of dietary decision making and of fish consumption in particular. Below we survey the commercial fish species for which FDA data, pricing data, and regional access data are currently available. Our aim is to inform future advisories and educational initiatives by identifying the products likely to have the greatest value for public health, in terms of their combined nutritional benefits, affordability, and accessibility.

Materials and methods

Leveraging the FDA's analysis, we considered only those fish species and market types for which the size of developmental benefits was known, and used the peak increase in childhood IQ by 9 years of age as a proxy for developmental benefits in general. As needed, these data were supplemented with independent studies identified on MEDLINE and PubMed. Of the species for which developmental benefit data was available, a smaller group showed significantly larger peak cognitive benefits and was further described by pricing data (multi-year average costs). A final selection of fish species from this smaller cohort was then directly compared, profiling six commercial fish categories as part of a dietary plan for a pregnant woman and listing cost and consumption rates for maximum benefit and adverse event occurrence. The analysis made no substantive modeling assumptions. In addition, notes on geographic distribution from surveys of food outlets in Orangeburg County, South Carolina, and in the U.S. North Central Region were included to profile regional availability. Orangeburg County was chosen because it covers a large land area containing a varied combination of rural, mixed, and urban Census Tracts. (Liese, 2007) Nielsen Holdings N.V., a global information company that assesses consumer behavior, provided data for multi-year trends for average retail price (ARP), polling on consumer attitudes toward seafood and regional availability. As needed, these data were supplemented by independent studies, identified on WebEc and other online resources.

Fish categories in the pricing data were not always aligned with "species or market type" categories in the FDA report, but in borderline cases a match was assumed. Following convention, we expressed weights of fish in ounces (1 oz = 28.35 g) and defined a fish meal as one serving of fish, which was a minimum of 4 oz. In addition, fish steaks were assumed to weigh 3 to 4 oz.

Results

Numerous fish species and market types are listed in ascending order of peak IQ benefit (Table 1). The 90 % confidence interval for Gulf tilefish, swordfish, shark, and king mackerel implies that zero consumption of these species may be advisable, but they are exceptions. Recommended consumption (8–12 oz of fish per week as stated in the 2010 Dietary Guidelines and reestablished in the 2015–2020 Dietary Guidelines) showed remarkably little variation across other fish types [24–26, 36]. While peak IQ benefit size ranged from 1.4 to 3.3 IQ points, consumption rate for net IQ detriment varied by nearly two orders of magnitude between the highest (3.3 IQ points) and lowest (1.4 IQ points) values.

Two features of Table 1 warrant special mention. First, when the four fish with the highest mean concentration of MeHg—gulf tilefish, swordfish, shark, and king mackerel—are excluded, the "best" and "worst" fish types differ in peak benefit by only 0.7 IQ points (2.6 to 3.3 IQ points), and therefore offer comparable developmental benefits. Second, the species with the highest mean concentration of MeHg (gulf tilefish), would need to be eaten at twice the rate predicted to achieve peak IQ benefit in order for adverse effects to be seen. For each other fish type, rates of consumption to experience adverse effects are more than three times greater than the rate needed to reach peak IQ benefit.

To assess the cost of consuming enough fish to achieve an IQ benefit, we reported the mean average cost of each fish variety per pound (ARP) converted to price per ounce over 2009–2013 or 2010–2013 (Table 2). Canned salmon and tuna were the least expensive with average cost per ounce of $0.20 and $0.26, respectively. All listed tuna products provide peak benefits between 2.8 and 3.1 IQ points, while maternal consumption of salmon provides 3.2 IQ points to a child.

We then calculated the number of meals per week and attendant costs of select fish species necessary to attain maximum nutritional benefit for a representative pregnant woman. Canned light tuna demonstrated the lowest cost per week for maximum benefit ($1.83), followed by canned salmon ($2.61) and canned albacore tuna ($2.72) (Table 3). These individual meal-per-week rates for maximum benefit are currently followed by only 5 to 25 % of U.S. men and women [17].

Finally, to briefly assess fish availability at food outlets in several U.S. regions, we report the availability of fresh and canned or pouched fish in common food outlets. Findings reveal that canned seafood is widely available in supermarkets, grocery stores, and convenience stores and found at a greater percentage at these locations than fresh seafood. Its data support the larger market presence of canned fish compared with fresh fish in more remote and rural areas especially.

Discussion

The results of this preliminary analysis indicated that canned and pouched fish products are low-cost options for consumers that can provide substantial cognitive benefits to the developing fetus. Because of the relatively

Table 1 Peak IQ benefits by 9 years of age[a]

Species or market type	Size of maximum benefit expressed as a number of IQ points, Estimate (CI)	Oz. per week to become adverse, Estimate (CI)	Oz. per week to reach maximum benefit, Estimate (CI)
Tilefish, Gulf	1.4 (0.0, 2.6)	16 (0, 30)	8 (0, 13)
Swordfish	2.0 (0.7, 3.0)	24 (12, 43)	8 (7, 13)
Shark	2.0 (0.7, 3.0)	24 (12, 44)	8 (7, 13)
Mackerel, King	2.4 (1.4, 3.2)	32 (16, 59)	8 (7, 13)
Orange Roughy	2.6 (1.7, 3.4)	41 (21, 76)	8 (8, 13)
Grouper	2.7 (1.9, 3.6)	54 (26, 94)	8 (8, 13)
Tuna, Fresh	2.8 (2.1, 3.7)	60 (31, 111)	9 (8, 13)
Mackerel, Spanish	2.8 (2.2, 3.7)	64 (33, 117)	9 (8, 13)
Sable Fish	2.8 (2.2, 3.7)	64 (33, 117)	9 (8, 13)
Bluefish	2.8 (2.2, 3.7)	64 (33, 117)	9 (8, 13)
Tuna, Albacore Canned	2.8 (2.2, 3.7)	67 (35, 123)	9 (8, 13)
Croaker, Pacific	2.9 (2.3, 3.8)	78 (40, 144)	9 (8, 13)
Lingcod & Scorpion Fish	2.9 (2.3, 3.9)	82 (42, 151)	9 (8, 13)
Trout, Saltwater	3.0 (2.3, 3.9)	91 (46, 166)	9 (8, 13)
Bass, Saltwater	3.0 (2.4, 3.9)	95 (49, 174)	9 (8, 13)
Halibut	3.0 (2.4, 3.9)	95 (49, 175)	9 (8, 13)
Carp & Buffalo Fish	3.1 (2.5, 4.0)	139 (71, 254)	9 (8, 13)
Snapper, Porgy & Sheepshead	3.1 (2.5, 4.1)	147 (76, 270)	9 (8, 13)
Perch (ocean), Rockfish, Mullet	3.1 (2.5, 4.1)	157 (81, 288)	9 (8, 13)
Skate	3.1 (2.5, 4.1)	172 (89, 315)	9 (8, 13)
Tuna, Light Canned	3.1 (2.6, 4.1)	296 (101, 360)	9 (8, 13)
Tilefish, Atlantic	3.2 (2.6, 4.1)	214 (110, 392)	9 (8, 13)
Whitefish	3.2 (2.6, 4.1)	235 (121, 432)	9 (8, 13)
Cod	3.2 (2.6, 4.1)	229 (118, 419)	9 (8, 13)
Mackerel, Chub	3.2 (2.6, 4.2)	268 (138, 490)	9 (8, 13)
Croaker, Atlantic	3.2 (2.6, 4.2)	302 (156, 553)	9 (8, 13)
Flatfish & Flounder	3.2 (2.6, 4.2)	310 (160, 568)	9 (8, 13)
Haddock, Hake & Monkfish	3.2 (2.6, 4.2)	351 (181, 644)	9 (8, 14)
Smelt	3.2 (2.6, 4.2)	351 (181, 644)	9 (8, 14)
Crabs	3.2 (2.6, 4.2)	374 (193, 685)	9 (8, 14)
Butterfish	3.2 (2.7, 4.2)	406 (209, 744)	9 (8, 14)
Anchovies, Herring, Shad	3.2 (2.7, 4.2)	471 (243, 863)	9 (8, 14)
Mackerel, Atlantic & Atka	3.2 (2.7, 4.2)	581 (248, 881)	9 (8, 14)
Pollock	3.2 (2.7, 4.2)	636 (328, 1166)	9 (8, 14)
Crawfish	3.2 (2.7, 4.2)	693 (357, 1269)	9 (8, 14)
Trout (freshwater)	3.2 (2.7, 4.2)	736 (379, 1349)	10 (8, 14)
Salmon	3.2 (2.7, 4.2)	1,024 (528, 1876)	10 (8, 14)
Clams	3.2 (2.7, 4.2)	1,024 (528, 1876)	10 (8, 14)
Sardines	3.2 (2.8, 4.3)	1,177 (607, 2158)	10 (8, 14)
Catfish & Pangasius	3.3 (2.7, 4.3)	1,385 (714, 2539)	10 (8, 14)

Abbreviations: *CI* 5 to 95 % confidence interval, *IQ* intelligent quotient, *oz.* ounces
[a]Excerpted from 2014 FDA Report (Table V-7)

Table 2 Multi-year average costs[a]

Species or market type	Average cost/ oz., fresh	Average cost/ oz., canned
Anchovy, Herring, Shad	–	$0.65
Bass, Saltwater	$1.11	–
Catfish, Pangasius	$0.26	–
Cod	$0.39	–
Flatfish, Flounder	$0.31	–
Haddock, Hake, Monkfish	$0.44	–
Halibut	$1.01	–
Perch, Ocean, Rockfish, Mullet	$0.33	–
Salmon	$0.45	$0.26
Sardines	–	$0.27
Snapper, Porgy, Sheepshead	$0.47	–
Trout, Freshwater	$0.42	$0.83
Trout, Saltwater	$0.42	$0.83
Tuna, Albacore	–	$0.30
Tuna, Fresh	$0.49	–
Tuna, Light	–	$0.20

[a]Excerpted from Nielsen 2014 [25]

low cost and wide distribution, canned tuna and other canned fish products could be eaten with regularity to provide peak cognitive benefits. By contrast, a large proportion of commercial fish are substantially more expensive, hindering consumer efforts to follow dietary guidance [12, 14–17]. Here we discuss each of these important sub-results, assessing validity and significance through relevant literature.

Developmental benefit

The FDA's peak cognitive benefit data list several fish species that, when part of a pregnant woman's diet, offer average childhood IQ increases of up to 3.3 points. This is a substantial increase, and all the more encouraging given that several of the most beneficial fish species are some of the most consumed [16, 17]. For example, fresh tuna was associated with a benefit of 2.8 IQ points at recommended consumption levels, while light canned tuna offers 3.1 points, the same value as for carp, skate, snapper, and perch (Table 3).

Table 3 Dietary plans for a pregnant woman

Species or market type	Meals per week for maximum benefit	Meals per week for possible adverse effects	Cost per week for maximum benefit	Cost per week as a multiple of cost for canned light tuna
Anchovies, Herring, Shad	3	~150	$5.82	3.18
Fresh Salmon	3–4	~330	$4.52	2.47
Fresh Cod	2–3	~70	$3.50	1.91
Canned Salmon	3–4	~330	$2.61	1.43
Canned Albacore Tuna	2–3	~20	$2.72	1.49
Canned Light Tuna	2–3	~90	$1.83	1

Such results are consistent with the well-characterized nutrition benefits of fish in general. There is a robust evidence base supporting the independent benefits of omega-3 fatty acids, which are essential structural components of neurons, among other cell types, and can only be obtained through dietary sources, including many commercial fish species[1]. Indeed, the FDA report separately considered the possibility that nutrition benefits for each fish type are due chiefly to omega-3 fatty acids and offered a preliminary analysis of developmental effects due to omega-3 fatty acids alone [17]. When omega-3 fatty acids are the sole source of the beneficial effect from fish consumption, a much larger serving size per week is needed to reach peak IQ benefit for most species [17]. Current literature also links omega-3 fatty acids and omega-3 fatty acid subtypes with various post-natal benefits, including longer gestation and increased birth weight; however, distinctions between dietary fish and fish oil supplements have yet to be confirmed [27]. Other nutrients found in fish such as vitamin D, selenium, and the essential amino acids found in protein offer developmental benefits that cannot be achieved with fish oil supplementation exclusively [28].

Regardless of the biochemical basis for the observed population-level cognitive benefits, the results complement an emerging consensus that early neurological development can be enhanced by dietary fish and that this enhancement probably reflects the full nutritional profile of fish [2, 29]. Indeed, a suite of studies have also linked greater maternal fish intake with improved neurological development on various measures. In a seminal study by Hibbeln et al., fish intake below 12 oz per week in pregnant women was associated with an elevated risk of having children in the lowest quartile of verbal development; similar results were obtained for prosocial behavior, fine motor skills, communication, and social development [19]. Independent studies have characterized a similar relationship for closely related measures of motor skills and vocabulary, and found marked benefits in verbal development at 15 months for infants of mothers who ate more than four fish meals per week [30, 31].

Cost and accessibility

The FDA analysis has quantified the developmental benefits of fish consumption, but economic factors are also key determinants of consumer choice. With this in mind, our results include economic data and an assessment of regional availability, which identify the fish species most likely to deliver population-wide cognitive benefits. The objective was to assess not just the nutrient value, but also the convenience of the food source.

Our analysis focused on cost and accessibility, which are both widely accepted determinants of food convenience [20]. The results presented here demonstrate that both cost and accessibility vary greatly among fish that provide strong cognitive benefits. The monthly cost of providing peak developmental benefits for a given commercial fish varied by a factor of more than 3. The substitution of canned tuna for fresh salmon, as a source of peak cognitive benefits, was shown to save an average adult nearly $3 per week in discretionary food spending—a figure whose social implications will be discussed below. Benchmarks for cost are readily available and can highlight its practical meaning for consumers. For example, the difference in cost between canned tuna and fresh salmon at recommended rates of consumption, is $130 annually, or nearly 6 % on average for the typical adult [32]. Similarly, recommended annual rates of canned tuna provide 6.5 g of protein per ounce, similar to the protein content of beef (6.0), less than chicken (8.3), and more than pork (3.5) [32]. This helps to make tuna not only metabolically, but financially practical as a dietary source of protein; a gram of protein from canned tuna costs roughly the same as a gram from beef and considerably less than a gram from pork [33]. In fact, roughly $100 per year, or 4.5 % of at-home food expenses for an average adult would be saved by substituting pork with canned tuna at recommended levels of consumption [33]. The savings are even more dramatic when the number of consumers per household is increased and the household income is decreased. Substituting canned tuna for fresh salmon based on cognitive benefits would save a family of four roughly 7.6 % of its annual food budget per year, while a substitution of canned tuna for pork based on protein content would save roughly 5.8 % per year.

The availability of fish products at food outlets showed similar disparities, particularly in rural areas. In a survey of food outlets in Orangeburg County, South Carolina, canned seafood was available in 100 % of supermarkets and grocery stores surveyed and in more stores than fresh seafood [14]. In a separate survey of food outlets in the U.S. North Central Region, 17 % of supermarket sales were pre-packaged/branded products, and 26 % of all surveyed rural supermarkets sold only pre-packaged/branded seafood [15].

Cost and availability does not, of course, preordain consumers' final selection of individual products. Other factors—including taste preferences and ease of cooking—also influence everyday dietary decision making. Still, the influence of both cost and local availability on the selection of food products generally, and of fish in particular, is thought to be strong. Prohibitive costs and sparse distribution present especially formidable barriers to fish consumption for low-income and rural consumers [11, 12, 14, 34].

These and other economic analyses underscore the potential benefits of public health advice and educational programs developed to educate consumers on optimal fish consumption. The results reported here suggest that fish products, specifically canned light tuna, with substantial nutritional benefits can be realistically adopted as dietary staples by most consumers. Addressing cost, availability, and other practical concerns could allow advisories to provide a broader heuristic framework to encourage consumers to increase their fish intake and meet the 12-ounce-per-week recommendation [18].

Behavioral rationale

Such recommendations could also serve to balance the consumer's tendency to use maladaptive shortcuts and overlook the context for dietary advice, such as avoiding foods with traces of contaminants to the detriment of overall health [4, 22, 23, 35]. This tendency is manifest in the bias against many fish products [4, 21, 23, 24]. In general, consumers deviate from health-optimal behavior because of the perception that there is a tradeoff between access and quality.

Environmental concerns may also contribute to lack of confidence and clarity surrounding fish consumption. Some advocacy groups have recommended avoiding consumption of certain types of fish, citing concerns about species depletion or habitat destruction. A focused perspective on reducing ecological harm can lead to contradictory advice; for example, farm-raised salmon in the diet is encouraged for its high omega-3 and low MeHg content, however some environmental groups suggest eliminating its consumption because of concern over how salmon aquaculture can affect the marine ecosystem [4]. The 2015 Dietary Guidelines for Americans Advisory Committee Report considered both the nutritional and sustainability aspects of seafood and concluded that farm-raised and wild versions of the same species are generally nutritionally similar, safe, and complement each other to meet demand for seafood now and moving forward. The Advisory Committee claim relies on the continuation of a projected 33 % increase in global aquaculture output by 2021, a rate which would raise the total supply of seafood by 15 % [36]. This increased supply would allow for global consumption to meet Dietary Guideline recommendations for consumption (at least 8 oz of seafood per week), if distributed evenly to the world population.

We submit that a strong commitment to effective messaging, with emphasis on the nutritional value of affordable fish products, can equip consumers with the necessary information to make health-optimal choices about the fish they eat. There are ample grounds for optimism about this approach; many pregnant women in focus groups reported

Table 4 Notes on geographic distribution

Market type	Relevant literature
Fresh Fish	In a survey of food outlets in Orangeburg County (OC), South Carolina, fresh seafood was available at 82, 63, and 0 % of supermarkets, grocery stores, and convenience stores, respectively [14].
	In a separate survey of food outlets in the U.S. North Central Region (NCR), 28 % of supermarket seafood sales were fresh products [15].
Canned Fish	Canned seafood was available at 100 %, 100 %, and ≥54 % of OC supermarkets, grocery stores, and convenience stores, respectively [14].
	17 % of NCR supermarket sales were pre-packaged/branded[a] products. 26 % of all surveyed NCR rural supermarkets sold *only* pre-packaged/branded seafood [15].
Canned Salmon	Canned salmon in water was available at 100, 100, and 23 % of OC supermarkets, grocery stores, and convenience stores, respectively [14].
Canned Tuna	Canned tuna in water was available at 100, 100, and 54 % of OC supermarkets, grocery stores, and convenience stores, respectively [14].

[a] Branded seafood products refer to pre-packaged items from companies such as Gorton's™ or Mrs. Paul's™

hearing no advice to eat fish while pregnant, and broader consumer surveys have revealed that the desire for health benefits is one of the main drivers of consumption behavior [3, 9, 13]. Low-income and rural consumers might stand especially to benefit, since their dietary options for fish are often limited to the fish species whose health benefits are rarely publicized [4, 14, 21]. An integrated health outreach strategy that incorporates the FDA's findings within their broader societal context would include advice stressing the nutritional benefits of affordable and accessible fish products and limiting the risk of developmental impairment from a low-fish diet or from harmful exposure to MeHg.

These findings help illustrate the benefits of a consumer-centric analysis, but are not without limitations. Their cost projections are simple averages over 4 to 5 years of recent data; sources of volatility in future pricing were beyond the scope of this analysis. Geographic resolution was also limited, relying on a handful of regional surveys to represent national trends in fish pricing and distribution (Table 4).

Conclusions

American consumers urgently need educational messages and materials that stress the healthful benefits of affordable and convenient fish. The under-consumption of fish, due partly to misconceptions about contaminant levels and due partly to perceived affordability barriers, can adversely affect the health and development of millions. An evidence-based approach to these unmet health needs should address the unintended consequences of the past and the decision making of real consumers. It would highlight the benefits of canned and pouched fish products, including canned and pouched tuna products, since, on several key indices, these products are most likely to deliver the developmental benefits that have so far eluded many Americans.

These products were found to offer high developmental and health benefits, while appearing in more food outlets for lower prices, ultimately saving individual consumers up to $130 per year in discretionary food spending. Such savings could improve the economic bottom line for low-income consumers and influence the dietary choices of nearly all consumers. Though the effect on individual purchasing choices may be subtle, these price differences may cumulatively favor the incorporation of fish products into a regular diet, ideally at levels where their health benefits can be fully realized.

Supplementing current nutrition data with research on consumer preferences and behavior is a likely first step in developing a new program for dietary guidance. A new dietary program rooted in empirical, market-based research could optimize health outcomes nationwide. These results suggest that a thorough consideration of market-based factors can provide dietary guidance based on the everyday considerations that influence consumer choice. In particular, they would likely reveal the need for a realignment of dietary guidance with a consumer-centric assessment of the risks and the benefits of fish consumption.

Endnotes

[1]Beyond development, the role of omega-3 fatty acids in maintaining cardiovascular health is well-documented. (13)

Abbreviations

ARP, average retail price; FDA, Food and Drug Administration; MeHg, methylmercury

Acknowledgments

We gratefully acknowledge support from various scientists with Inventiv Health and the National Fisheries Institute.

Authors' contributions

JM, RK, JL and JK each contributed significantly to the drafting of this manuscript. All authors read and approved the final manuscript.

Competing interests

JM and RK are consultants for the National Fisheries Institute. JL and JK are employed by inVentiv Medical Communications. This work was funded by the National Fisheries Institute.

Author details

[1]National Fisheries Institute, 7918 Jones Branch Dr #700, McLean, VA 22102, USA. [2]inVentiv Medical Communications, 450 West 15th Street, Suite 405, New York, NY 10011, USA.

References

1. Mahaffey KR, Sunderland EM, Chan HM, Choi AL, Grandjean P, Marien K, Oken E, Sakamoto M, Schoeny R, Weihe P. Balancing the benefits of n-3 polyunsaturated fatty acids and the risks of methylmercury exposure from fish consumption. Nutr Rev. 2011;69:493–508.
2. Nesheim MC, Yaktine AL. Committee on Nutrient Relationships in Seafood: Selections to Balance Benefits and Risks. In: Seafood Choices: Balancing Benefits and Risks. National Academies Press. 2007
3. Verbeke W, Sioen I, Pieniak Z, Van Camp J, De Henauw S. Consumer perception versus scientific evidence about health benefits and safety risks from fish consumption. Public Health Nutr. 2005;8:422–9.
4. Oken E, Choi AL, Karagas MR, Marien K, Rheinberger CM, Schoeny R, Sunderland E, Korrick S. Which fish should I eat? Perspectives influencing fish consumption choices. Environ Health Perspect. 2012;120:790–8.
5. Kris-Etherton PM. Fish consumption, fish oil, omega-3 fatty acids, and cardiovascular disease. Circulation. 2002;106:2747–57.
6. Kris-Etherton PM. Position of the American Dietetic Association and Dietitians of Canada: dietary fatty acids. J Am Diet Assoc. 2007;107:1599–611.
7. Monterey Bay Aquarium. Monterey Bay Aquarium Seafood Watch. https://www.seafoodwatch.org/-/m/sfw/pdf/guides/mba-seafoodwatch-northeast-guide.pdf. 2011.
8. Hughner RS, Maher JK, Childs NM. Review of food policy and consumer issues of mercury in fish. J Am Coll Nutr. 2008;27:185–94.
9. Bloomingdale A, Guthrie LB, Price S, Wright RO, Platek D, Haines J, Oken E. A qualitative study of fish consumption during pregnancy. Am J Clin Nutr. 2010;92:1234–40.
10. Lando AM, Fein SB, Choiniere CJ. Awareness of methylmercury in fish and fish consumption among pregnant and postpartum women and women of childbearing age in the United States. Environ Res. 2012;116: 85–92.
11. Verbeke W, Vackier I. Individual determinants of fish consumption: application of the theory of planned behaviour. Appetite. 2005;44:67–82.
12. Altintzoglou T. Translating barriers into potential improvements: the case of new healthy seafood product development. J Consum Mark. 2010;27:224–35.
13. Birch D, Lawley MA. A conceptual framework for investigating fish consumption in Australia. Proceedings of ANZMAC 2010. Australian and New Zealand Marketing Academy. 2010; 1-10.
14. Liese AD. Food Store Types, Availability, and Cost of Foods in a Rural Environment. J Acad Nutr Diet. 2007;107:1916–23.
15. Riepe JR. Supermarkets and Seafood in the North Central Region. Ames: Iowa State University; 1999.
16. Burger J, Stern AH, Dixon C, Jeitner C, Shukla S, Burke S, Gochfeld M. Fish availability in supermarkets and fish markets in New Jersey. Sci Total Environ. 2004;333:89–97.
17. FDA. A Quantitative Assessment of the Net Effects on Fetal Neurodevelopment from Eating Commercial Fish (As Measured by IQ and also by Early Age Verbal Development in Children). Food and Drug Administration. Silver Spring, Maryland. 2014.
18. USDA. Dietary Guidelines for Americans 2010. In: Agriculture USDo, editor. USDOHAHS. Washington: U.S. Government Printing Office; 2010.
19. Hibbeln JR, Davis JM, Steer C, Emmett P, Rogers I, Williams C, et al. Maternal seafood consumption in pregnancy and neurodevelopmental outcomes in childhood (ALSPAC study): an observational cohort study. Lancet. 2007;369:578–85.
20. Drewnowski A, Eichelsdoerfer P. Can Low-Income Americans Afford a Healthy Diet? Nutr Today. 2010;44:246–9.
21. Shimshack JP, Ward MB, Beatty TKM. Mercury advisories: Information, education, and fish consumption. Journal of Health Economics. 2007; 50:158-179.
22. Kahneman D. Maps of Bounded Rationality: Psychology for Behavioral Economics. Am Econ Rev. 2003;93:1449–75.
23. McFadden D. Economic Choices. Am Econ Rev. 2001;91:351–78.
24. Engelberth H, Teisl MF, Frohmberg E, Butts K, Bell KP, Stableford S, Smith AE. Can fish consumption advisories do better? Providing benefit and risk information to increase knowledge. Environ Res. 2013;126:232–9.
25. Nielsen. General Population Survey of Attitudes Towards Seafood and Impact of FDA and NFI "Dream" Advisory Statements, Presentation edition. 2014.
26. Neale EP: Effectiveness of dietary advice to increase fish consumption over a 12-month period. Food and Nutrition Sciences 2012. DOI: 10. 4236/fns.2012.34065
27. Olsen SF. Low consumption of seafood in early pregnancy as a risk factor for preterm delivery: prospective cohort study. BMJ. 2002;324:447.
28. European Food Safety Authority. Guidance on human health risk-benefit assesment of foods. EFSA Journal. 2010; 8:25.
29. Harvard School of Public Health. Fish: Friend or Foe?
30. Oken E, Radesky JS, Wright RO, Bellinger DC, Amarasiriwardena CJ, Kleinman KP, et al. Maternal fish intake during pregnancy, blood mercury levels, and child cognition at age 3 years in a US cohort. Am J Epidemiol. 2008;167:1171–81.
31. Daniels JL. Fish Intake During Pregnancy and Early Cognitive Development of Offspring. Epidemiology. 2004;15:394–402.
32. Economic Reasearch Service. Table 13-Per Capita Food Expenditures. US Department of Agriculture. Online: USDA.GOV; 2014.
33. US Department of Agriculture. Quarterly Food-at-Home Price Database. US Department of Agriculture. http://www.ers.usda.gov/data-products/quarterly-food-at-home-price-database.aspx: Economic Research Service. 2010.
34. Herrmann RO. Identifying Frequent Seafood Purchasers in the Northeastern U.S. Agric Resour Econo Rev. 1994;23:226–35.
35. Shimshack JP, Ward MB. Mercury advisories and household health trade-offs. J Health Econ. 2010;29:674–85.
36. US Department of Agriculture. Scientific Report of the 2015 Dietary Guidelines Advisory Committee. US Department of Agriculture. 2015.

7

Several grain dietary patterns are associated with better diet quality and improved shortfall nutrient intakes in US children and adolescents: a study focusing on the 2015–2020 Dietary Guidelines for Americans

Yanni Papanikolaou[1*], Julie Miller Jones[2] and Victor L. Fulgoni III[3]

Abstract

Background: The present study identified the most commonly consumed grain food patterns in US children and adolescents (2–18 years-old; $N = 8{,}367$) relative to those not consuming grains and compared diet quality and nutrient intakes, with focus on 2015–2020 Dietary Guidelines for Americans (2015–2020 DGA) shortfall nutrients.

Methods: Cluster analysis using data from the National Health and Nutrition Examination Survey 2005–2010, identified 8 unique grain food patterns: a) no consumption of main grain groups, b) cakes, cookies and pies, c) yeast bread and rolls, d) cereals, e) pasta, cooked cereals and rice, f) crackers and salty snacks, g) pancakes, waffles and French toast and other grains, and h) quick breads.

Results: Energy intake was higher for all grain cluster patterns examined, except 'cereals', compared to no grains. Children and adolescents in the 'yeast bread and rolls', 'cereals', 'pasta, cooked cereals and rice', and 'crackers and salty snacks' patterns had a higher diet quality relative to no grains (all $p < 0.01$). Energy adjusted (EA) dietary fiber intake was greater in five of the seven grain patterns, ranging from 1.8 – 2.8 g more per day (all $p < 0.01$), as compared to those consuming no grains. All grain patterns, except cakes, cookies and pies had higher EA daily folate relative to children in the no grains pattern (all $p < 0.0001$). EA total fat was lower in 'cereals', 'pasta, cooked cereals and rice', and 'pancakes, waffles, French toast and other grains' in comparison to the no grains food pattern (all $p < 0.01$). EA magnesium intakes were greater in children and adolescents consuming 'yeast bread and rolls', 'pasta, cooked cereals and rice', and 'quick breads', while EA iron was higher in all grain patterns relative to no grains (all $p < 0.01$). EA vitamin D intake was higher only in children consuming 'cereals' vs. no grain group ($p < 0.0001$). There were no significant differences in total or added sugar intake across all grain clusters as compared to no grains.

Conclusions: Consumption of several, but not all, grain food patterns in children and adolescents were associated with improved 2015–2020 DGA shortfall nutrient intakes and diet quality as compared to those consuming no grains.

Keywords: NHANES, Grains, Children, Adolescents, Nutrient intakes, Diet quality

* Correspondence: papanikolaou.yanni@gmail.com
[1]Nutritional Strategies Inc., 59 Marriott Place, Paris, ON N3L 0A3, Canada
Full list of author information is available at the end of the article

Background

The 2015–2020 Dietary Guidelines for Americans (2015–2020 DGA) policy report states that several nutrients are under-consumed relative to requirement levels set by the Institute of Medicine (IOM). These have been characterized as shortfall nutrients and include vitamin A, vitamin D, vitamin E, vitamin C, folate, calcium, magnesium, fiber, and potassium. For adolescent, premenopausal females and women who are pregnant, iron is also deemed an under-consumed nutrient of public health concern largely due to increased risk of iron-deficiency in these populations. Of the shortfall nutrients, calcium, vitamin D, fiber, and potassium also are classified as nutrients of public health concern because their under-consumption has been linked in the scientific literature to adverse health outcomes [1]. The report further identified that a healthy dietary pattern is higher in fruits, vegetables, whole grains, low- and non-fat dairy, seafood, legumes, and nuts; and lower in red and processed meat, sugar-sweetened foods and beverages and refined grains. However, a variety of grain-based food products, of which include refined/enriched grains, are sources for several shortfall nutrients identified by the DGA, including dietary fiber, folate, iron, and magnesium [1]. With mandatory folic acid fortification commencing in 1998 by the Food and Drug Administration [2], specific grain foods became leading sources for folate; breads, rolls, and crackers are the largest contributor of total folate to the US diet, contributing nearly 16% of total intake, which exceeds contribution of folate from vegetables [3]. Similarly, using data from the National Health and Nutrition Examination Survey (NHANES) 2003–2006, researchers have reported that fortification of grain foods substantially contributes nutrient adequacy for U.S. children and adolescents aged 2–18 years-old, without excessive intakes for most vitamins and minerals [4].

While certain grain food products are contributors of nutrients to limit in the diet, including added sugar, total and saturated fat [5, 6], grain foods also contribute positive nutrients to the diet, including dietary fiber, iron, magnesium, and B vitamins (thiamin, riboflavin, niacin and folate). Food sources of energy and nutrients data in children showed that while three of the top ten ranking foods for calorie contribution to the diet were grain-based foods, the top ten ranking food sources of dietary fiber included six grain-based products, collectively contributing 40% of total daily dietary fiber intake [4]. Others have argued that while three of the top ten sources of energy provided no nutritional value, the remaining sources of energy, including milk, beef, poultry, cheese and baked goods are significant contributors of nutrients of concern and other essential nutrients, postulating the premise that elimination of these foods from food patterns could potential have inadvertent effects on diet quality in the US population [6].

Recent NHANES data in adults showed that some, but not all, grain food patterns were associated with better nutrient intakes, improved diet quality and beneficial obesity-related parameters [7]. While 2015–2020 DGA identify several healthy dietary food patterns, and encourage increased whole grain consumption and reduced refined grain intake, at present, there are no data that evaluate the association of different grain food patterns on nutrient intakes and diet quality outcomes in children and adolescents. Further, some popular diet plans encourage diet patterns that omit gluten- containing or grain-based foods (e.g. Paleolithic diet) as healthier patterns [8, 9]. As such, the objective of the current analyses was to isolate the most commonly consumed grain food patterns in U.S. children and adolescents and compare nutrient intakes and diet quality of those consuming various grain food patterns to those not consuming grain foods using data from the National Health and Nutrition Examination Survey (NHANES) 2005–2010. The hypothesis for the present analysis was that certain grain food patterns are associated with improved diet quality and can significantly contribute nutrients, including shortfall nutrients, while concurrently lowering nutrients to limit in the diet.

Methods

Data were obtained from What We Eat in America, the dietary intake component of NHANES. NHANES is a government-directed program led by the Center for Disease Control and Prevention in collaboration with US Department of Agriculture. Written informed consent was obtained for all participants or proxies, and the survey protocol was approved by the Research Ethics Review Board at the National Center for Health Statistics. **The distribution of the civilian non-institutionalized US population, as well as response rate percentages and population totals in NHANES 2005–2010 data by age and gender, can be viewed at www.cdc.gov/nchs/nhanes/response_rates_cps.htm.** Data from the current NHANES are released every two years and for the current analyses, we used three data releases, namely 2005–2006, 2007–2008, and 2009–2010 [10, 11].

The dietary intake data were obtained from an in-person 24-hour dietary recall (Day 1) by trained specialists using the Automated Multiple-Pass Method [12] as a means to reduce bias in reporting energy and nutrient intakes in the Mobile Examination Center. The Multiple-Pass Method consisted of five steps: (1) the quick list, which included an uninterrupted list of foods and beverages consumed by the subject; (2) the forgotten foods list, which queried the subject on categories of foods that have been documented as frequently forgotten; (3) a time and occasion where foods were consumed; (4) the detail cycle, which elicited descriptions of foods and amounts consumed with the

aid of an interactive Food Model Booklet and measuring guides; and (5) final probe review. USDA's Food and Nutrient Database for Dietary Studies, 3.0, 4.1, and 5.0 was used to code dietary intake data and calculate nutrient intakes [13–15].

Cluster analysis was used to develop patterns of grain consumption—a statistical procedure that analyses large data sets to identify various patterns while trying to maximize differences among the patterns. **Cluster analysis allows for the focus on a specifically defined aspect (i.e., grain food consumption) and then forces maximal differences in clusters for assessments. Cluster analysis also allows for group comparisons rather than factor analysis which are generally associations.** The USDA food coding system was used to define categories of grain foods [15]. Grain foods intake patterns were identified using SAS 9.2 (SAS Institute, Cary, NC, 2013) PROC CLUSTER using a single 24-hour dietary recall in NHANES 2005–2010. **SUDAAN v.11.0 (Research Triangle Institute; Raleigh, NC) was used to adjust analyses for sampling weights and the sampling units and strata information as provided by NHANES.** Clusters were developed based on the percentage of calories consumed from the grain products as the centroid for each cluster. Grains from flour and dry mixes, mixed dishes, and meat substitutes were not included in development of grain clusters. Cluster analyses provides the ability to focus on a particular defined aspect (e.g. calories from grains) and then forces maximal differences in clusters for assessment. For these analyses, the USDA grains products main categories were used to identify the grain cluster patterns of intake (see Table 1).

All main grain food codes fit into one and only one of the grain foods groupings. The patterns identified by the cluster analysis were then identified by percent calories within each grain food grouping (only groups that contributed 5% or more of calories were used to define the clusters) at the centroid of each cluster. Using this method resulted in seven readily identifiable grain food patterns and a no consumption of main grain groups (i.e., no grains group); creating eight unique patterns of **grain food** consumption. With grain food cluster patterns identified, and using the output from the cluster procedure, each subject was then placed in the cluster that matched most closely to the pattern of calories across the food categories.

Adjusted **least-square means ± SE** values for subjects were determined in each cluster using PROC REGRESS and LOGREGRESS in SUDAAN 11.0 **for dietary intakes and diet quality [Healthy Eating Index (HEI)-2010]** with various sets of covariates. Covariates for analyses of energy intake, HEI-2010 and HEI sub-components [16] were age, gender, and ethnicity. **The poverty income ratio (PIR) grouped into three categories (<1.25, 1.25–3.49, and >3.49) and physical activity (sedentary, moderate or vigorous based on questionnaire responses), current smoking status, alcohol intake (g/d), and energy intake for nutrient-related variables (with the exception of energy intake itself or HEI-2010) also served as covariates. The PIR values reflected the federally established poverty criteria, thus a PIR of <1.25 equated to below 125% of poverty, while higher values represented the subject was from a higher income status.** The HEI-2010 provides a measure of diet quality and measures conformance to federal dietary guidance and has been predominantly used to monitor dietary practices of the US population and the low-income subpopulation. Nutrient intakes were also adjusted for energy intakes. The main comparison of interest was to compare results between the no consumption of main grain groups (cluster 0) and all other clusters. A conservative *P*-value of $p < 0.01$ was set for significance.

Table 1 Grain cluster pattern based on percentage of calories from grains in children and adolescents 2–18 years-old of age using data from NHANES 2005–2010

Cluster Number	Grain Foods Pattern	Description
0	No Grains	4.0% of the population
1	Cakes, Cookies and Pies	(5.1% of the population) with approximately 92% of grains coming from this grain group)
2	Yeast Breads and Rolls	(33.8% of the population) with over 68% of grains coming from this grain group;
3	Cereals	(4.0% of the population) with over 95% of grains coming from this grain group;
4	Pasta, Cooked Cereals and Rice	(4.9% of the population) with over 67% of grains coming from this grain group;
5	Crackers and Salty Snacks	(26.1% of the population) with over 53% of grains coming from this grain group;
6	Pancakes, Waffles, French Toast and Other Grains	(9.4% of the population) with over 51% of grains coming from this grain group and approximately 23% of grains coming from yeast bread and rolls.
7	Quick Breads	(12.8% of the population) with approximately 57% of grains coming from this group.

Results

Eight grain clusters were identified, one of which included isolating a group of children and adolescents that did not consume any of the identified grains (4.0% of the population). The eight clusters are defined as outlined in Table 1, namely: 1) no consumption of main grain groups, 2) cakes, cookies and pies 3) yeast breads and rolls, 4) cereals, 5) pasta, cooked cereal and rice, 6) crackers and salty snacks, 7) pancakes, waffles, French toast, and 8) quick breads.

Energy and nutrient intakes

Energy intake was significantly higher for children and adolescents in all grain pattern clusters, with the exception of 'cereals' ($p = 0.089$), when compared to the no grains group. The higher energy intake ranged from 416 - 524 kcal/d with 'pancakes, waffles, French toast and other grains' and 'quick breads' clusters representing the greatest increase in kcal/day (Table 2).

Energy adjusted nutrient intakes in the eight grain food patterns are presented in Table 2. When examining nutrients of concern, as outlined by the 2015–2010 DGA [1], no differences in calcium intake was observed in children all of the grain clusters compared to those not consuming grain foods, while dietary fiber was higher in children consuming 'yeast breads and rolls', 'cereals', 'pasta, cooked cereals and rice', 'crackers and salty snacks', and 'quick breads', ranging from 1.8 - 2.8 g/day greater daily fiber than children and adolescents in the no grains group.

In terms of nutrients (i.e., vitamins and minerals) present naturally or added to grain foods, via either enrichment or fortification practices, nutrient intakes were higher for those in certain grain clusters. Iron intake was greater across all seven grain clusters examined, thus demonstrating the relevance of both the naturally occurring and added iron in contributing to this 2015–2020 DGA shortfall nutrient. Daily vitamin D (D2 + D3) was significantly greater only in children and adolescents consuming a 'cereals' grain pattern, while no significant differences were observed with potassium intakes in any of the grain clusters as compared to those not consuming grain food products. Intakes of thiamin were significantly higher for children and adolescents consuming all grain clusters, except for 'cakes, cookies and pies', while daily intakes of riboflavin were significantly greater all grain patterns, with the exception of 'cakes, cookies and pies', 'pasta, cooked cereals and rice' and 'crackers and salty snacks' when compared to those not consuming grain foods. Similarly, folate was higher (76 - 411 µg/d; all $p < 0.0001$) in those in all grain food clusters, except 'cakes, cookies and pies', relative to the no grains cluster. Zinc intake was higher only in children and adolescents consuming 'yeast breads and rolls', 'cereals' and 'pasta, cooked cereals and rice' and significantly lower in those consuming 'cakes, cookies and pies' compared to those in the no grains cluster. Magnesium intakes were greater in children and adolescents consuming 'yeast bread and rolls', 'pasta, cooked cereals and rice', and 'quick breads' relative to the no grains group (Table 2).

Regarding nutrients to limit, daily saturated fat intake was significantly lower in all grain patterns examined, with the exception of 'yeast breads and rolls' and 'quick breads', compared to those not consuming grain foods, with a range of difference in saturated fat ranging from 1.5 - 4.8 g less per day. Daily sodium intake was only lower (approximately 350 mg/day) in children and adolescents consuming 'cakes, cookies and pies' compared to the no grains cluster pattern. There were no significant differences in total and added sugar intake across all grain clusters as compared to the no grain cluster (Table 2).

Diet quality assessment

Diet quality, as measured by USDA's HEI-2010 is depicted in Table 3. Four of the grain clusters had significantly greater scores when compared to the no grains cluster. Specifically, those in the 'pasta, cooked cereals and rice' had the greatest score at 50.6 ± 1.0, while children and adolescents consuming 'yeast breads and rolls', 'cereals' and 'crackers and salty snacks' had scores of 46.1 ± 0.5, 48.5 ± 1.2, and 46.0 ± 0.4, respectively (all $p < 0.001$) compared to the no grains cluster (42.7 ± 0.9).

When examining the subcomponents of HEI-2010 (Table 3), children and adolescents in the 'crackers, salty snacks', 'pancakes, waffles, French toast and other grains' and 'quick breads' had significantly lower total vegetable scores than subjects in the no grains pattern. Children and adolescents in all grain clusters examined had significantly greater scores for whole grains as compared to those not consuming grain foods, which indicated higher consumption of whole grains (see Table 3). Children and adolescents in the 'cakes, cookies and pies' grain cluster were the only cluster to show significantly higher scores for sodium intake relative to individuals not consuming grains. The lower HEI-2010 sub-component scores were more than offset with increased scores for those in the 'yeast breads and rolls', 'cereal', 'pasta, cooked cereals and rice' and 'crackers and salty snacks' clusters for total fruit, whole fruit and whole grains as compared to those not consuming grain foods. Additionally, children and adolescents consuming 'yeast breads and rolls', 'pasta, cooked cereals, and rice', 'crackers and salty snacks' and 'quick breads' had significantly higher scores for greens and beans, while the 'cereals' cluster showed higher dairy scores in comparison to children and adolescents in the no grains pattern. The significantly greater score for empty calories in the 'pasta, cooked cereals, and rice' cluster translates as fewer calories from solid fats, alcohol and added sugars), while those consuming 'cakes, cookies and pies' ingested more calories from solid fats, alcohol and added sugars relative to the no grains dietary pattern.

Discussion

This is the first study that has identified various grain food patterns in US children and adolescents with

Table 2 Adjusted mean (SE) nutrient and energy intake for all grain clusters using NHANES 2005–2010, 2–18 years of age

Energy or Nutrient	No Grains		Cakes, Cookies & Pies			Yeast Breads and Rolls			Cereals			Pasta, Cooked Cereals & Rice			Crackers & Salty Snacks			Pancakes, Waffles, French Toast and Other Grains			Quick Breads		
	Cluster 0		Cluster 1			Cluster 2			Cluster 3			Cluster 4			Cluster 5			Cluster 6			Cluster 7		
	LSM	SE	LSM	SE	P	LSM	SE	P	LSM	SE	P	LSM	SE	P	LSM	SE	P	LSM	SE	P	LSM	SE	P
Energy (kcal)	1497	90	1931	65	0.0009	1961	22	<0.0001	1694	65	0.0887	1913	62	0.0005	1946	29	<0.0001	2021	39	<0.0001	2021	36	<0.0001
Carbohydrate (g)	245	6.0	268	3.4	0.0016	256	1.2	0.0679	269	4.2	0.0012	272	3.4	0.0004	262	1.4	0.0046	265	2.2	0.0014	255	2.1	0.1542
Total sugars (g)	134	6.7	149	3.6	0.0594	130	1.4	0.6016	139	4.9	0.5190	130	4.4	0.6484	128	1.7	0.3738	130	2.3	0.6479	124	1.9	0.1674
Added sugars (tsp eq)	22	2.0	25	0.5	0.1791	20	0.3	0.2535	21	1.0	0.7195	19	1.1	0.1331	20	0.4	0.2152	20	0.6	0.3609	18	0.4	0.0874
Protein (g)	72	2.2	59	1.1	<0.0001	72	0.5	0.7474	70	1.5	0.2823	72	1.7	0.9931	65	0.6	0.0004	67	1.3	0.0301	68	0.9	0.0685
Total fat (g)	76	1.9	72	1.2	0.0958	71	0.4	0.0296	67	1.5	0.0004	64	1.3	<0.0001	72	0.5	0.0727	70	0.8	0.0022	74	0.8	0.4128
Total monounsaturated fatty acids (g)	27	0.8	28	0.6	0.7623	26	0.2	0.0648	24	0.7	0.0003	23	0.5	<0.0001	26	0.3	0.1789	26	0.4	0.0958	27	0.4	0.7836
Total saturated fatty acids (g)	27	0.7	25	0.5	0.0080	26	0.2	0.0313	25	0.6	0.0049	22	0.7	<0.0001	25	0.2	0.0001	24	0.5	0.0001	26	0.4	0.0311
Cholesterol (mg)	261	23.5	184	8.0	0.0018	229	4.5	0.1745	198	9.4	0.0163	211	8.1	0.0771	189	4.2	0.0074	240	9.7	0.4133	233	9.9	0.2342
Dietary fiber (g)	11	0.5	12	0.4	0.4815	13	0.2	0.0007	13	0.6	0.0052	13	0.5	<0.0001	13	0.2	0.0006	12	0.3	0.1014	14	0.3	<0.0001
Calcium (mg)	962	53.5	863	28.2	0.1005	1054	12.6	0.0898	1092	31.5	0.0388	964	31.0	0.9737	968	13.6	0.8987	1056	32.4	0.1635	1043	19.1	0.1526
Magnesium (mg)	208	8.7	204	5.0	0.6863	232	2.1	0.0089	231	4.9	0.0158	257	6.7	<0.0001	230	2.3	0.0141	209	2.9	0.8743	237	4.5	0.0009
Iron (mg)	10.6	0.3	11.8	0.3	0.0097	14.17	0.15	<0.0001	19.03	0.67	<0.0001	15.45	0.39	<0.0001	14.16	0.21	<0.0001	13.34	0.23	<0.0001	13.44	0.25	<0.0001
Zinc (mg)	9.4	0.3	8.2	0.2	0.0016	10.97	0.16	0.0001	12.74	0.41	<0.0001	11.00	0.37	0.0050	10.12	0.12	0.0322	9.23	0.22	0.7165	9.93	0.19	0.2085
Sodium (mg)	2996	87.24	2645	44.20	0.0018	3137	23.94	0.1432	3004	71.10	0.9403	3429	150.37	0.0107	3066	38.87	0.4346	3129	45.06	0.2079	3118	55.97	0.2002
Potassium (mg)	2148	91.60	2021	69.94	0.2406	2243	21.46	0.3103	2333	46.88	0.0663	2365	51.12	0.0385	2070	23.24	0.3637	2044	33.81	0.3037	2209	39.34	0.5443
Folate, DFE (μg)	361	12.60	393	13.48	0.0694	526	10.60	<0.0001	772	36.39	<0.0001	636	29.86	<0.0001	523	11.21	<0.0001	438	9.85	<0.0001	498	12.04	<0.0001
Riboflavin (Vitamin B2) (mg)	1.8	0.1	1.8	0.0	0.9836	2.1	0.03	0.0001	2.6	0.04	<0.0001	2.0	0.05	0.0171	2.0	0.03	0.0154	2.1	0.04	0.0014	2.1	0.05	0.0031
Thiamin (Vitamin B1) (mg)	1.3	0.0	1.3	0.1	0.7019	1.6	0.02	<0.0001	1.9	0.04	<0.0001	1.7	0.04	<0.0001	1.5	0.03	0.0003	1.5	0.03	0.0024	1.5	0.03	<0.0001
Total choline (mg)	266	14.4	215	5.5	0.0007	260	3.4	0.6977	245	7.7	0.2363	264	6.9	0.9240	225	2.7	0.0053	260	7.4	0.6825	256	5.8	0.5145
Vitamin A, RAE (μg)	481	34.5	536	29.2	0.1948	599	9.8	0.0016	736	21.5	<0.0001	666	39.2	0.0008	551	12.2	0.0592	650	21.7	0.0001	578	18.6	0.0192
Vitamin B12 (μg)	4.2	0.2	3.8	0.1	0.1470	5.3	0.1	0.0001	6.8	0.3	<0.0001	4.7	0.2	0.1237	4.7	0.1	0.0246	4.9	0.1	0.0255	4.8	0.2	0.0529
Vitamin B6 (mg)	1.4	0.1	1.4	0.0	0.7590	1.7	0.03	0.0004	2.2	0.1	<0.0001	1.9	0.1	<0.0001	1.6	0.03	0.0059	1.7	0.04	0.0031	1.7	0.1	0.0045

Table 2 Adjusted mean (SE) nutrient and energy intake for all grain clusters using NHANES 2005–2010, 2–18 years of age *(Continued)*

Vitamin C (mg)	70.0	5.0	78.0	6.0	0.2829	80.0	2.0	0.0690	83.9	6.1	0.0575	103.6	9.0	0.0025	80.0	2.6	0.0846	72.3	3.1	0.7126	78.7	3.0	0.1833
Vitamin D (D2 + D3) (µg)	5.0	0.5	4.7	0.3	0.5028	6.0	0.2	0.0753	7.6	0.4	<0.0001	6.0	0.2	0.1363	5.3	0.1	0.5640	5.3	0.3	0.6946	5.8	0.2	0.1939
Vitamin E as alpha-tocopherol (mg)	5.8	0.3	5.6	0.2	0.6583	5.9	0.2	0.6465	5.1	0.1	0.0198	5.9	0.4	0.7239	6.2	0.1	0.1437	5.4	0.1	0.1511	6.1	0.2	0.3859
Vitamin K (µg)	52.7	4.0	57.4	5.4	0.4934	58.2	2.6	0.3003	52.2	5.5	0.9396	76.7	9.8	0.0277	52.4	1.9	0.9567	55.9	3.3	0.5779	55.4	1.7	0.5403

NHANES 2005–2010, $N = 8{,}367$

LSM: least square mean; *SE*: standard error; $P = p$ value of difference as compared to cluster 0 (No grains)

Covariates include age, gender, ethnicity, poverty income ratio, physical activity, current smoking status, alcohol and for all variables except Energy, the covariate of energy (kcal)

Table 3 Adjusted mean (SE) Total healthy eating index-2010 (HEI) and component scores for all grain clusters using NHANES 2005–2010, 2–18 years of age

	No Grains		Cakes, Cookies & Pies			Yeast Breads and Rolls			Cereals			Pasta, Cooked Cereals & Rice			Crackers & Salty Snacks			Pancakes, Waffles, French Toast and Other Grains			Quick Breads		
HEI-2010 Component	Cluster 0		Cluster 1			Cluster 2			Cluster 3			Cluster 4			Cluster 5			Cluster 6			Cluster 7		
	LSM	SE	LSM	SE	P	LSM	SE	P	LSM	SE	P	LSM	SE	P	LSM	SE	P	LSM	SE	P	LSM	SE	P
Total Vegetables	2.52	0.13	2.13	0.10	0.0327	2.16	0.05	0.0121	2.44	0.16	0.7002	2.56	0.17	0.8395	1.93	0.06	0.0001	1.74	0.10	<0.0001	2.06	0.07	0.0024
Greens and Beans	0.30	0.07	0.50	0.10	0.0784	0.62	0.05	0.0002	0.61	0.16	0.0617	1.32	0.20	<0.0001	0.54	0.04	0.0064	0.52	0.09	0.0808	0.77	0.08	0.0004
Total Fruit	1.97	0.11	2.28	0.14	0.0468	2.58	0.07	<0.0001	2.51	0.17	0.0039	2.72	0.16	0.0007	2.55	0.06	<0.0001	2.60	0.12	0.0002	2.57	0.10	0.0003
Whole Fruit	1.72	0.17	1.96	0.19	0.3720	2.31	0.08	0.0004	2.38	0.23	0.0073	2.51	0.18	0.0081	2.21	0.07	0.0038	2.33	0.14	0.0079	2.25	0.09	0.0087
Whole Grains	0.26	0.06	0.57	0.10	0.0033	2.11	0.08	<0.0001	2.24	0.17	<0.0001	2.58	0.28	<0.0001	2.36	0.12	<0.0001	1.44	0.15	<0.0001	1.66	0.12	<0.0001
Dairy	6.84	0.26	6.53	0.25	0.3773	7.20	0.09	0.2028	8.09	0.29	0.0029	6.78	0.22	0.8751	6.76	0.11	0.7361	6.89	0.21	0.8796	7.12	0.16	0.3282
Total Protein Foods	3.65	0.14	3.03	0.14	0.0002	3.74	0.05	0.4854	3.38	0.16	0.1844	3.66	0.15	0.9260	3.36	0.05	0.0363	3.59	0.09	0.7878	3.47	0.08	0.3256
Seafood and Plant Protein	0.98	0.13	1.10	0.16	0.4806	1.46	0.08	<0.0001	0.98	0.18	0.9839	1.45	0.21	0.1112	1.37	0.06	0.0161	1.14	0.09	0.2582	1.47	0.09	0.0018
Fatty Acid Ratio	3.31	0.23	3.84	0.23	0.1020	3.30	0.08	0.9556	3.06	0.34	0.5560	4.15	0.31	0.0378	4.34	0.11	0.0001	3.74	0.18	0.1540	3.81	0.16	0.1028
Sodium	4.98	0.34	6.78	0.23	0.0002	4.69	0.09	0.4418	4.98	0.35	1.0000	3.97	0.34	0.0330	5.00	0.14	0.9503	4.69	0.20	0.4555	4.93	0.18	0.8815
Refined Grains	6.78	0.30	5.72	0.23	0.0054	5.40	0.12	0.0001	7.02	0.33	0.5979	6.55	0.26	0.5711	4.95	0.08	<0.0001	4.63	0.21	<0.0001	4.20	0.16	<0.0001
SoFAAS Calories	9.42	0.58	6.46	0.41	0.0003	10.50	0.21	0.0992	10.80	0.63	0.1216	12.33	0.54	0.0004	10.65	0.16	0.0250	10.19	0.36	0.2374	10.00	0.34	0.3755
HEI-2010 Total Score	42.72	0.85	40.90	0.92	0.1926	46.06	0.48	0.0003	48.48	1.19	0.0005	50.58	1.02	<0.0001	46.02	0.44	0.0009	43.49	0.60	0.4102	44.33	0.65	0.1534

NHANES 2005–2010, $N = 8{,}367$

LSM: least square mean; *SE*: standard error; $P = p$: value of difference as compared to cluster 0 (no grains)

SoFAAS: solid fat, alcohol, added sugars

Covariates include age, gender, ethnicity, poverty income ratio, physical activity, current smoking status, and alcohol

reported associations between grain pattern consumption, energy and nutrient intakes and diet quality. The current data support that a variety of grain food patterns, including those recommended by dietary guidance and those that focus on enriched and fortified grain staples, are associated with greater nutrient intakes, including higher consumption of shortfall nutrients and nutrients of public health concern as identified by the 2015–2020 DGA [1], in comparison to an alternative dietary pattern that does not emphasize grain-based foods in children and adolescents. The findings from the present study are aligned with recently published data in American adults, where consumption of specific grain foods were associated with greater nutrient intakes, including greater consumption of shortfall nutrients and nutrients of public health concern. Several, but not all grain food patterns, were associated with improved diet quality compared to adults not consuming main grain groups. Adults consuming pasta, cooked cereals and rice also had lower body weights and smaller waist circumferences when compared to individuals not consuming grain foods [7].

Several nutrients contributed by grain foods naturally or via fortification/enrichment, including folate, calcium, magnesium, fiber and iron are under consumed relative to IOM nutrition standards [17]. Dietary patterns that encourage nutrient-dense grain foods, with the concept of limiting sodium, total fat and sugar, may help shift population consumption in children and adolescents toward recommended intake levels for several shortfall nutrients identified by 2015 DGAC [17]. Additionally, creating positive habits including nutrient-dense dietary patterns that include whole and enriched grain consumption in earlier years may benefit health outcomes into adulthood [18, 19]. Indeed, the current research in children and adolescents provides a sound rationale to support more specific dietary guidance for American children and adolescents about grain consumption rather than simply having two broad categories of recommended intakes that revolve around refined/enriched and whole grains. The current data illustrates how various enriched grain products contribute to daily nutrient intakes and overall diet quality. For example, we observed that children and adolescents consuming 'yeast breads and rolls,' 'cereals,' 'pasta, cooked cereals and rice,' and 'crackers and salty snacks' grain patterns had a significantly higher diet quality, as measured by USDA's HEI-2010 and dietary fiber intake was significantly greater in five of the eight patterns, ranging from 1.8 – 2.8 g more daily fiber, as compared to those consuming no grain foods. It is rationale to suggest that these daily increases in dietary fiber can have a meaningful impact on public health initiatives by helping to minimize gaps in fiber consumption in children and adolescents. In fact, a recent study evaluating ten-year trends in fiber intakes using NHANES data from 2001–2010 in children and adolescents reported mean fiber intake to be 13.2 ± 0.1 g/day [20]. Thus, dietary fiber intake levels in children and adolescents continue to fall short of meeting dietary guidance based on recommendations set forth by the Institute of Medicine where fiber Adequate Intake in children 1 – 8 years and children and adolescents 9–18 years is set at 19 – 25 g/day and 26 – 38 g/day, respectively [21].

Collaborative efforts from the American Heart Association, American College of Cardiology and The Obesity Society state that nearly one-third of children and youth are overweight or obese, further exacerbating poor health profiles and increasing risks for chronic diseases and their co-morbidities [22, 23]. In the current analyses, total fat intake was lower in, 'cereals' and 'pasta, cooked cereals and rice,' and daily saturated fat intake was lower in many of the grain patterns examined, in comparison to the no grains food pattern. The range of saturated fat lowering per day translates to meaningful reductions when considering the U.S. Food and Drug Administration's Daily Value (DV) for saturated fat; the mean lowering of saturated fat ranged from 1.5 – 4.8 g per day which represents 7.5 – 24% of the DV for adults and children ≥4 years of age consuming 2000 kcal/day. Taken collectively, some grain food patterns, comprised of both whole and enriched grains, can be beneficial in children and adolescents when considering dietary guidance and health outcomes.

Our results are aligned with previous observational findings that considered sources of nutrients in the US diet. When identifying the top food sources of nutrients, including both intrinsic and added to foods via fortification, results showed that grain foods represented the top five ranking food sources for folate, such that ready-to-eat cereals, yeast breads and rolls, pizza, pasta and crackers, popcorn, pretzels, and chips contributed 56.7 and 54.4% of folate to the diet of children and adolescents, respectively. Results were similar another shortfall nutrient, such that grain foods represented the top five food sources for iron in the diet of US children and adolescents, with ready-to eat cereals, yeast breads, pizza, cakes, cookies, and pies, and crackers, popcorn, pretzels, and chips cumulatively contributing 52.1 and 48.7% of iron [24].

The 2015–2020 DGA and 2015 Dietary Guidelines Advisory Committee (2015 DGAC) report further states 'of the shortfall nutrients, calcium, vitamin D, fiber, and potassium also are classified as nutrients of public health concern because their under consumption has been linked in the scientific literature to adverse health outcomes" [21], a principle carried forward from the DGA 2010 policy document [25]. The 2015 DGAC [17] also reports that "if whole grains were consumed in the amounts recommended in the recommended food patterns, whole grains would provide substantial percentages of several key nutrients, such as about 32% of dietary fiber, 42% of iron, 35% of folate, 29% of magnesium and 16% of vitamin A". While these nutrients levels represent significant contributions from whole grains, whole grain consumption alone can still leave a gap between consumption and recommendation levels. The 2005 DGAC reported that refined grains contribute substantial levels of key nutrients to food patterns, naming folate, iron, calcium, dietary fiber, thiamin, riboflavin and niacin [26], thus demonstrating the importance of consuming both enriched and whole grains. The committee further acknowledged that including only three ounce equivalents of whole grains daily with no refined grains in recommended food patterns would lower intake of many of key nutrients and potentially place specific populations at risk for nutrient inadequacy [26]; an argument which led the 2015 DGAC to conclude that consumption of whole grains with no substitutions would result in nutrient shortfalls [17]. The current analysis provides data linking different grain food patterns with nutrient intakes and concurrently we observe the adverse nutrient- and health-related outcomes when grain foods as a whole are eliminated from the diet. In many of the grain patterns examined, we see a better overall nutrient intake profile, which demonstrates the important dietary contributions made by different grain foods and emphasizes the importance of consuming a balance of whole grains, enriched and fortified grain products. Indeed, while some of the grain food clusters contributed nutrients to limit in the diet as identified by the 2015–2020 DGA [1], including saturated fat, added sugars, and sodium, several of the grain food patterns were associated with lower intakes of these nutrients and improved shortfall nutrients and diet quality. Such findings provide a rationale for more specific, evidence-based dietary guidance around grain consumption.

There are several limitations to the present analysis that deserve recognition. Data for energy and nutrient intakes, including values reported for diet quality, were obtained using 24-hour dietary recalls, which rely on study participant memory. While validated procedures are used to collect the data, recalled information may be inaccurate and biased from misreporting or memory challenges [27]. In addition, the current evidence, being observational, cannot establish a causal link between the different grain foods patterns examined and improvements in nutrient intakes and diet quality. However, a large strength of the current work stems from the use of NHANES, which is a large continuous survey that examines a nationally representative sample of about 5,000 individuals yearly by highly-trained medical personnel. Additionally, numerous covariates were used to adjust the data in an attempt to remove potential confounding scenarios. However, residual confounding may still exist and may explain some of the results reported. Lastly, we identified a small percentage of the population with no consumption of the main grain groups investigated, which served as the comparison group. While the comparison group was relevant for research purposes, it only represented 4% of the population, suggesting that further research is required.

Conclusions

Several grain food dietary patterns in U.S. children and adolescents are associated with greater nutrient intakes, including greater consumption of shortfall nutrients and nutrients of public health concern as identified by the 2015–2020 DGA. Improved diet quality, as measured by USDA's HEI-2010 was also linked to consumption of specific grain food patterns, including 'pasta, cooked cereals and rice, 'cereals', 'yeast breads and rolls' and 'crackers and salty snacks', when compared to those children and adolescents not consuming grain food dietary pattern. Improved diet quality was due not only to the contribution of nutrients inherent in the grain, but also to those added through enrichment and fortification practices and those provided by natural food pairings such as cereal and dairy foods (i.e., milk). Overall, while some grain food patterns were associated with elevated sodium and added sugar, the present data also support that several grain food patterns can serve as part of a healthy dietary food pattern in children and adolescents, that accounts for 2015–2020 DGA dietary recommendations to reduce total fat, saturated fat and added sugar consumption, while concurrently increasing intake of shortfall nutrients and/or nutrients of concern, including iron, magnesium, dietary fiber, vitamin D, potassium and folate.

Acknowledgments
Not Applicable.

Funding
This project has been funded by the Grain Foods Foundation. The funding group had no role in the design of the study and collection, analysis and interpretation of the data, nor in the writing of the manuscript.

Availability of data and materials
The NHANES datasets during and/or analysed during the current study are available from the corresponding author on reasonable request.

Authors' contributions
YP and JMJ collaborated on the intellectual conception and interpretation of the research. VLF directed the intellectual conception and design of the research, conducted the analyses and provided interpretation. YP drafted the manuscript and all authors approved the final manuscript version of the present research.

Competing interests
YP as Vice President of Nutritional Strategies Inc. provides food, nutrition and regulatory affairs consulting services for numerous food and beverage companies and food-related associations and collaborates with VLF on NHANES analyses; JMJ as Professor Emerita of Food and Nutrition at St. Catherine University provides nutrition science research consulting to food companies and not-for-profit organizations. VLF as Senior Vice President of Nutrition Impact, LLC provides food and nutrition consulting services for numerous food and beverage companies. VLF also conducts analyses of NHANES data for members of the food industry.

Consent for publication
Not Applicable.

Ethics approval and consent to participate

Ethics approval/consents have been previously conducted via the Centers for Disease Control and Prevention and the Research Ethics Review Board at the National Center for Health Statistics.

Author details

[1]Nutritional Strategies Inc., 59 Marriott Place, Paris, ON N3L 0A3, Canada. [2]Distinguished Scholar and Professor Emerita of Food and Nutrition, Department of Foods and Nutrition, St. Catherine University, 4030 Valentine Ct. Arden Hills, Minnesota, MN 55112, USA. [3]Nutrition Impact, LLC, 9725 D Drive North, Battle Creek, MI, USA.

References

1. United States Department of Health and Human Services and United States Department of Agriculture, "2015 – 2020 Dietary Guidelines for Americans, 8th Edition," U.S. Government Printing Office, December 2015. https://health.gov/dietaryguidelines/2015/resources/2015-2020_Dietary_Guidelines.pdf. Accessed 28 June 2016.
2. U.S. Food and Drug Administration. Food standards: amendment of standards of identity for enriched grain products to require addition of folic acid. Fed Reg. 1996;61(44). http://www.gpo.gov/fdsys/pkg/FR-1996-03-05/pdf/96-5014.pdf. Accessed 22 May 2016.
3. Dietrich M, Brown CJ, Block G. The effect of folate fortification of cereal-grain products on blood folate status, dietary folate intake, and dietary folate sources among adult non-supplement users in the United States. J Am Coll Nutr. 2005;24:266–74.
4. Keast DR, Fulgoni VL, Nicklas TA, O'Neil CE. Food sources of energy and nutrients among children in the United States: NHANES 2003–2006. Nutrients. 2013;5:283–301.
5. Reedy J, Krebs-Smith SM. Dietary sources of energy, solid fats, and added sugars among children and adolescents in the United States. J Am Diet Assoc. 2010;110:1477–84.
6. Huth PJ, Fulgoni VL, Keast DR, Park K, Auestad N. Major food sources of calories, added sugars, and saturated fat and their contribution to essential nutrient intakes in the U.S. Diet: data from the national health and nutrition examination survey (2003–2006). Nutr J. 2013;12:116. doi:10.1186/1475-2891-12-116.
7. Papanikolaou Y, Fulgoni VLF. Certain grain food patterns are associated with improved 2015 dietary guidelines shortfall nutrient intakes, diet quality, and lower body weight in US adults: results from the national health and nutrition examination survey, 2005–2010. Food Nutr Sci. 2016;7:772–81.
8. Jönsson T1, Granfeldt Y, Lindeberg S, Hallberg AC. Subjective satiety and other experiences of a Paleolithic diet compared to a diabetes diet in patients with type 2 diabetes. Nutr J. 2013;12. doi:10.1186/1475-2891-12-105.
9. Manheimer EW, van Zuuren EJ, Fedorowicz Z, Pijl H. Paleolithic nutrition for metabolic syndrome: systematic review and meta-analysis. Am J Clin Nutr. 2015;102:922–32.
10. National Health and Nutrition Examination Survey. Analytic and Reporting Guidelines. Available at http://www.cdc.gov/nchs/data/nhanes/nhanes_03_04/nhanes_analytic_guidelines_dec 2005.pdf. Accessed 17 June 2016.
11. National Health and Nutrition Examination Survey. Analytic Note Regarding 2007–2010 Survey Design Changes and Combining Data Across other Survey Cycles. Available at http://www.cdc.gov/nchs/data/nhanes/analyticnote_2007-2010.pdf. Accessed 17 June 2016.
12. Moshfegh AJ, Rhodes DG, Baer DJ, Murayi T, Clemens JC, Rumpler WV, Paul DR, Sebastian RS, Kuczynski KJ, Ingwersen LA, Staples RC, Cleveland LE. The US department of agriculture automated multiple-pass method reduces bias in the collection of energy intakes. Am J Clin Nutr. 2008;88:324–32.
13. USDA Food and Nutrient Database for Dietary Studies, 3.0. 2008. Beltsville: U.S. Department of Agriculture, Agricultural Research Service, Food Surveys Research Group. https://www.ars.usda.gov/ARSUserFiles/80400530/pdf/fndds/fndds3_doc.pdf. Accessed 17 June 2016.
14. USDA Food and Nutrient Database for Dietary Studies, 4.1. 2010. Beltsville: U.S. Department of Agriculture, Agricultural Research Service, Food Surveys Research Group. https://www.ars.usda.gov/ARSUserFiles/80400530/pdf/fndds/fndds4_doc.pdf. Accessed 17 June 2016.
15. Ahuja JKA, Montville JB, Omolewa-Tomobi G, Heendeniya KY, Martin CL, Steinfeldt LC, et al. USDA food and nutrient database for dietary studies, 5.0. Beltsville: U.S. Department of Agriculture, Agricultural Research Service, Food Surveys Research Group; 2012.
16. Guenther PM, Casavale KO, Reedy J, Kirkpatrick SI, Hiza HA, Kahle LL, Krebs-Smith SM. Update of the healthy eating index: HEI-2010. J Acad Nutr Diet. 2013;113:569–80.
17. U.S. Department of Agriculture and U.S. Department of Health and Human Services (USDA/HHS). Scientific Report of the 2015 Dietary Guidelines Advisory Committee: Advisory Report to the Secretary of Health and Human Services and Secretary of Agriculture. 2015. Washington: USDA, Agricultural Research Service; 2015. http://health.gov/dietaryguidelines/2015-scientific-report/PDFs/Scientific-Report-of-the-2015-Dietary-Guidelines-Advisory-Committee.pdf. Accessed 17 June 2016.
18. Jaaskelainen P, Magnussen CG, Pahkala K, Mikkila V, Kahonen M, Sabin MA, Fogelholm M, Hutri-Kahonen N, Taittonen L, Telama R, Laitinen T, Jokinen E, Lehtimaki T, Viikari JS, Raitakari OT, Juonala M. Childhood nutrition in predicting metabolic syndrome in adults: the cardiovascular risk in young Finns study. Diabetes Care. 2012;35:1937–43.
19. Qi Y, Niu J. Does childhood nutrition predict health outcomes during adulthood? evidence from a population-based study in china. J Biosoc Sci. 2015;47:650–66.
20. McGill CR, Fulgoni 3rd VL, Devareddy L. Ten-year trends in fiber and whole grain intakes and food sources for the united states population: national health and nutrition examination survey 2001–2010. Nutrients. 2015;7:1119–30.
21. Institute of Medicine of the National Academies, Food and Nutrition Board. Dietary reference intakes for energy, carbohydrate, fiber, Fat, fatty acids, cholesterol, protein, and amino acids. Washington: The National Academies Press; 2005.
22. Eckel RH, Jakicic JM, Ard JD, de Jesus JM, Houston Miller N, Hubbard VS, et al. AHA/ACC guideline on lifestyle management to reduce cardiovascular risk: a report of the american college of cardiology/american heart association task force on practice guidelines. J Am Coll Cardiol. 2014;63(25 Pt B):2960–84.
23. Jensen MD, Ryan DH, Apovian CM, Ard JD, Comuzzie AG, Donato KA, et al. American college of cardiology/american heart association task force on practice guidelines; obesity society. 2013 AHA/ACC/TOS guideline for the management of overweight and obesity in adults: a report of the american college of cardiology/american heart association task force on practice guidelines and the obesity society. J Am Coll Cardiol. 2014;63(25 Pt B):2985–3023.
24. Berner LA, Keast DR, Bailey RL, Dwyer JT. Fortified foods are major contributors to nutrient intakes in diets of US children and adolescents. J Acad Nutr Diet. 2014;114:1009–22.
25. U.S. Department of Agriculture and U.S. Department of Health and Human Services (USDA/HHS). Scientific report of the 2010 dietary guidelines advisory committee: advisory report to the secretary of health and human services and secretary of agriculture. Washington: USDA, Agricultural Research Service; 2010.
26. U.S. Department of Agriculture and U.S. Department of Health and Human Services (USDA/HHS). Scientific report of the 2005 dietary guidelines advisory committee: advisory report to the secretary of health and human services and secretary of agriculture. Washington: USDA, Agricultural Research Service; 2005.
27. Dwyer J, Picciano MF, Raiten DJ. Members of the steering committee; national health and nutrition examination survey. Collection of food and dietary supplement intake data: what We Eat in america-NHANES. J Nutr. 2003;133:590S–600S.

8

Masquelier's grape seed extract: from basic flavonoid research to a well-characterized food supplement with health benefits

Antje R. Weseler* and Aalt Bast

Abstract

Careful characterization and standardization of the composition of plant-derived food supplements is essential to establish a cause-effect relationship between the intake of that product and its health effect. In this review we follow a specific grape seed extract containing monomeric and oligomeric flavan-3-ols from its creation by Jack Masquelier in 1947 towards a botanical remedy and nutraceutical with proven health benefits. The preparation's research history parallels the advancing insights in the fields of molecular biology, medicine, plant and nutritional sciences during the last 70 years. Analysis of the extract's flavanol composition emerged from unspecific colorimetric assays to precise high performance liquid chromatography - mass spectrometry and proton nuclear magnetic resonance fingerprinting techniques. The early recognition of the preparation's auspicious effects on the permeability of vascular capillaries directed research to unravel the underlying cellular and molecular mechanisms. Recent clinical data revealed a multitude of favorable alterations in the vasculature upon an 8 weeks supplementation which summed up in a health benefit of the extract in healthy humans. Changes in gene expression of inflammatory pathways in the volunteers' leukocytes were suggested to be involved in this benefit. The historically grown scientific evidence for the preparation's health effects paves the way to further elucidate its metabolic fate and molecular action in humans.

Keywords: Flavanols, Proanthocyanidins, Grape seed, Masquelier, Cardiovascular, Health, Inflammation, Oxidative stress, Nutraceutical, Food

Introduction

In scientifically evaluating the health benefit of a food-derived product, three major rules have to be followed: 1) The product for which a health claim is made should be well characterized; 2) the (claimed) effect should be well defined and of physiological benefit; 3) a cause-and-effect relationship between the intake of the food product and the claimed effect on human health is substantiated by human (observational and intervention) studies. In this review we will follow a specific botanical preparation, i.e. a mixture of monomeric and oligomeric flavan-3-ols from the seeds of grapes, on its travel from its creation in 1947 towards a botanical remedy and nutraceutical with proven health benefits.

The authentic mixture of monomeric and oligomeric flavan-3-ols extracted from the seeds of grapes (*Vitis vinifera* L.) is commercially available as the herbal remedy Endotélon® and as Masquelier's® Original OPCs (Anthogenol®) in various food supplements. This plant extract forms an interesting example of how product-specific research followed and contributed to the scientific evolution of botanical, biochemical and physiological insights during the post-WWII period. In this time, grape seed extracts constantly remained at the forefront of successive innovations in scientific investigation [1]. Applications have been found in the treatment of chemo- and radiotherapy-induced toxicity [2], in chemoprevention [3–5], in cardiovascular diseases [6] and neurodegenerative diseases [7, 8], in oral health [9] or as cosmeceutical [10]. In the early development some focus

* Correspondence: a.weseler@maastrichtuniversity.nl
Department of Pharmacology and Toxicology; Faculty of Health, Medicine and Life Sciences, P.O. Box 6166200, MD, Maastricht, The Netherlands

was given to the effect of grape seed extracts as phlebotonics for venous insufficiency [11].

Research on the bioactive components of grape seeds extracts, i.e. in flavonoids, started in the beginning of the 20th century, when nutritional scientists were dedicated to the isolation and identification of compounds we came to define as "vitamins." The Hungarian scientist Albert Szent-Györgyi isolated vitamins C and P from citrus fruits. In contrast to vitamin C, the chemical characterization of vitamin P appeared to be difficult. As a result, it was not possible to attribute the vitamin P effect to a specific compound or preparation. Moreover, the notion of such a vitamin was abandoned since no deficiency disease could be linked to Szent-Györgyi's citrus extract. However, the biological effect of "vitamin P", i.e. its influence on vascular permeability was established as well as its enforcing influence on the anti-scurvy effect of vitamin C. Efforts to identify this putative vitamin P were directed to yellow colored plant pigments, the flavonoids (*flavus* (Latin) means yellow).

In 1947 the French researcher Jack Masquelier extracted during his work for his PhD thesis a colorless fraction from the red-brown skin of peanuts. He found this fraction to be responsible for the vitamin P effect in animals and proposed its major components as oligomers of flavan-3-ol units (i.e. (+)-catechin or (-)-epicatechin; Fig. 1). Nowadays, these polyphenolic compounds are commonly classified as monomeric and oligomeric flavan-3-ols. Condensed flavanols (oligomers and polymers) are also designated as proanthocyanidins. Oligomers of proanthocyanidins are well-known by the abbreviation "OPCs." As the name suggests, proanthocyanidins are the precursors (*pro*) of anthocyani(di)ns (*anthos* (ancient Greek) means flower and *kyanos* (ancient Greek) means blue), which are water-soluble pigments being responsible for the blue, violet or red color of many flowers and fruits. In plants, anthocyanins are usually present as glycosides, i.e. bound to one or several

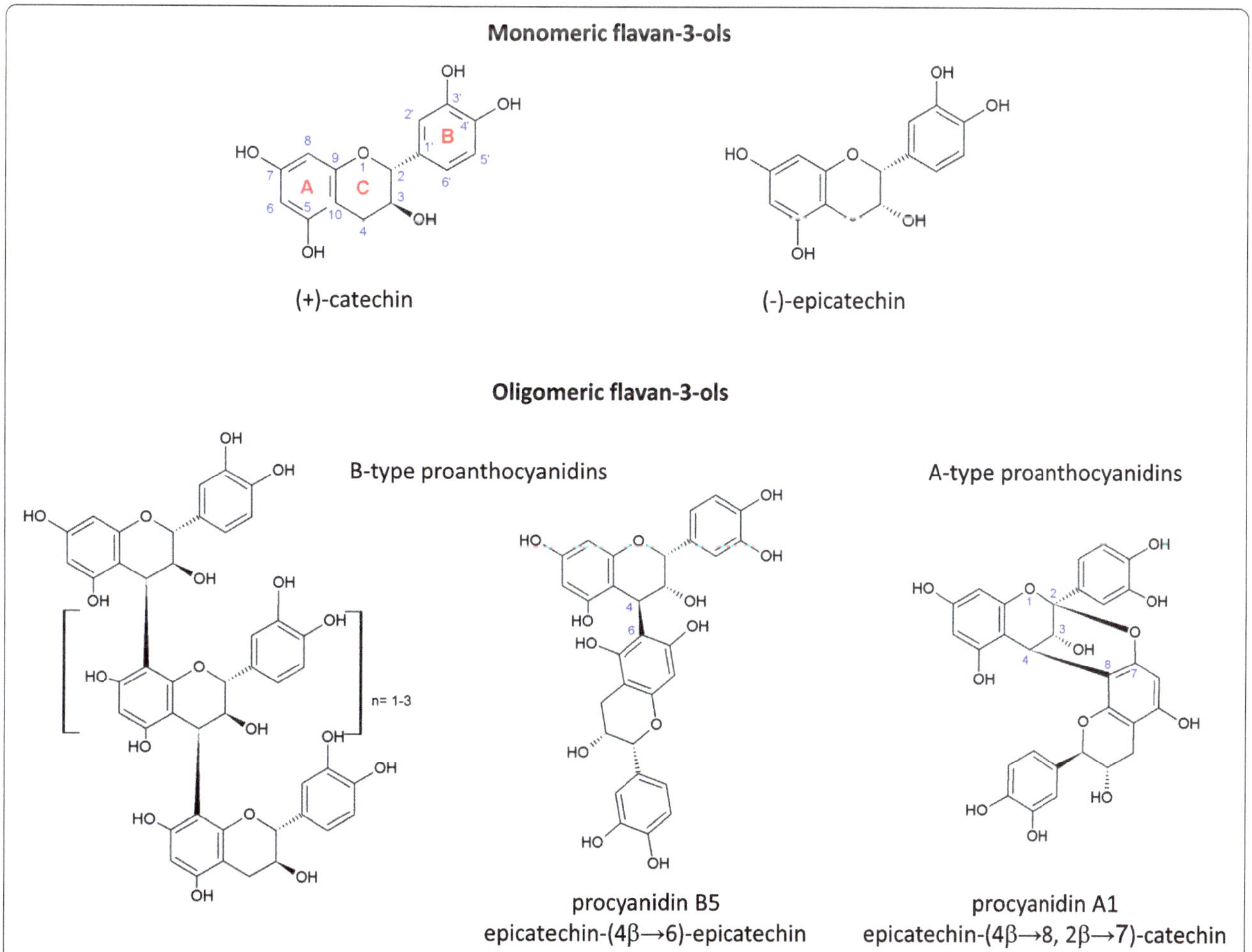

Fig. 1 Molecular structure of monomeric and oligomeric flavan-3-ols

sugar moieties. Their color depends on the pH of their environment changing from red/pinkish at acidic conditions to blue—purple at neutral conditions and yellowish at alkaline conditions.

In any case, the scientific journey in the field of extracts consisting of monomeric and oligomeric flavanols begins in the early attempt to classify these compounds as a vitamin amidst all other vitamins that were discovered in those days. As nutrients that are essential to prevent symptoms of deficiency, vitamins were realized to ensure and procure health. In this context, the first discovered health effects of Masquelier's flavanol-preparations fitted well in the, at that time, new WHO definition of health as "a state of complete physical, mental and social well-being and not merely the absence of disease or infirmity" [12].

Besides developing synthetic routes [13] and improving methods for the extraction of monomeric and oligomeric flavanols from different plant sources, Jack Masquelier also directed much of his and his colleagues' efforts to elucidate the biological activities of the extracts produced. In recent years, quite some scientific data have been generated that provide insights in the presumed effects of all sorts of more or less well defined grape seed extracts on human health. However, in contrast to drugs, which are mostly single chemical compounds, the evaluation of the biological effects of phytochemicals produced by extraction is challenging. The fact that most plant extracts contain a wide variety of individual chemical entities bedevils the establishment of a relationship between an effect in a biological test system and an individual, chemically-defined molecule which is part of the extract. For this reason, the extract as a whole has to be regarded as the biologically active entity. Therefore, to maintain and assure physiological consistency, it is essential to have a well-characterized and standardized plant extract available, of which each batch possesses the qualitative and quantitative composition of the researched preparation. Monomeric and oligomeric flavanols are heterogeneous phytochemicals that differ in their polymerization degree, stereochemistry and linkage of the monomeric units. As described later in detail, particular (parts of) plants are rich in these flavanols such as pine bark and grape seeds. A recently performed literature search in PubMed (http://www.ncbi.nlm.nih.gov/pubmed; search performed on 8 July 2016) using the search terms "grape" and "seed" and "extract" yielded 995 hits. However, a clear picture on the bioactivity and health effects of the category of extracts loosely defined as "grape seed-derived flavanols" can hardly be obtained, since data on the qualitative and quantitative composition of the investigated extracts are either missing, imprecise or incomparable. Therefore, in this review, we decided to focus on Masquelier's grape seed-derived monomeric and oligomeric flavanols extract (Masquelier's Original OPCs®), since it has a well-defined, consistent composition (*vide infra*) and an over decades established pool of in vitro, in vivo and clinical data unravelling health benefits of monomeric and oligomeric flavanols (Fig. 2).

Many plant products originate from traditional use. Historical findings and concepts that come with it are a valuable source to get insides into the origin and potential health effects of these products. The data on Masquelier's flavanol preparation suggest a vitamin-like action on capillary function, which can be associated with the monomeric and oligomeric flavanols present in this extract. A closer look at the biosynthetic origin of flavanols in plants may help to better understand their chemical nature and biological activity.

Flavanol biosynthesis in plants

Monomeric flavan-3-ols like (-)-epicatechin and (+)-catechin are enzymatically synthesized by plants via a combination of the shikimate and the acetate pathway [14]. The first step towards the synthesis of shikimic acid consists of the condensation of phosphoenolpyruvate (PEP; produced in glycolysis) and D-erythrose-4-phosphate (produced in pentose phosphate cycle) to 3-deoxy-D-arabinose-heptulosonic acid-7-phosphate (DAHP; Fig. 3a). Intramolecular aldol-type condensation and NADH-mediated redox reactions result in dephosphorylation and cyclization to 3-dehydroquinic acid. Dehydration and reduction of the latter give shikimic acid which is eventually converted to chorismic acid. Chorismic acid serves as the precursor of the amino acids L-tyrosine and L-phenylalanine. From both amino acids 4-hydroxycinnamic acid (*p*-coumaric acid) is generated. Upon esterification with coenzyme A 4-hydroxycinnamoyl-CoA is extended by 3 malonyl-CoA units which are derived from the acetate pathway (Fig. 3b). This reaction is catalyzed by the enzyme chalcone synthase and leads via a polyketide intermediate to naringenin-chalcone. A Michael-type nucleophilic attack of one of the phenolic OH-groups on the α,β-unsaturated ketone results in the C-ring formation and yields the flavanone naringenin (Fig. 3b). Naringenin is the basic molecule from which all different flavonoid subclasses are synthesized including flavan-3-ols. Hydroxylation of naringenin by flavanone-3-hydroxylase (F3H) and subsequent NADPH-dependent reduction by dihydroflavanol-4-reductase (DFR) produces leucoanthocyanidins such as leucocyanidin. Leucoanthocyanidins can be converted by leucoanthocyanidin reductase (LAR) to 2,3-*trans*-(+)-flavan-3-ols like (+)-catechin. Moreover, they are oxidized by anthocyanidin synthase (ANS) to anthocyanidins which are reduced by anthocyanidin reductase (ANR) into 2,3-*cis*(-)-flavan-3-ols like (-)-epicatechin (Fig. 3b). The formation of 2,3-*cis* configured flavan-3-ols is remarkable because all chiral intermediates in the flavonoid biosynthesis pathway have a 2,3-*trans* configuration. Since the majority of proanthocyanidins are

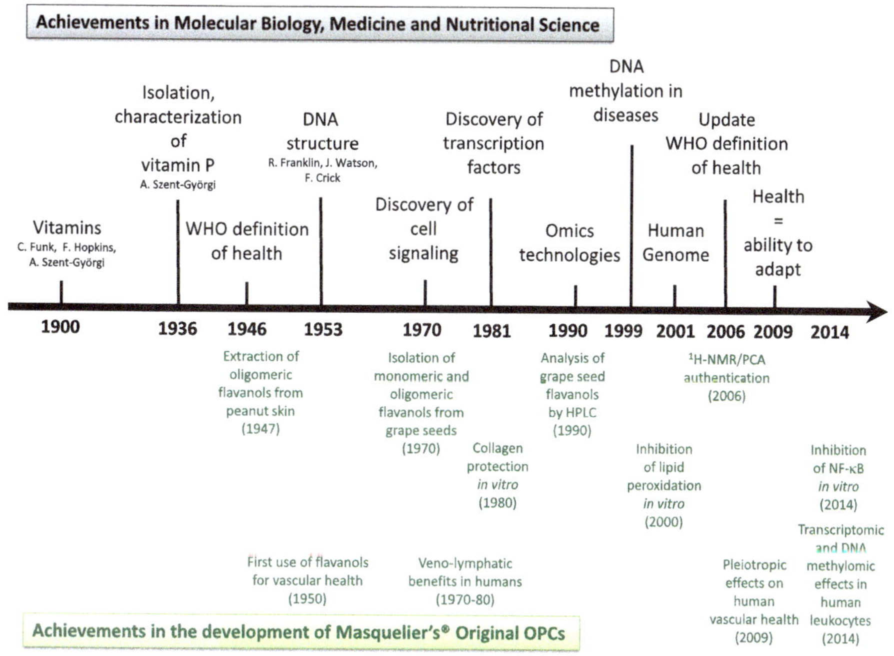

Fig. 2 Timeline of achievements in the field of molecular biology, medicine and nutritional science during the last decade which are paralleled by achievements in the development and investigation of a grape seed extract by the French scientist Jack Masquelier. Today this preparation of monomeric and oligomeric flavan-3-ols is commercially available in the herbal remedy Endotélon® and as Masquelier's® Original OPCs in nutraceuticals and food supplements

condensed products of (-)-epicatechin and (+)-catechin, it is obvious that the stereochemistry of the oligomers varies depending on the number and position of the (-)-epicatechin and (+)-catechin units. It is an ongoing debate if the polymerization of (-)-epicatechin and (+)-catechin units is facilitated by enzymes or occurs non-enzymatically [15]. Efforts to identify an enzyme that controls the condensation of the precursor units to proanthocyanidins have yet not been successful [16]. Polyphenol oxidase (PPO) has been suggested as a possible candidate (Fig. 3c) since it can catalyze the conversion of (-)-epicatechin and (+)-catechin to their corresponding quinone methides [17]. However, the physiological relevance of this mechanism remains doubtful because oligomeric flavanols are formed in the vacuole while PPO is usually located on plastids or chloroplasts [18]. An oxidase with similar catalytic activity in the vacuole has not been found until now.

Under acidic conditions in vitro proanthocyanidins could be synthesized from leucoanthocyanidins which condensate with (-)-epicatechin or (+)-catechin via the formation of a quinone methide and carbocation (flavylium cation) at the C4 position [19] (Fig. 3c). The electrophilic C4 of the leucoanthocyanidin (flavan-3,4-diol, i.e. the extension (upper) unit) reacts with the nucleophilic C6 or C8 position of the flavan-3-ol (i.e. the starter/terminal (lower) unit). However, the existence of an acidic compartment in plant cells was controversial until recent findings in *Arabidopsis thaliana* showed that gene disruption of the plasma membrane H^+-ATPase AHA10 caused a substantial loss of proanthocyanidin accumulation in the seed coat endothelium [20]. Assuming that AHA10 or other plant H^+-ATPases contribute to the acidification of cytoplasmic or vacuolar compartments, non-enzymatic condensation reactions in an acidic environment may occur in plants (Fig. 3c).

Despite many unresolved questions on the precise molecular processes leading to the proanthocyanidins formation in plants, a wealth of different structures has been identified so far. Based on their hydroxylation pattern oligomeric flavan-3-ols are classified in subgroups like procyanidins that have a 3′,4′-dihydroxylation pattern in the B-ring ((+)-catechin and (-)-epicatechin extension units), propelargonidins with 4′-hydroxylation pattern in the B-ring ((+)-afzelechin and (-)-epiafzelechin extension units) and prodelphinidins with 3′,4′,5′-trihydroxylation pattern ((+)-gallocatechin and (-)-epigallocatechin extension units). The hydroxylation pattern of the A and C-ring is identical in these 3 subgroups and comprises OH-groups at C3, C5 and C7. However, more proanthocyanidin-subgroups have been isolated from plants or chemically synthesized that differ in their positions of OH-groups in the A and C ring [16]. In accordance to the interflavan linkage procyanidins are classified in A- and B-type. Oligomers (and polymers) of the B-type are linked via 1 bond which is usually located between C4 of the extension (upper) unit and the C6 or

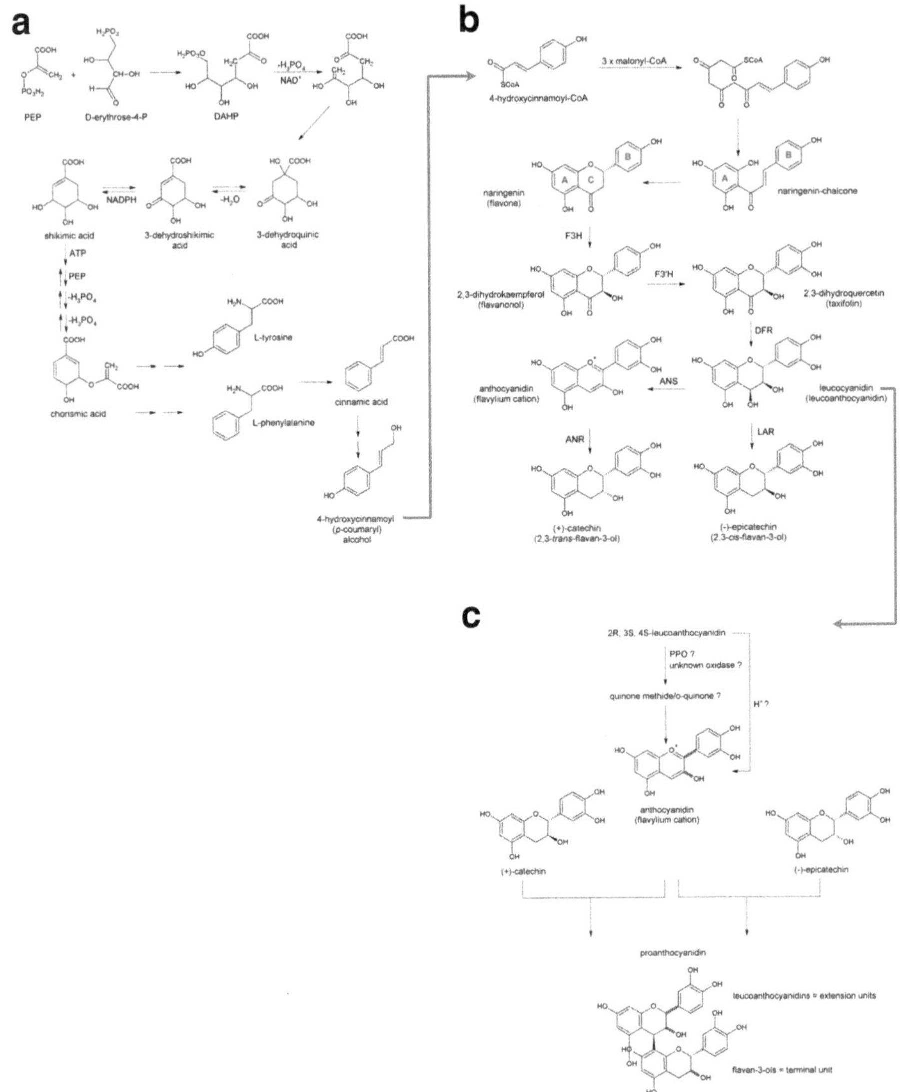

Fig. 3 a-c Biosynthesis of monomeric and oligomeric flavan-3-ols in plants (panel **a**-**c**). **a** Shikimate pathway starting from phosphoenol pyruvate (PEP) and D-erythrose-4-phosphate (D-erythrose-4-P) leading to the formation of 4-hydroxycinnamoyl alcohol, DHAP = 3-deoxy-D-arabinose-heptulosonic acid-7-phosphate, NAD = nicotine-adenine dinucleotide, NADPH = reduced nicotine-adenine dinucleotide phosphate; **b** Formation of monomeric flavan-3-ols (+)-catechin and (-)-epicatechin from 4-hydroxycinnamoyl-CoA and 3 molecules of malonyl-CoA, F3H = flavanone-3-hydroxylase, F3′H = flavanone-3′-hydroxylase, DFR = dihydroflavanol-4-reductase, ANS = anthocyanidin synthase, ANR = anthocyanidin reductase, LAR = leucoanthocyanidin reductase; **c** Polymerization of monomeric flavan-3-ols to oligomeric proanthocyanidins, PPO = polyphenol oxidase, ? indicates uncertainty in existence/role of (intermediate) compound/enzyme

C8 of the starting/terminating (lower) unit (e.g. procyanidin B5, Fig. 1). In addition to this C-C-linkage, A-type proanthocyanidins possess an ether bond between the C2 of the upper flavan-3-ol unit and the O at the C5 or C7 position of the lower unit (e.g. procyanidin A1, Fig. 1). In both types, the stereochemistry of the linking bond(s) between two and more flavan-3-ol units can be either α (denoted as hashed wedge in the molecular structural formula) or β (denoted as solid wedge). In order to cope with the increasing numbers of individual proanthocyanidins structurally elucidated in plants, a novel nomenclature has been introduced to unequivocally designate the complex molecular structures with higher polymerization degree [21]. The building units of the oligomers are named according to their names as monomeric flavan-3-ols framing parenthesis which specify the C-position and direction of the interflavan linkage indicated as an arrow. For example, the dimer procyanidin B1 is designated as epicatechin-(4β → 8)-catechin, the dimer procyanidin A1 (Fig. 1) is given as epicatechin-(4β → 8, 2β → 7)-catechin and the trimer procyanidin C1 is denoted as [epicatechin-(4β → 8)]$_2$-epicatechin.

Unravelling the biosynthesis of monomeric and oligomeric flavanols provides knowledge on the nature of the phytochemicals. In the case of monomeric and oligomeric flavanols it becomes obvious why they are not glycosylated in plants and why there exists a large variety of different oligomeric flavanols. These insights also clarify why it is an absolute necessity to carefully characterize commercially available flavanolic preparations used in medicines, food supplements and cosmetics. Batch-to-batch consistency allows establishing the cause-and-effect relationship between the product and its physiological effect, i.e. the physiological consistency of the preparation. Therefore, scientific data of a well-characterized flavanolic preparation cannot be extrapolated to or associated with the daily consumption of flavanols via *ordinary foods, because foods contain a wide and unspecific variety of all kinds of flavanols. Dietary intake of flavanols is relevant only in the context of epidemiological studies in which average and mean intakes are associated with the health status of certain populations. In this respect the association between the consumption of red wine and cardiovascular mortality may serve as an example* [22]. *On top of that, during the past 30 years many more epidemiological data have become available on the dietary intake of flavanols and the health of populations.*

World-wide daily flavan-3-ol and total flavonoid intake

Monomeric, oligomeric and polymeric flavanols form one of the most abundant classes of flavonoids and are almost ubiquitous in the plant kingdom. As such they are present in a wide variety of vegetables and plant-derived food products including wine, fruit juices, tea leafs, cocoa beans, fruits, cereal grains and legume seeds [23–25]. Among fruits, berries like blackcurrants, blueberries, chokeberries, strawberries have been found to contain the highest amounts of monomeric and oligomeric flavanols. Also apples and plums are sources of monomeric and oligomeric flavanols and are suggested to contribute to their dietary amount daily consumed [25]. By combining the latest food composition databases on polyphenols and using dietary recall data of large population cohort studies estimations of the habitual intake of monomeric and oligomeric flavanols in Europe were recently published [26–28]. Considerable differences in the dietary flavanol intake among European countries and geographic regions were observed. The average total flavan-3-ol intake in Europe was reported to be 369 mg/d [27] with the highest intake in Ireland (mean: 793 mg/d; median: 701 mg/d) and the lowest intake in the Czech Republic (mean: 181 mg/d; median: 69 mg/d). The mean and median intake of proanthocyanidins (both, oligomers (i.e. 2–10 flavanol units) and polymers (i.e. > 10 flavanol units)) in Mediterranean countries was calculated to 160 mg/d and 30 mg/d (highest intake in Spain; mean: 175 mg/d, median: 36 mg/d), respectively. This exceeded the mean and median intake of countries in central Europe (114 and 26 mg/d, respectively) and northern (Scandinavian) countries (110 and 25 mg/d, respectively). The lowest averaged proanthocyanidin intake of all European countries was found in The Netherlands with 96 mg/d (median: 19.6 mg/d). Tea, wine, cocoa products, pome (in particular apples and pears) and stone fruits as well as berries could be identified as major dietary sources of proanthocyanidins [26–28]. It was also observed that the proanthocyanidin intake within populations seems to depend on socio-demographic, anthropometric and lifestyle characteristics. Subjects with a higher level of education, increasing age (44–64 years), being moderately active and without obesity (i.e. body mass index (BMI) < 30 kg/m^2) appeared to consume more proanthocyanidins than subjects without formal schooling, younger than 44 years, being inactive and having an BMI > 30 kg/m^2 [28].

In contrast to Europe, adults in the USA seem to daily consume on average lower amounts of total flavonoids, flavan-3-ols and proanthocyanidins, respectively. Latest data from a 24 h food recall in a cohort of 5420 people above 20 years old indicated a mean total flavonoid intake of 251 mg/d of which 81% comprised flavanols mainly derived from tea [29]. The oligomeric proanthocyanidin intake was estimated to range between 60 and 95 mg/d [25, 30]. Apples, chocolate products, grapes, tea, legumes and wine could be identified as major food sources. As in Europe, differences in the habitual intake of proanthocyanidins among adult subgroups appeared to be associated with sociodemographic factors [30].

Whereas the isoflavonoid intake from soy products by Asian populations is relatively well documented [31–34], data on the consumption of monomeric and oligomeric flavanols in Asian countries are lacking. A few studies report daily amounts of total flavonoids in specific Asian countries without specifying the intake of oligomeric flavan-3-ols. For example, in a population of almost 1400 adult Chinese total flavonoid intake was assessed as 166 mg/d [35]. A case-control study in Korea middle-aged men revealed that on average 105 mg total flavonoids were daily consumed of which 20–23 mg were flavan-3-ols [36]. However, these data do not provide an estimate of the ingested proanthocyanidin quantities, because the reported flavan-3-ols only comprised monomers. Similarly, a cross-sectional cohort study including 569 middle-aged Japanese women estimated flavan-3-ol monomer consumption by means of 24 h food records as 386 mg flavan-3-ols (i.e. (-)-epicatechin, catechin and epicatechingallate) [37]. Ninety-eight percent of these flavanols were ingested by tea.

Australian adults were found to daily consume on average 454 mg total flavonoids of which 92% are flavan-

3-ols (without any subclass specification) predominantly derived from tea consumption [38]. A prospective clinical study in 948 Australian women above 75 years assessed by means of food frequency questionnaires an average total proanthocyanidin (sum of dimers, trimers, 4–6 mers, 7–10 mers, polymers) intake of 215 mg/d (range: 18–1728 mg/d) which was mainly associated with the consumption of fruits, chocolate and alcoholic beverages [39].

Proanthocyanidin intake data for Middle and South America can hardly be found. Arabbi et al. determined the flavonoid content of commonly consumed Brazilian fruits and vegetables [40]. They also gave an overview on 4 epidemiological studies that indicate that the total habitual flavonoid intake in Brazilians ranges between 60 and 106 mg/d. They concluded from these studies that dietary flavonoid sources in Brazil are not very diverse since more than 70% of flavonoids are derived from oranges, 12% from lettuce and about 3% from tomatoes [40]. A recent survey estimates total average flavonoid intakes of 139 mg/d [41]. Despite a lack of data on quantities of subclasses, the identified major flavonoid food sources included legumes, fruits and beverages which are known to be rich in proanthocyanidins [24, 25, 42]. However, the total habitual intake of fruits and vegetables in Brazil appears to be much lower than in other countries world-wide. Less than 10% of the Brazilian population daily consumes 400 g fruits and vegetables as recommended by the WHO [40, 43]. Data on dietary flavonoid intake in African countries are not available in literature. In view of the discrepancies in chemical nomenclature, the size and anthropometric composition of the cohorts, the dietary assessment of food intake, the estimation of flavonoid and proanthocyanidin content of national food products by the use of different flavonoid databases, it is obvious that the reviewed data provide only rough estimates of the actual dietary intake of monomeric and oligomeric proanthocyanidins around the globe. However, it can be concluded with confidence that monomeric and oligomeric flavan-3-ols are present in human diets world-wide. Regular consumption of pome and stone fruits, berries, legumes, tea, wine and dark chocolate products leads to an intake of several hundreds of mg per day.

Due to the methodological limitation being associated with the quantitative assessment of the daily consumption of specific dietary constituents within populations, it is likely that individual's intake may be above or below the population's average. Since the daily dietary intake of monomeric and oligomeric flavanols fluctuates in and between individuals the attribution of health benefits to daily intakes remains problematic. Therefore, a nutraceutical with a well-defined monomeric and oligomeric composition, such as Masquelier's® Original OPCs, constitutes a relevant alternative since its recommended use will provide the health benefits that were established in preparation-specific research.

Chemical composition of Masquelier's grape seed extract

In order to warrant safety and efficacy of a plant extract, i.e. pharmaceutical quality and physiological consistency, the same criteria as for synthetic substances apply, i.e. identity, purity and content of the material must be established batch-to-batch [44]. Quality assurance of plant extracts is challenging since the raw materials from which they are obtained are prone to a number of variables that cannot always be controlled. The spectrum of constituents of natural materials relies on environmental factors under which the plant is grown (e.g. soil composition, climate, pest) as well as processing procedures (e.g. harvesting, transportation, drying, storage). Masquelier's® Original OPCs exemplify how pharmaceutical-grade quality of a plant extract can be achieved. Table 1 provides an overview on the properties and methods used to assess the identity, composition and purity of the extract. The preparation's identity is established by organoleptic and spectrophotometric characteristics, e.g. the polyphenols' absorbance maxima of $\lambda = 220–280$ nm. The purity of the preparation is determined by moisture, ash, physical constants, solvent residues, microbiological contaminations, foreign materials (e.g. heavy metals, pesticide residues, aflatoxins) and adulterations (Table 1).

The extract's specification of the content requires the qualitative and quantitative analysis of the phytochemicals. Various colorimetric though unspecific assays have a long tradition to determine the presence of polyphenols in general. The Folin-Denis and the Folin-Ciocalteau reagents, respectively are largely used to quantify total polyphenolic content of plant materials [45]. Both reagents rely on the oxidation of phenolic compounds in alkaline solution and subsequent reaction to blue colored phosphotungstic-phosphomolybdenum complexes which absorb at a wavelength of around $\lambda = 760$ nm. By means of the reference polyphenol gallic acid total polyphenolics are quantified as gallic acid equivalents (GAE) per kg or liter extract. As shown in Table 2 the total polyphenolic content of Masquelier's grape seed extract amounts to 90–95% according to spectrophotometry and the Folin-Ciocalteau method. Drawbacks of this method are that not all plant phenolics are detected with the same sensitivity and that with regard to mono- and/or oligomeric flavanols, it is useless since it is unspecific and cannot provide any information in terms of the various flavanolic fractions in extracts. Moreover, sugars, aromatic amines and ascorbic acid can interfere with the color reaction [46].

The commonly used colorimetric method to determine the presence of proanthocyanidins is n-butanol/HCl hydrolysis to red colored anthocyanidins which

Table 1 Properties to control identity and purity of Masquelier's grape seed extract. The data were provided by the extract's manufacturer

Property	Standard	Method
Organoleptic characteristics		
Aspect	Fine powder	
Color	Light brown/pinkish	
Odor	Characteristic woody	
Taste	Astringent, bitter	
Identification		In house
UV spectrum (approx. 40 mg/L in ethanol 96%)	λ max = 280 ± 5 nm	
	λ min = 256 ± 5 nm	
Bate-Smith reaction (approx. 100 mg/L)	λ max = 540–550 nm	
Loss on drying	≤10%	Ph. Eur. 01/2005: 20817
Sulphated ashes	≤0.5%	Ph. Eur. 01/2005: 20414
Solubility	conform	Ph. Eur. 6.7: 51100
1% (w/v) in water	insoluble < 5%	
2% (w/v) in methanol	Soluble	
1% (w/v) in isopropanol	Soluble	
0.01% (w/v) in chloroform	Insoluble	
pH (4% (w/v) in water)	2.5–4.5	In house
Residual solvents	conform	Ph. Eur. 6.7: 20424
acetone	≤10 ppm	
chloroform	≤10 ppm	
ethanol	≤10 ppm	
ethyl acetate	≤10 ppm	
n-butanol	≤10 ppm	
Microbiology	conform	Ph. Eur. 6.7: 50104
Bacteria	<10000 cfu/g	
Enterobacteria	<100 cfu/g	
Escherichia coli	0 cfu/g	
Staphylococcus aureus	0 cfu/g	
Salmonella	0 cfu/10 g	
Pseudomonas aeruginosa	0 cfu/g	
Yeasts and moulds	<100 cfu/g	
Mycotoxins	Comply with Reg. EC 1881/2006	In house
Pesticide/phytosanitary products [a]	≤0.05 ppm	Ph. Eur. 6.7: 20813
Heavy metals (Fe, Cd, Hg, Pb, As)	<1 ppm	Ph. Eur. 6.7: 20408
Polychlorinated biphenyls and dioxins	Comply with Reg. EC 1881/2006	In house

[a] The EU has established Maximum Residue Limits (MRL) of pesticides for *"certain products of plant origin"* (Directive 90/642/EC incl. amendments and corrections). The investigated phytosanitary products include aldrin; 4,4′-dichlorodiphenyldichloroethane; 4,4′- dichlorodiphenyldichloroethylene; 2,4′-dichlorodiphenyltrichloroethane; 4,4′- dichlorodiphenyltrichloroethane; dieldrin; α-endosulfan; β-endosulfan; endrin; α-hexachlorocyclohexane; β-hexachlorocyclohexane; γ-hexachlorocyclohexane; heptachlor; trans-heptachlor epoxide; hexachlorobenzene; methoxychlor

have an absorbance maximum at around $\lambda = 550$ nm [47, 48]. Due to numerous technical limitations it was recommended to use this assay to detect the presence of oligomeric flavanols rather than to quantify them [49]. Another limitation is that the Bate-Smith reaction does not differentiate between specific fractions of proanthocyanidins. The coloration is produced by all proanthocyanidins, oligomers and polymers, i.e. irrespective of their level of polymerisation. For the purpose of quantifying total proanthocyanidins in a preparation, the vanillin assay

Table 2 Analysis of the flavanol content of Masquelier's grape seed extract. The data were provided by the extract's manufacturer

Compound	Analytical method	Content
Total polyphenols	Spectrophotometric (GAE), $n = 3$	90–95%
	Folin-Ciocalteau reagent (GAE), $n = 3$	
Flavan-3-ols	Vanillin-H_2SO_4 (Sun et al., [50]), $n = 9$	60–70%
	HPLC, $n = 14$	
Monomeric flavanols	HPLC (every batch)	25–30%
Oligomeric flavanols (2–5 units)	HPLC (every batch)	35–40%
Polymeric flavanols (>6 units)	HPLC (every batch)	1–5%

GAE gallic acid equivalence, *HPLC* high performance liquid chromatography

might be a slightly better colorimetric alternative. In the presence of sulfuric acid vanillin reacts with condensed flavan-3-ols (oligomers and polymers) to a red colored complex that can be measured at a wavelength of $\lambda =$ 500 nm. Usually, catechin is used as a reference substance although for the quantification of polymerized flavanols internal standards would be more advantageous to account for different reaction rates of monomers and oligomers [50]. Various factors influencing the outcomes of the vanillin assay were identified [49], and led to a meticulous reexamination of the assay [50]. By means of this vanillin method the total proanthocyanidins content of Masquelier's Original OPCs amount to 60–70% (Table 2). Nonetheless, the major disadvantage of all these spectrophotometric assays is that they solely provide an estimation of the total polyphenolic and/or proanthocyanidin content of extracts. Individual fractions cannot be qualified or quantified by these methods. For this purpose, high performance liquid chromatography (HPLC) is the preferred technique. Several excellent reviews have been published over the last years that provide an overview on HPLC methods for the quantification of polyphenols as wells as a critical appraisal of factors that are essential to take into account for reliable measurements [46, 51–53]. In 1990, Masquelier and his team developed an HPLC method to analyze the monomeric and oligomeric flavanol content in grape seed and pine bark extracts [54]. To isolate and identify the individual monomeric and oligomeric flavanols the crude plant extract was first purified by solid phase extraction (SPE) on Sephadex G25 and LH20 columns and by semi-preparative HPLC. Fifteen flavanol monomers and oligomers could be identified by chemical (acidic degradation in the presence of α-toluenethiol) and spectroscopic techniques like nuclear magnetic resonance (NMR), ultraviolet-visible (UV/VIS) and infrared (IR) [55]. Next to the monomers (+)-catechin, (-)-epicatechin and (-)-epicatechin gallate, 6 dimers of the B-series were found, i.e. proanthocyanidin B1, B2, B3, B4, B5 and B7 and 1 dimer of the A-series, i.e. proanthocyanidin A2. Moreover 4 trimers have been identified, i.e. (+)-catechin - (+)-catechin - (+)-catechin, (-)-epicatechin - (-)-epicatechin - (-)-epicatechin, (-)-epicatechin - (-)-epicatechin - (+) catechin and (-)-epicatechin - (-)-epicatechin - (-)-epicatechin-gallate (EEEg) as well as a tetramer consisting of (-)-epicatechin - (-)-epicatechin - (-)-epicatechin - (-)-epicatechin [54]. Later, the preparation's manufacturer (Berkem SA; Gardonne; France) in collaboration with the University of Bordeaux repeated and modified Masquelier's analyses by using a C18 base-deactivated reversed-phase column (e.g. ProntoSIL 120-5-C18H, Bischoff Chromatography, Leonberg, Germany) with a gradient elution system of water/trifluoroacetic acid (TFA) 0.005% (v/v) and acetonitrile 65% (v/v)/TFA 0.005% (v/v) at a flow rate of 0.7 ml/min, at ambient column temperature and with UV detection at a wavelength of $\lambda = 280$ nm. In the chromatogram obtained mainly the monomeric and dimeric compounds are identified (Fig. 4), although centrifugal partition chromatography (CPC), preparative HPLC, NMR and mass spectrometry allowed the identification of 14 monomeric, dimeric and trimeric flavan-3-ols in addition to gallic acid. This HPLC analysis can be used to routinely monitor the composition of the grape seed extract next to ^{1}H-NMR spectroscopy followed by principle component analysis (PCA) as described below. Batch-to-batch analyses revealed that approximately a fourth of the grape seed extract's flavanols is made up by monomers, a second fourth are dimers and half of the extract consists of trimers, tetra- and pentamers (Table 3). Normal phase (NP)-HPLC demonstrated the absence of higher polymerized flavanols [56]. The qualitative and quantitative analysis of the grape seed extract is an important prerequisite to control and achieve a constant, standardized phytochemical composition. The HPLC data revealed that the Masquelier's extract is a complex mixture of individual flavanols of various polymerization degrees ($n = 2$–5). Monitoring batch-to-batch variations of the preparation based on only one flavanol would be inadequate because changes in one specific flavanol might not be representative for all the different individual flavanolic fractions. Since the physiologically active principle of a plant extract is the entire mixture of individual phytochemicals and not a single compound, profiling the whole spectrum of phytochemicals in the grape seed extract is necessary to guarantee a stable composition and ultimately consistent

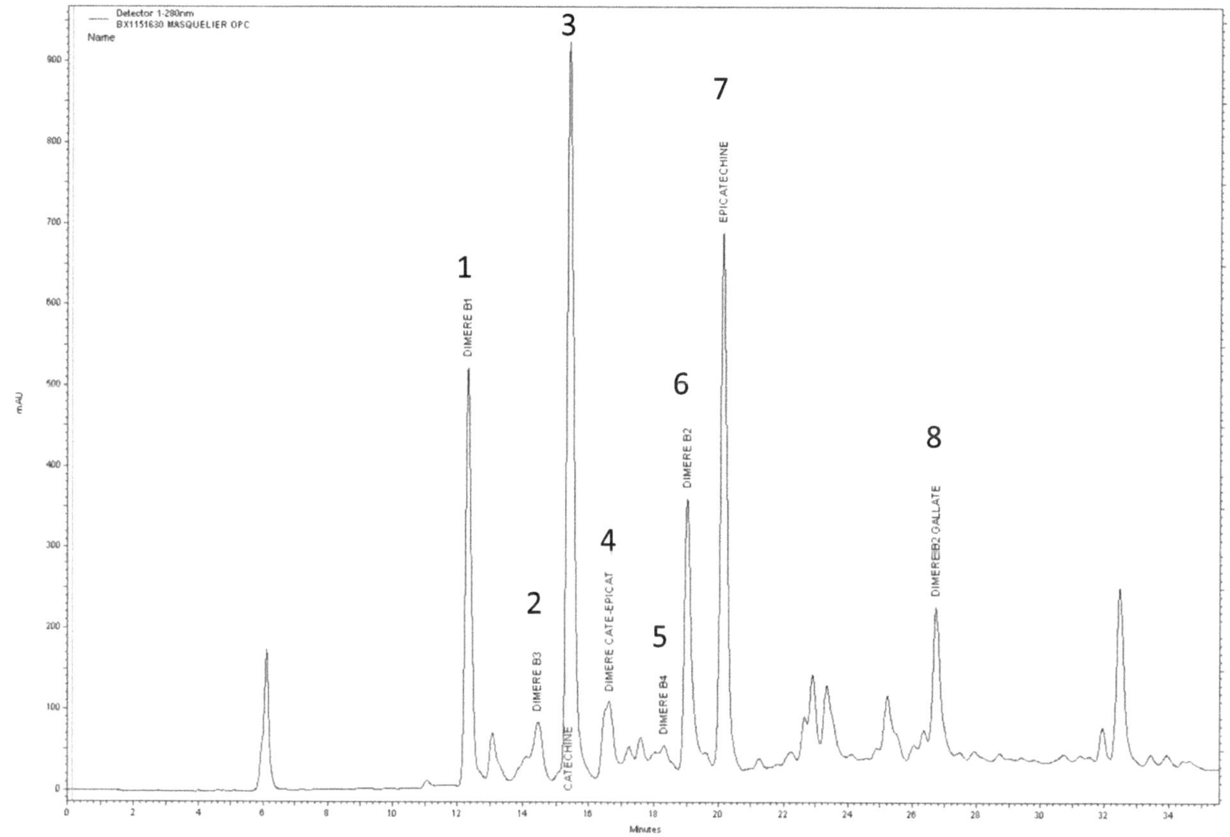

Fig. 4 Representative chromatogram of Masquelier's grape seed extract measured by high performance liquid chromatography (HPLC) using a C18 base-deactivated reversed-phase column (e.g. ProntoSIL 120-5-C18H, Bischoff Chromatography, Leonberg, Germany) with a gradient elution system of water/trifluoroacetic acid (TFA) 0.005% (v/v) and acetonitrile 65% (v/v)/TFA 0.005% (v/v) at a flow rate of 0.7 ml/min, at ambient column temperature and with UV detection at a wavelength of $\lambda = 280$ nm. The peaks in the chromatogram have been identified as the following individual monomeric and oligomeric flavan-3-ols: 1 = procyanidin B1, 2 = procyanidin B3, 3 = (+)-catechin, 4 = dimeric procyanidin consisting of (+)-catechin-(-)-epicatechin, 5 = procyanidin B4, 6 = procyanidin B2, 7 = (-)-epicatechin, 8 = prodcyanidin B2 gallate. The data were provided by the extract's manufacturer

bioactivity. NMR spectroscopy is a versatile analytical technique to screen complex composed samples with minimal and non-destructive sample preparation. Standard ^{1}H- or ^{13}C-NMR spectra provide a wealth of information on both, chemical structures of individual compounds and chemical profiles of compound mixtures. That makes it increasingly popular for elucidation of novel plant-derived compounds as well as for characterization of plant extracts and food products [52]. All molecules containing atoms with a non-zero magnetic moment (e.g. ^{1}H, ^{13}C, ^{14}N, ^{15}N, ^{19}F, ^{31}P) give an unique NMR signal which originates from the structural location of these atoms in the molecule. NMR analysis of an extract with a complex mixture of plant metabolites provides a unique spectrum of signals, i.e. a fingerprint, depending on its molecular composition (Fig. 5a). Multivariate analysis of such unassigned fingerprint NMR-spectra is a convenient and accurate tool to compare the phytochemical content of different plant extracts e.g. from distinct manufacturers or from different batches [57]. Therefore, ^{1}H-NMR spectroscopy followed by PCA [58] is used to control batch-to-batch consistency of Masquelier's grape seed extract. The yellow dots in the three-dimensional plot (Fig. 5b) represent the 95% confidence intervals of each batch analysis and form a clearly separated cloud indicating high similarity of the phytochemical NMR-profile of the individual batches. This cluster of Masquelier`s grape seed extract batches (Anthogenol®, yellow) clearly distinguishes from the cluster of French pine bark extracts (M-PM, red) and other grape seed extracts (GSEs, magenta). Samples of the Endotélon extract (red) and samples of Masquelier's extract from 1985 (VV-OPC 1985, yellow) are located within the "Anthogenol" cluster proving the qualitative and quantitative equality of these extracts and its consistency throughout the years. The application of NMR fingerprinting enables to continuously authenticate the extract and allows for the production of a genuinely standardized product. Eventually, this is essential for safeguarding the preparation's physiological consistency.

Lacking standardization and characterization of the phytochemical composition of herbal extracts makes

Table 3 Mean quantities ± standard deviation (SD) of monomeric and oligomeric flavan-3-ols of 10 batches of Masquelier's grape seed extract measured by high performance liquid chromatography (HPLC, see also Fig. 4). The data were provided by the extract's manufacturer

Compound	Mean quantity ± SD (% (w/w))
Total monomers	*25.6 ± 2.2*
(+)-catechin	10.9 ± 1.6
(-)-epicatechin	12.2 ± 1.6
(-)-epicatechin-3-O-gallate	2.5 ± 1.6
Total dimers	*27.5 ± 1.6*
Procyanidin B1	7.7 ± 1.6
(-)-epicatechin-(4 β → 8)-(+)-catechin	
Procyanidin B2	8.3 ± 1.6
(-)-epicatechin-(4β → 8)-(-)-epicatechin	
Procyanidin B3	2.8 ± 1.6
(+)-catechin-(4α → 8)-(+)-catechin	
Procyanidin B4	1.6 ± 1.6
(+)-catechin-(4α → 8)-(-)-epicatechin	
Procyanidin B2-gallate	7.1 ± 1.6
Total tri-, tetra- and pentameric proanthocyanidins	*46.9 ± 1.6*

studying the in vivo *biotransformation of the plant-derived constituents cumbersome. With a meticulously defined product, such as Masquelier's flavanol blend, it becomes feasible to study the bioavailability and metabolism.*

Bioavailability and metabolism of Masqulier's grape seed extract

Knowledge on the bioavailability, biotransformation and kinetics of grape-seed derived flavan-3-ols is important for the elucidation of their mechanism of action. In addition, these data strengthen the cause-effect relationship between the (recommended) dietary intake and the observed health effect of these compounds. In order to shed more light on the fate of orally ingested monomeric and oligomeric flavan-3-ols, animal experiments were conducted in the late 70ies of the last century. Radiolabeled monomeric and oligomeric flavan-3-ols (0.6 μCi (0.2 × 10^3 Bq)/mg) could be obtained from the seeds of grapes (*Vitis vinifera* L. of the Cabernet and Merlot variety) grown during grape formation in a $^{14}CO_2$ atmosphere for 40 days. After oral administration of a single dose of 2 μCi (approximately 3.3 mg grape seed extract) radioactivity in blood of mice ($n = 5$) was measured at 9 consecutive time points between 10 min and 7 h [59, 60]. Following a rapid increase in the blood's radioactivity, maximal plasma levels were reached 45 min. after ingestion. The plasma half-life was estimated to 5 h. The distribution of the flavanols in the mice was determined in various types of tissue collected at 1, 3, 6 and 24 h after intake of a single oral dose (5 mg) [59, 60]. During the first 6 h most of the radioactivity was located in the gastro-intestinal tract including gall-bladder and bladder. Lower levels of radioactivity could be detected in the liver, kidneys, skin, cartilage tissue, arteries, cardiac muscle and blood. After 24 h the gastro-intestinal tract was free of any radioactivity. In contrast, radioactivity was markedly elevated in the gastro-intestinal vasculature, arteries, skin, and cartilage tissue. Decreasing levels of radioactivity were seen in liver, spleen, venous tunica, periost, kidneys, lungs, bones and blood. Repeated daily dosages over 5 consecutive days did not seem to lead to an accumulation of the flavanols in mice [59, 60]. In rats ($n = 5$) bile was found to be essentially involved in the elimination of monomeric and oligomeric flavanols [59, 60]. The use of semi-synthetically produced ^3H-labeled flavan-3,4-diol monomer confirmed the tissue distribution of the ^{14}C-labeled grape seed flavanols. Since ^3H-radioactivity remained measurable in mice tissue sections, especially in collagen-rich types of tissue, it was suggested that tissue binding of flavanols neither involves the hydroxyl-group in the C4-position of the flavan-moeity (C-ring) nor *in situ* polymerization of flavanol-monomers via the C4-position [59, 60]. Although these early experimental data indicate that grape-seed-derived monomeric and oligomeric flavanols become bioavailable upon oral ingestion, it remained unknown in which form, i.e. as parent compounds or metabolites, they are distributed in the body. Moreover, it remains to be elucidated whether bioavailability and biotransformation routes differ between rodents and humans as reported for other types of flavonoids [61].

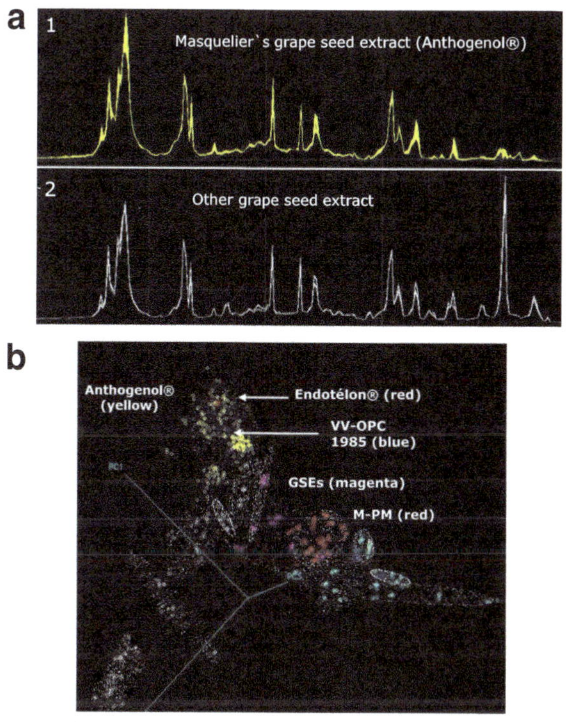

Fig. 5 **a** Typical examples of an unassigned fingerprint proton nuclear magnetic resonance (^{1}H-NMR) spectra of Masquelier's grape seed extract (1) and another grape seed extract (2). **b** Three-dimensional plot of the principle component analysis (PCA) using unassigned fingerprint proton nuclear magnetic resonance (^{1}H-NMR) spectra to compare the phytochemical content of different plant extracts e.g. from distinct manufacturers or from different batches. The small white dotted lines indicate the 95% confidence interval per cluster. The cluster of Masquelier's grape seed extract (Anthogenol®, *yellow*) clearly distinguish from the cluster of French pine bark extract (M-PM, *red*) and other grape seed extracts (GSEs, magenta). Samples of the Endotélon extract (*red*) and samples of Masquelier's extract from 1985 (VV-OPC 1985, *yellow*) are located within the cluster of Masquelier's grape seed extract proofing the qualitative and quantitative equality of these extracts. The green-blue lines represent the 3 strongest principal components (PC), i.e. the variables derived from the ^{1}H-NMR spectra which define the biggest differences between all the samples. The farther 2 samples are apart from each other in respect of one particular axis, the more different they are in this particular aspect. The data were provided by the extract's manufacturer

In a preliminary human pharmacokinetic study with ^{14}C labelled grape seed mono- and oligomeric flavanols (Endotélon®), 6 healthy volunteers received a single oral dose of 150 mg in the morning under fasting conditions [62]. Plasma radioactivity was in general low and found to be in the range of ng equivalents of the administered dose. Despite considerable inter-individual differences maximal radioactivity plasma levels were observed at approximately 14 h after flavanol administration with a slow decrease over the subsequent 144 h. During 96 h after intake between 11 and 27% (mean ± SD = 22.09 ± 5.99%) of the oral dose was eliminated via urine and between 22 and 67% (mean ± SD = 45.61 ± 14.92%) via feces. On average approximately 6% of the flavanols was measured in breath as $^{14}CO_2$ with the majority exhaled during the first 24 h [62].

One major drawback of those studies is that they do not provide any information on the origin of the ^{14}C labelled radioactivity in tissue, i.e. whether it derives from the ingested parent compounds or from metabolites. Thereby it remains unclear in which form flavanols reach target tissue and may be responsible for putative health effects. The development of highly sensitive analytical techniques such as HPLC coupled to mass spectrometric (MS) detection has considerably increased insights in the metabolic fate of monomeric and oligomeric flavanols. Today it is possible to quantify flavanols in the fmolar range in various types of matrices and at the same time to elucidate their molecular structure. This has considerably advanced the knowledge on the absorption, distribution, metabolism and excretion of flavanols. Animal studies reported flavanolic monomers, dimers and trimers in plasma, urine and feces of rats orally administered with grape seed extracts [63–66]. In these in vivo studies the major biotransformation routes comprised methylation, glucuronidation and sulphation of both, monomeric and oligomeric flavanols [64–66]. Data on the bioavailability and metabolism of grape seed derived flavanols in humans are scarce. A recent perfusion study revealed that the absorption of a single 50 mg dose of the flavanolic monomer (-)-epicatechin varies between healthy persons ranging between 31 and 90% [67]. Glucuronidation, sulphation and methylation produce the major epicatechin metabolites that can be found in plasma approximately 2 h after oral ingestion [68] and which are excreted in bile and in urine [67]. Plasma concentrations of untransformed epicatechin have been reported to be around 1% of the epicatechin sulfate metabolites and amount to approximately 4 nM 1 h after ingestion of a cocoa dairy-based drink providing 1.8 mg epicatechin per kg body weight [68]. In contrast to monomers human data on the fate of oligomers are less consistent. Dimeric B-type proanthocyanidins have been detected in nmolar quantities in the circulation after a single dose of 323 mg cocoa-derived monomers and 256 mg dimers [69] and 2 g of a grape-seed extract [70], respectively. However, higher condensation products are assumed not to be absorbed due to their molecular weight, although in vitro and in vivo studies showed the absorption of the proanthocyanidins trimer C2 [64, 66, 71]. Trimeric and larger condensation products are generally suggested to undergo colonic degradation to phenolic acids [72] and valerolactones [73, 74], rather than to serve as monomer precursors [68, 75]. Therefore, based on the current data it needs to be presumed that the intake of grape seed extract containing both, monomeric and oligomeric flavan-3-ols, will lead to monomeric phase II conjugates and colonic biotransformation products in the human circulation. It remains to be elucidated in how far these metabolites contribute to the observed health effects.

Over the past decades, the state of the art of analytical-chemical techniques increased considerably. These technical advances revealed that the historical data using radioactive-labelled grape seed flavanols lacks specificity. Thereby, the precise metabolic fate and kinetic profile of Masquelier's grape seed extract is still incomplete. Whether flavanol-tissue binding takes place as concluded by Laparra et al. [59, 60], *remains questionable. Still, the fact that proanthocyanidins bind to collagen-rich tissues has been well established. Polymers of proanthocyanidins are called tannins because of their "tanning" properties. Tannins strongly bind to collagen-rich tissue (leather). This millenia-old knowledge forms an indication that part of the oligomers' protective mode of action may stem from their affinity to collagen. In this regard, separate from the kinetic profiling of flavanolic plant extracts, their physiological mode of action is key in developing the product as a nutraceutical.*

Mechanisms of action of Masquelier's grape seed extract

Effects on collagen and elastin fibers in vitro and in vivo

The time-journey of Masquelier's monomeric and oligomeric flavan-3-ols extract started with the observation of their effect in vascular tissue. With other grape seed extracts many other, often similar studies have been done. It is, however, known that grape seed extract may vary widely in the way they are composed (*vide supra*) as nicely illustrated by Nakamura et al. [76]. It is therefore important to use a well-characterized grape seed extract with a stable composition. Since composition affects biological activity, in the description of the mechanisms of action we limit this review to the available data on Masquelier's extract. The microcirculatory effect of Masquelier's monomeric and oligomeric flavanol extract was correlated to the original findings that the preparation protects collagen. The stability of collagen depends on the cross-linking of the peptic chain in the molecule. Denaturation of the molecule, for example by increased temperature or oxidative stress, leads to shortening of the collagen fibers. In vitro, Masquelier's® Original OPCs have been shown to protect against the thermal contraction of the collagen [77]. Of all bioflavonoids only the proanthocyanidins (oligomeric flavanols) seem to exert this protecting effect which might be due to the variation in their cross-linking effect. Oligomeric flavanols show strong collagen protection and isotopic labelling of monomeric and oligomeric flavan-3-ols can be interpreted as a confirmation of the oligomers' affinity for the vascular wall (*vide supra*) [60]. This was also confirmed in 1982 by A. Pfister et al. who studied the localization of monomeric and oligomeric flavanols in cell membranes of endothelial cells and pneumocytes [78].

Similarly, the risk of vascular damage can be reduced by Masquelier's grape seed extract through the protection of elastin from degradation by elastase in vitro and in vivo. In vitro, the solubilization of elastin obtained from calf articular ligament by either elastase from porcine pancreas or human leukocyte was inhibited by incubating the elastin with the extract. Also in vivo, after intradermal injections of the flavanols in the skin of rabbits, it was shown that this pretreatment protected the elastin [79]. The inhibition of the hydrolysis of elastin by elastase and of collagen by collagenase has been confirmed in other in vitro models [80]. There are even indications that the synthesis of collagen and elastonectin fibers is promoted by the extract in vitro [80] and in vivo [78].

This antiproteolytic activity offered by the oligomeric flavan-3-ols present in the preparation has been classified as 'substrate protection', because the compounds do not primarily inhibit the proteinases that degrade the matrix-components but rather bind to the matrix macromolecules thus preventing degradation by various triggers such as temperature, oxidative stress, inflammation, proteinases among others [81].

In Wistar rats, collagenase-induced vascular capillary hyperpermeability was inhibited by the grape seed derived monomeric and oligomeric flavanols [80]. The flavanols' strengthening effect on collagen- and elastin-rich tissues like blood vessels and the venous system has also been demonstrated in various human intervention studies as reviewed in 2003 [82].

Antioxidant effects in vitro and in vivo

With the discovery that reactive oxygen species play a pivotal role in the aging physiology a lot of attention was given to this research area [83]. Also vascular function is strongly influenced by oxidative stress [84]. The imaginative studies in the early fifties of the previous century already demonstrated that the oxidation of the antioxidant vitamin C could be prevented by Masquelier's extract [85]. The established action of the flavanols on vascular function directed the research to the field of prevention and attenuation of oxidative stress and ever since the antioxidant action of monomeric and oligomeric flavan-3-ols has indeed been widely studied. In 1987, the US Patent Office granted Jack Masquelier a patent for the use of proanthocyanidins as antioxidants in various fields of human physiology [86].

Polyphenolic structures are known to be good antioxidants [87]. Monomeric and oligomeric flavanols have been shown to have radical scavenging activity, e.g.

scavenging of the 2,2-diphenyl-1-picrylhydrazyl (DPPH) radical [88] and the superoxide anion radical [89, 90]. Moreover, monomeric and oligomeric flavan-3-ols protect against hydrogen peroxide [91] and organic peroxide (*i.e.* cumene hydroperoxide)-induced damage of fetal bovine vascular endothelial cells [92]. Iron (Fe^{2+}- adenosine diphosphate (ADP)) in combination with ascorbic acid leads to lipid peroxidation in rat liver microsomes, which is inhibited by monomeric and oligomeric flavan-3-ols [89, 93].

Monomeric and oligomeric flavan-3-ols are clearly and not unexpectedly (based on the molecular structure of the constituents) able to scavenge reactive oxygen and nitrogen species and inhibit lipid peroxidation. Due to the low concentrations that are found in the human circulation after flavanol supplementations (*vide supra*), the relevance of direct antioxidant effects of these compounds under physiological conditions is increasingly debated. However, we recently demonstrated that also epicatechin phase II metabolites attenuate intracellular oxidative stress in primary human umbilical vein endothelial cells (HUVECs) in concentrations as low as 0.5 μM [94].

With the progressing insights into redox regulation of cell signaling during the last decades, studies aimed at unraveling the effects of monomeric and oligomeric flavanols on redox-sensitive transcription factors like nuclear factor (erythroid-derived 2)-like 2 (Nrf2). Nrf2 is critical in the transcriptional regulation of genes coding enzymes that facilitate cellular protection against oxidative stress. In hepatocytes it was recently shown that epicatechin transiently activates, among other redox-sensitive transcription factors, Nrf2 [95]. Similarly, procyanidin B2 activated redox-sensitive signaling cascades involved in the activation of Nrf2, induced the translocation of Nrf2 from the cytoplasm into the nucleus and activated the transcription of the detoxifying enzyme glutathione S-transferase pi 1 (GSTP1) in in epithelial colon cells [96]. Interestingly, Nrf2 activation and modulation of Nrf2-mediate gene transcription was reported in various in vitro and in vivo models by monomeric and oligomeric flavanol-rich extracts of different plants sources [97–99] including grape seeds [100, 101].

Nowadays, it is well established that diminishing oxidative stress also reduces the inflammatory response. A vicious interplay between oxidative stress and inflammation is apparent. In fact, inflammation is probably fundamental in many pathologies and maintaining health is achieved by keeping the inflammation low.

Anti-inflammatory effects in vitro and in vivo

Monomeric and oligomeric flavan-3-ols inhibit the inflammatory response also in a more direct way. Leukocyte-induced luminescence stimulated with either zymosan or the phorbol ester phorbol12-myristate 13-acetate (PMA) was dose-dependently inhibited by the monomeric and oligomeric flavanols preparation [88]. Also in animal experiments the anti-inflammatory effect of Masquelier's extract has been demonstrated. Blaszò et al. reported that in a carrageenan-induced rat paw oedema model the intraperitoneally administered preparation in dosages of 10, 20, 40 mg/kg displayed an anti-inflammatory action [102]. Oral administration of rats with 500 mg/kg Masquelier's Original OPCs® also gave protection against the carrageenan paw oedema effect [88].

More than 20 years later, the anti-inflammatory effects of the grape-seed derived monomeric and oligomeric flavanols were further explored on a cellular and subcellular level. The transcription factor nuclear factor kappa-light-chain enhancer of activated B cells (NF-κB) is the key regulator of the transcription and synthesis of inflammatory mediators in immune cells [103]. In human monocytes (U937 cells) which were stably transfected with a luciferase-reporter gene construct containing NF-κB binding sites and which were differentiated into macrophage-like cells the inhibition of NF-κB-mediated gene expression by the grape-seed derived monomeric and oligomeric flavanols was demonstrated [104]. That this subcellular effect has consequences for the function of human monocytes was proven in an assay that allows studying the chemotaxis and adhesion of monocytes to vascular endothelial cells [104]. Preincubation of the monocytes with the grape-seed derived monomeric and oligomeric flavanols for 24 h reduced the number of adhering cells at the endothelial cells by approximately one third [104]. These data shed light on a molecular mechanism of the grape-seed derived flavanolic preparation that may help to explain their anti-inflammatory activity observed in humans (*vide infra*).

Moreover, (-)-epicatechin was recently suggested to enhance the anti-inflammatory effects of the endogenous glucocorticoid cortisol in human macrophage-like cells under oxidative stress [105]. Next to the parent compound also epicatechin phase II metabolites exhibit capacity to preserve the anti-inflammatory effects of cortisol in this model [106]. This mechanism is an eminent example of the intertwined link between oxidative stress and the development of inflammation by a compromised endogenous cortisol response. In how far Masquelier's extract exert similar protection of the cortisol response must be demonstrated.

As illustrated here, Masquelier's flavanol blend show a multitude of biological effects. This is distinctive from most pharmaceuticals that are generally selected for their strong effect on a well-defined single molecular target. The efficacy of drugs in humans is determined in clinical trials by a statistical change in a primary outcome parameter indicative for an improvement of a disease. In contrast, to capture the multiple - pleiotropic - effects of botanical extracts a broad panel of biomarkers is required. Moreover, effects on human health are characterized by the ability to withstand a stressor in the physiological system and maintain or restore homeostasis [107]. *The relevance of results from human intervention studies should therefore be judged from this perspective, i.e. whether the observed effects are the result of integrated physiological phenomena.*

Effects of Masquelier's grape seed extract on human health

Initially, several clinical studies on the protective effect of Endotélon® (the French herbal remedy consisting of Masquelier's grape seed extract) on capillary fragility were performed. Dartenuc et al. reported in an open-label study using 100 – 150 mg/d of Endotélon® for 30 – 45 days a reduction in capillary fragility in 39 out of 46 subjects assessed by a cupping glass method [108]. To confirm these findings, the researchers performed a second study which was placebo-controlled. The daily intake of Masquelier's grape seed preparation for 15 days improved capillary fragility in 10 of 21 volunteers, whereas in the placebo-group a similar effect was only seen in 3 out of 12 subjects [108]. The capillary resistance defined as the property of capillaries to counteract the forces of rupture was improved by the intake of 100–150 mg after 15–30 day of intervention [109]. The protection of capillary resistance by Endotélon® was also demonstrated in a double-blind placebo-controlled study in subjects with either spontaneous capillary fragility or acetylsalicylic acid-induced capillary fragility [109]. In a double-blind placebo-controlled trial the measurement of skin temperature as a measure of dermal circulation and rheographic parameters were used to show an improved venous tone in subjects who daily took 150 mg of Masquelier's preparation (Endotélon®) for 45 days [110]. During 15–90 days Beylot C. and Bioulac P. administered patients with a variety of problems related to capillary fragility 150 mg Endotélon® per day and observed a decrease in fragility in 62 out of 78 subjects [111]. In patients with varying phlebologic disorders the influence of Endotélon® on edema, varicose veins, hypodermitis, capillaries and petechies was investigated by a placebo-controlled randomized clinical trial [112]. The daily intake of 150 mg Endotélon® over 4 weeks improved edema and varicose veins compared to the placebo treatment. In a homogenous study population of 92 patients with a mean age of 40 years and a venous pathology of in average 7 years obtained 300 mg Endotélon® for 4 weeks [113]. Clinical scoring of the amelioration was achieved in 75% of the patients (versus 41% in the placebo group, $P < 0.01$). Also, edema reduction was apparent.

The most recent clinical data of Masquelier's grape seed extract (embodied in the food supplement Anthogenol®) were obtained in a double-blind randomized placebo-controlled clinical study in healthy volunteers [114]. This study aimed at capturing the diverse effects of the grape seed-derived monomeric and oligomeric flavanols observed in all the previous studies by a broad panel of outcome parameters reflecting vascular function as well as cellular and subcellular processes in the human vasculature associated with cardiovascular pathologies. For this purpose, 28 male healthy smokers were daily supplemented for 8 weeks with 200 mg Masquelier's® Original OPCs. Neither macrovascular function (assessed as flow mediated dilation of the brachial artery) nor microvascular function (measured by laser-Doppler flowmetry) changed significantly during the 8 weeks intervention compared with the placebo-supplemented group. Individuals with elevated total cholesterol and low density lipoprotein (LDL) serum concentrations in the beginning of the trial revealed a 5% and 7% reduction ($P < 0.05$ vs. baseline), respectively after 8 weeks supplementation with Masquelier's preparation. These effects could not be observed in a similar subgroup on placebo. Whereas platelet aggregability remained unaffected, a significant attenuation of the inflammatory responsiveness of leukocytes to *ex vivo* added bacterial endotoxin (compared to baseline and compared to the placebo intervention) was found in blood from volunteers after the 8 weeks supplementation with Masquelier's® Original OPCs. While total antioxidant capacity of plasma and the lipid peroxidation marker 8-iso-prostglandin F2α did not change during the intervention, erythrocytes' ratio of reduced to oxidized glutathione appeared to increase in the supplemented group compared to baseline. Integration of all the effects assessed by the meticulously selected parameter panel into a global vascular health index revealed a significant increase upon the 8 weeks supplementation with Masquelier's grape seed extract compared to placebo. In order to elucidate the underlying molecular pathways which might be involved in the observed changes, RNA and DNA was isolated from leukocytes of a subset of the volunteers to determine genome wide changes in gene expression and DNA methylation [104]. The dietary intervention with Masquelier's extract seemed to affect in particular the expression of genes associated with pathways involved in the regulation of inflammation and chemotaxis, adhesion and transendothelial migration of leukocytes. Experimental models substantiate these findings by demonstrating the extract-mediated inhibition of the inflammatory transcription factor NF-κB [104]. This mechanism may also contribute to the reduced adhesion of monocytes exposed to the grape seed-derived flavanols to vascular endothelial cells in vitro [104]. Despite clear effects of the daily supplementation with 200 mg Masquelier's® Original OPCs over 8 weeks on the expression of genes associated with pathophysiological mechanisms in the cardiovascular system, the transcriptomic changes could not be related to alterations in the DNA methylation state due to high inter-individual variability in leukocytes DNA methylation [104].

This beneficial modulation of inflammatory, metabolic and redox pathways in the vasculature and the very recently reported effects of a grape seed extract on liver nicotine adenine dinucleotide (NAD^+)-metabolism and expression of the protein deacetylase sirtuin 1 [115] may hold promise to extend the clinical investigations on this extract in the future also to hepatic, endocrine and cognitive health.

Conclusion

The three requirements to substantiate the health benefit of a food product include 1) the characterization of the product, 2) the clear definition and understandable wording of the physiological benefit and 3) the plausible cause-effect relationship between the food product's intake and the health effect.

Ad 1) In contrast to many commercially plant extracts Masquelier's grape seed preparation is rigidly defined and standardized by HPLC and ^{1}H-NMR/PCA fingerprinting. This combination of methods is optimal for monitoring the quality of plant extracts and is superior to the analysis of one or more individual "target" components of an extract.

Ad 2) The numerous human intervention studies that became available over time formed the basis for designing an intervention study that employed innovative biomolecular techniques and reflects conceptual advances in nutritional science. This novel approach enabled to capture the pleiotropic effects of Masqulier's grape seed extract on vascular health in humans [114]. This physiological benefit can be briefly worded as "maintenance of vascular homeostasis".

Ad 3) Understanding the consistency, dose–response and biological plausibility of the association between the vascular health effects and Masquelier's grape seed extract is based on the totality of the human intervention studies. These outcomes are substantiated by experimental studies that elucidate the molecular mechanisms of the herbal extract and some of its individual components. In this regard, the knowledge on the mode of action of flavanols in general parallels and supports the more refined and preparation-specific insights into the physiological processes described in the studies on the products that embody the specific monomeric and oligomeric flavanols extract developed by Jack Masquelier. In the quest for unravelling the molecular action of complex botanical preparations such as Masquelier's® Original OPCs, studies are ongoing to enhance our existing knowledge and understanding in the intricately related fields of nutrition, physiology, health and disease. The preparation's pleiotropic effects explain why and how it can be applied as an herbal remedy as well as a nutraceutical in the field of vascular health.

Abbreviations

^{1}H-NMR: Proton nuclear magnetic resonance; ADP: Adenosine diphosphate; ANR: Anthocyanidin reductase; ANS: Anthocyanidin synthase; BMI: Body mass index; CPC: Centrifugal partition chromatography; DAHP: 3-deoxy-D-arabinose-heptulosonic acid-7-phosphate; D-erythrose-P: D-erythrose-4-phosphate; DFR: Dihydroflavanol-4-reductase; DPPH: 2,2-diphenyl-1-picrylhydrazyl; F3'H: Flavanone-3'-hydroxylase; F3H: Flavanone-3-hydroxylase; GAE: Gallic acid equivalence; GSTP1: Glutathione S-transferase pi 1; HPLC: High performance liquid chromatography; HUVECs: Human umbilical vein endothelial cells; IR: Infrared; LAR: Leucoanthocyanidin reductase; LDL: Low density lipoprotein; MS: Mass spectrometry; NAD: Nicotine-adenine dinucleotide; NADPH: Reduced nicotine-adenine dinucleotide phosphate; NF-kB: Nuclear factor kappa-light-chain enhancer of activated B cells; Nrf2: Nuclear factor (erythroid-derived 2)-like 2; OPCs: Oligomeric proanthocyanidins; PC: Principle components; PCA: Principle component analysis; PEP: Phosphoenol pyruvate; PMA: Phorbol12-myristate 13-acetate; PPO: Polyphenol oxidase; SPE: Solid phase extraction; TFA: Trifluoroacetic acid; UV/VIS: Ultraviolet-visible

Acknowlegements

Not applicable

Funding

This work was financially supported by International Nutrition Company (INC) BV, Loosdrecht, The Netherlands.

Availability of data and material

Not applicable.

Authors' contributions

ARW and AB equally contributed to writing and editing the manuscript. All authors read and approved the final manuscript.

Competing interest

Both authors declare no competing interest.

Consent for publication

Not applicable

Ethics approval and consent to participate

Not applicable

References

1. Nassiri-Asl M, Hosseinzadeh H. Review of the pharmacological effects of *Vitis vinifera* (grape) and its bioactive constituents: an update. Phytother Res. 2016;30(9):1392–403.
2. Olaku OO, Ojukwu MO, Zia FZ, White JD. The role of grape seed extract in the treatment of chemo/radiotherapy induced toxicity: a systematic review of preclinical studies. Nutr Cancer. 2015;67:730–40.
3. Kasdagly M, Radhakrishnan S, Reddivari L, Veeramachaneni DN, Vanamala J. Colon carcinogenesis: influence of Western diet-induced obesity and targeting stem cells using dietary bioactive compounds. Nutrition. 2014;30:1242–56.
4. Ting H, Deep G, Agarwal C, Agarwal R. The strategies to control prostate cancer by chemoprevention approaches. Mutat Res. 2014;760:1–15.
5. Tong LX, Young LC. Nutrition: the future of melanoma prevention? J Am Acad Dermatol. 2014;71:151–60.
6. Feringa HH, Laskey DA, Dickson JE, Coleman CI. The effect of grape seed extract on cardiovascular risk markers: a meta-analysis of randomized controlled trials. J Am Diet Assoc. 2011;111:1173–81.

7. Ho L, Pasinetti GM. Polyphenolic compounds for treating neurodegenerative disorders involving protein misfolding. Expert Rev Proteomics. 2010;7:579–89.
8. Pasinetti GM, Ho L. Role of grape seed polyphenols in Alzheimer's disease neuropathology. Nutr Diet Suppl. 2010;2010:97–103.
9. Wu CD. Grape products and oral health. J Nutr. 2009;139:1818S–23S.
10. Baumann LS. Less-known botanical cosmeceuticals. Dermatol Ther. 2007;20: 330–42.
11. Martinez-Zapata MJ, Vernooij RW, Uriona Tuma SM, Stein AT, Moreno RM, Vargas E, Capella D, Bonfill Cosp X. Phlebotonics for venous insufficiency. Cochrane Database Syst Rev. 2016;4:CD003229.
12. World Health Organization (WHO). Constitution of the World Health Organization - basic documents, vol. Supplement. 45th ed. 2006.
13. Michaud JMJRAM. Synthèse des procyanidines naturelles. Ann Pharm Fr. 1973;31:385–95.
14. Dewick PM. The Shikimate Pathway: Aromatic Amino Acids and Phenylpropanoids. In: Medicinal Natural Products. Hoboken: Wiley; 2009. p. 137–86.
15. Xie D-Y, Dixon RA. Proanthocyanidin biosynthesis – still more questions than answers? Phytochemistry. 2005;66:2127–44.
16. He F, Pan QH, Shi Y, Duan CQ. Biosynthesis and genetic regulation of proanthocyanidins in plants. Molecules. 2008;13:2674–703.
17. Dixon RA, Xie D-Y, Sharma SB. Proanthocyanidins – a final frontier in flavonoid research? New Phytol. 2005;165:9–28.
18. Vaughn KC, Lax AR, Duke SO. Polyphenol oxidase: The chloroplast oxidase with no established function. Physiol Plant. 1988;72:659–65.
19. Creasy LL, Swain T. Structure of condensed tannins. Nature. 1965;208:151–3.
20. Baxter IR, Young JC, Armstrong G, Foster N, Bogenschutz N, Cordova T, Peer WA, Hazen SP, Murphy AS, Harper JF. A plasma membrane H^+-ATPase is required for the formation of proanthocyanidins in the seed coat endothelium of Arabidopsis thaliana. Proc Natl Acad Sci U S A. 2005;102: 2649–54.
21. Hemingway RW, Foo LY, Porter LJ. Linkage isomerism in trimeric and polymeric 2,3-cis-procyanidins. J Chem Soc, Perkin Trans. 1982;1:1209–16.
22. St Leger AS, Cochrane AL, Moore F. Factors associated with cardiac mortality in developed countries with particular reference to the consumption of wine. Lancet. 1979;1:1017–20.
23. Prior RL, Gu L. Occurrence and biological significance of proanthocyanidins in the American diet. Phytochemistry. 2005;66:2264–80.
24. USDA database for the proanthocyanidin content of selected foods - 2004, available at https://www.ars.usda.gov/northeast-area/beltsville-md/beltsville-human-nutrition-research-center/nutrient-data-laboratory/docs/usda-database-for-the-proanthocyanidin-content-of-selected-foods-2004/ accessed. Accessed 30 June 2016.
25. Gu L, Kelm MA, Hammerstone JF, Beecher G, Holden J, Haytowitz D, Gebhardt S, Prior RL. Concentrations of proanthocyanidins in common foods and estimations of normal consumption. J Nutr. 2004;134:613–7.
26. Zamora-Ros R, Knaze V, Rothwell J, Hémon B, Moskal A, Overvad K, Tjønneland A, Kyrø C, Fagherazzi G, Boutron-Ruault M-C, et al. Dietary polyphenol intake in Europe: the European Prospective Investigation into Cancer and Nutrition (EPIC) study. Eur J Nutr. 2015;55:1–17.
27. Vogiatzoglou A, Mulligan AA, Luben RN, Lentjes MAH, Heiss C, Kelm M, Merx MW, Spencer JPE, Schroeter H, Kuhnle GGC. Assessment of the dietary intake of total flavan-3-ols, monomeric flavan-3-ols, proanthocyanidins and theaflavins in the European Union. Br J Nutr. 2014;111:1463–73.
28. Knaze V, Zamora-Ros R, Lujan-Barroso L, Romieu I, Scalbert A, Slimani N, Riboli E, van Rossum CT, Bueno-de-Mesquita HB, Trichopoulou A, et al. Intake estimation of total and individual flavan-3-ols, proanthocyanidins and theaflavins, their food sources and determinants in the European Prospective Investigation into Cancer and Nutrition (EPIC) study. Br J Nutr. 2012;108:1095–108.
29. Sebastian RS, Wilkinson Enns C, Goldman JD, Martin CL, Steinfeldt LC, Murayi T, Moshfegh AJ. A New database facilitates characterization of flavonoid intake, sources, and positive associations with diet quality among US adults. J Nutr. 2015;145:1239–48.
30. Wang Y, Chung S-J, Song WO, Chun OK. Estimation of daily proanthocyanidin intake and major food sources in the U.S. diet. J Nutr. 2011;141:447–52.
31. Messina M, Nagata C, Wu AH. Estimated Asian adult soy protein and isoflavone intakes. Nutr Cancer. 2006;55:1–12.
32. Chan SG, Ho SC, Kreiger N, Darlington G, Adlaf EM, So KF, Chong PY. Validation of a food frequency questionnaire for assessing dietary soy isoflavone intake among midlife Chinese women in Hong Kong. J Nutr. 2008;138:567–73.
33. Chan SG, Ho SC, Kreiger N, Darlington G, So KF, Chong PY. Dietary sources and determinants of soy isoflavone intake among midlife Chinese Women in Hong Kong. J Nutr. 2007;137:2451–5.
34. Kim J-S, Kwon C-S. Estimated dietary isoflavone intake of Korean population based on National Nutrition Survey. Nutr Res. 2001;21:947–53.
35. Li G, Zhu Y, Zhang Y, Lang J, Chen Y, Ling W. Estimated daily flavonoid and stilbene intake from fruits, vegetables, and nuts and associations with lipid profiles in Chinese adults. J Acad Nutr Diet. 2013;113:786–94.
36. Woo H, Lee J, Choi I, Kim C, Lee J, Kwon O, Kim J. Dietary flavonoids and gastric cancer risk in a Korean population. Nutrients. 2014;6:4961–73.
37. Otaki N, Kimira M, Katsumata S-i, Uehara M, Watanabe S, Suzuki K. Distribution and major sources of flavonoid intakes in the middle-aged Japanese women. J Clin Biochem Nutr. 2009;44:231–8.
38. Johannot L, Somerset SM. Age-related variations in flavonoid intake and sources in the Australian population. Public Health Nutr. 2006;9:1045–54.
39. Ivey KL, Lewis JR, Lim WH, Lim EM, Hodgson JM, Prince RL. Associations of proanthocyanidin intake with renal function and clinical outcomes in elderly women. PLoS One. 2013;8:e71166.
40. Arabbi PR, Genovese MI, Lajolo FM. Flavonoids in vegetable foods commonly consumed in brazil and estimated ingestion by the Brazilian Population. J Agric Food Chem. 2004;52:1124–31.
41. Corrêa VG, Tureck C, Locateli G, Peralta RM, Koehnlein EA. Estimate of consumption of phenolic compounds by Brazilian population. Rev Nutr. 2015;28:185–96.
42. Neveu V, Perez-Jiménez J, Vos F, Crespy V, du Chaffaut L, Mennen L, Knox C, Eisner R, Cruz J, Wishart D, Scalbert A. Phenol-Explorer: an online comprehensive database on polyphenol contents in foods. Database (Oxford). 2010;2010:bap024.
43. World Health Organization (WHO). Diet, nutrition and the prevention of chronic diseases In: WHO Tech Rep Ser, vol. No. 916 (TRS 916). Geneva: WHO; 2003.
44. Bauer R. Quality criteria and standardization of phytopharmaceuticals: Can acceptable drug standards be achieved? Drug Inf J. 1998;32:101–10.
45. Singleton VL, Rossi JA. Colorimetry of total phenolics with phosphomolybdic-phosphotungstic acid reagents. Am J Enol Vitic. 1965;16:144–58.
46. Stalikas CD. Extraction, separation, and detection methods for phenolic acids and flavonoids. J Sep Sci. 2007;30:3268–95.
47. Bate-Smith EC. Phytochemistry of proanthocyanidins. Phytochemistry. 1975; 14:1107–13.
48. Porter LJ, Hrstich LN, Chan BG. The conversion of procyanidins and prodelphinidins to cyanidin and delphinidin. Phytochemistry. 1985;25:223–30.
49. Schofield P, Mbugua DM, Pell AN. Analysis of condensed tannins: a review. Anim Feed Sci Technol. 2001;91:21–40.
50. Sun B, Ricardo-da-Silva JM, Spranger I. Critical factors of vanillin assay for catechins and proanthocyanidins. J Agric Food Chem. 1998;46:4267–74.
51. Naczk M, Shahidi F. Phenolics in cereals, fruits and vegetables: occurrence, extraction and analysis. J Pharm Biomed Anal. 2006;41:1523–42.
52. Ignat I, Volf I, Popa VI. A critical review of methods for characterisation of polyphenolic compounds in fruits and vegetables. Food Chem. 2011;126:1821–35.
53. Khoddami A, Wilkes MA, Roberts TH. Techniques for analysis of plant phenolic compounds. Molecules. 2013;18:2328–75.
54. Dumon M, Michaud J, Masquelier J. Dosages des procyanidols dans les extraits végétaux destinés a la préparation de médicaments. Bull Soc Pharm Bord. 1990;129:51–65.
55. Dumon M. Recherches analytiques sur les pycnogenols. PhD thesis. Bordeaux: Université de Bordeaux II, UFR des Sciences Pharmaceutiques; 1990.
56. de Haan B, Achanta G, Post JA. A potential role for oligomeric proanthocyanidins (OPCs) in delaying senescence in human endothelial cells. Free Radic Biol Med. 2008;45:S78.
57. Krishnan P, Kruger NJ, Ratcliffe RG. Metabolite fingerprinting and profiling in plants using NMR. J Exp Bot. 2005;56:255–65.
58. Hylands PJN, JK, Holmes E, Dunn MJ. Process for quality control and standardization of medicinal plant products. In Google patent, vol. US6806090 B1. USA; 2004.
59. Laparra J, Michaud J, Masquelier J. Étude pharmacocinétique des oligomères flavanoliques. Plantes Medicinales Phytotherapie. 1977;9:133–42.
60. Laparra J, Michaud J, Lesca MF, Blanquet P, Masquelier J. Étude pharmacocinetique des oligomeres procyanidoliques totaux du raisin. Acta Ther. 1978;4:233–46.

61. Jacobs H, Koek GH, Peters R, Moalin M, Tack J, van der Vijgh WJ, Bast A, Haenen GR. Differences in pharmacological activities of the antioxidant flavonoid monoHER in humans and mice are caused by variations in its metabolic profile. Clin Pharmacol Ther. 2011;90:852–9.
62. Benakis A, Schopfer C, Ritschard J. Disposition of 14C-labelled ENDOTELON in humans. Eur J Drug Metab Pharmacokinet. 2008;33:37–43.
63. Choy YY, Jaggers GK, Oteiza PI, Waterhouse AL. Bioavailability of intact proanthocyanidins in the rat colon after ingestion of grape seed extract. J Agric Food Chem. 2013;61:121–7.
64. Prasain JK, Peng N, Dai Y, Moore R, Arabshahi A, Wilson L, Barnes S, Michael Wyss J, Kim H, Watts RL. Liquid chromatography tandem mass spectrometry identification of proanthocyanidins in rat plasma after oral administration of grape seed extract. Phytomedicine. 2009;16:233–43.
65. Serra A, Macia A, Romero MP, Salvado MJ, Bustos M, Fernandez-Larrea J, Motilva MJ. Determination of procyanidins and their metabolites in plasma samples by improved liquid chromatography-tandem mass spectrometry. J Chromatogr B Analyt Technol Biomed Life Sci. 2009;877:1169–76.
66. Tsang C, Auger C, Mullen W, Bornet A, Rouanet JM, Crozier A, Teissedre PL. The absorption, metabolism and excretion of flavan-3-ols and procyanidins following the ingestion of a grape seed extract by rats. Br J Nutr. 2005;94:170–81.
67. Actis-Goretta L, Leveques A, Rein M, Teml A, Schafer C, Hofmann U, Li H, Schwab M, Eichelbaum M, Williamson G. Intestinal absorption, metabolism, and excretion of (-)-epicatechin in healthy humans assessed by using an intestinal perfusion technique. Am J Clin Nutr. 2013;98:924–33.
68. Ottaviani JI, Momma TY, Kuhnle GK, Keen CL, Schroeter H. Structurally related (−)-epicatechin metabolites in humans: Assessment using de novo chemically synthesized authentic standards. Free Radic Biol Med. 2012;52:1403–12.
69. Holt RR, Lazarus SA, Sullards MC, Zhu QY, Schramm DD, Hammerstone JF, Fraga CG, Schmitz HH, Keen CL. Procyanidin dimer B2 [epicatechin-(4β-8)-epicatechin] in human plasma after the consumption of a flavanol-rich cocoa. Am J Clin Nutr. 2002;76:798–804.
70. Sano A, Yamakoshi J, Tokutake S, Tobe K, Kubota Y, Kikuchi M. Procyanidin B1 is detected in human serum after intake of proanthocyanidin-rich grape seed extract. Biosci Biotechnol Biochem. 2003;67:1140–3.
71. Deprez S, Mila I, Huneau JF, Tome D, Scalbert A. Transport of proanthocyanidin dimer, trimer, and polymer across monolayers of human intestinal epithelial Caco-2 cells. Antioxid Redox Signal. 2001;3:957–67.
72. Rios LY, Gonthier M P, Rémésy C, Mila I, Lapierre C, Lazarus SA, Williamson G, Scalbert A. Chocolate intake increases urinary excretion of polyphenol-derived phenolic acids in healthy human subjects. Am J Clin Nutr. 2003;77:912–8.
73. Appeldoorn MM, Vincken JP, Aura AM, Hollman PC, Gruppen H. Procyanidin dimers are metabolized by human microbiota with 2-(3,4-dihydroxyphenyl)acetic acid and 5-(3,4-dihydroxyphenyl)-gamma-valerolactone as the major metabolites. J Agric Food Chem. 2009;57:1084–92.
74. Stoupi S, Williamson G, Drynan JW, Barron D, Clifford MN. Procyanidin B2 catabolism by human fecal microflora: Partial characterization of 'dimeric' intermediates. Arch Biochem Biophys. 2010;501:73–8.
75. Wiese S, Esatbeyoglu T, Winterhalter P, Kruse H-P, Winkler S, Bub A, Kulling SE. Comparative biokinetics and metabolism of pure monomeric, dimeric, and polymeric flavan-3-ols: A randomized cross-over study in humans. Mol Nutr Food Res. 2015;59:610–21.
76. Nakamura Y, Tsuji S, Tonogai Y. Analysis of proanthocyanidins in grape seed extracts, health foods and grape seed oils. J Health Sci. 2003;49:45–54.
77. Masquelier J, Dumon M, Dumas J. Stabilisation du collagene par les oligomeres procyanidoliques. Acta Ther. 1981;7:101–5.
78. Pfister A, Simon M, Gazave J. Sites de fixation des oligomeres procyanidoliques dans la paroi des capillaires sanguins du poumon de cobaye. Acta Ther. 1982;8:223–37.
79. Tixier JM, Godeau G, Robert AM, Hornebeck W. Evidence by in vivo and in vitro studies that binding of pycnogenols to elastin affects its rate of degradation by elastases. Biochem Pharmacol. 1984;33:3933–9.
80. Gavignet-Jeannin C, Groult N, Godeau G, Robert A, Robert L. Mode d'action des oligomeres procyanidoliques sur la paroi vasculaire. Toulouse: Congrès International d'Angiologie, symposium satellite Endotelon et unite circulatoire; 1988.
81. Robert AM. Substrate-protecting antiproteolytic agents for the prevention of pathological degradation of connective tissues. A review. Pathol Biol (Paris). 2012;60:48–57.
82. Oligomeric proanthocyanidins (OPCs). Monograph Altern Med Rev 2003, 8:442-450.
83. Bast A, Haenen GRMM. Ten misconceptions about antioxidants. Trends Pharmacol Sci. 2013;34:430–6.
84. Weseler AR, Bast A. Oxidative stress and vascular function: implications for pharmacologic treatments. Curr Hypertens Rep. 2010;12:154–61.
85. Masquelier J. Action comparee de divers facteurs vitaminiques P sur l'oxydation de l'acide ascorbique par les ions cuivriques. Bull Soc Chim Biol (Paris). 1951;33:302–5.
86. Masquelier J. Plant extract with a proanthocyanidins content as therapeutic agent having radical scavenger effect and use thereof, vol. US4698360 A. USA; 1987.
87. van Acker SA, de Groot MJ, van den Berg DJ, Tromp MN, Donne-Op den Kelder G, van der Vijgh WJ, Bast A. A quantum chemical explanation of the antioxidant activity of flavonoids. Chem Res Toxicol. 1996;9:1305–12.
88. Barbier AM, JP, Savi P, Unkovic J, Vilain P. Activité angioprotectrice des oligomères procyanidoliques chez l'animal. Toulouse: Congrès International d'Angiologie; 1988.
89. Meunier M, Duroux E, Bastide P. Activite antiradicalaire d'oligomeres procyanidolique et d'anthocyanosides vis-a-vis de l'anion superoxyde et vis-a-vis de la lipoperoxydation. Plantes Medicinales Phytotherapie. 1989;13:267–74.
90. Masquelier J. Effets physiologiques du vin - Sa part dans l'alcoolisme. Bulletin de l'OIV. 1988;689:555–78.
91. de Haan B, Babat S, Post JA. Protection of vascular endothelial cells from oxidative damage by oligomeric proanthocyanidins. In: Oxidants and antioxidants in biology. Santa Barbara: Oxygen Club of California; 2006.
92. de Haan B, Babat S, Post JA. Oligomeric proanthocyanidins protect vascular endothelial cells from lipid oxidation. Inflamm Res. 2006;Supplement 2:S116.
93. Bos MA, Vennat B, Meunier MT, Pouget MP, Pourrat A, Fialip J. Procyanidins from tormentil: antioxidant properties towards lipoperoxidation and anti-elastase activity. Biol Pharm Bull. 1996;19:146–8.
94. Ruijters EJ, Weseler AR, Kicken C, Haenen GR, Bast A. The flavanol (-)-epicatechin and its metabolites protect against oxidative stress in primary endothelial cells via a direct antioxidant effect. Eur J Pharmacol. 2013;715:147–53.
95. Granado-Serrano AB, Martin MA, Haegeman G, Goya L, Bravo L, Ramos S. Epicatechin induces NF-kappaB, activator protein-1 (AP-1) and nuclear transcription factor erythroid 2p45-related factor-2 (Nrf2) via phosphatidylinositol-3-kinase/protein kinase B (PI3K/AKT) and extracellular regulated kinase (ERK) signalling in HepG2 cells. Br J Nutr. 2010;103:168–79.
96. Rodriguez-Ramiro I, Ramos S, Bravo L, Goya L, Martin MA. Procyanidin B2 induces Nrf2 translocation and glutathione S-transferase P1 expression via ERKs and p38-MAPK pathways and protect human colonic cells against oxidative stress. Eur J Nutr. 2012;51:881–92.
97. Ohnuma T, Anzai E, Suzuki Y, Shimoda M, Saito S, Nishiyama T, Ogura K, Hiratsuka A. Selective antagonization of activated Nrf2 and inhibition of cancer cell proliferation by procyanidins from Cinnamomi Cortex extract. Arch Biochem Biophys. 2015;585:17–24.
98. Krajka-Kuzniak V, Paluszczak J, Oszmianski J, Baer-Dubowska W. Hawthorn (Crataegus oxyacantha L.) bark extract regulates antioxidant response element (ARE)-mediated enzyme expression via Nrf2 pathway activation in normal hepatocyte cell line. Phytother Res. 2014;28:593–602.
99. Bak MJ, Jun M, Jeong WS. Procyanidins from wild grape (Vitis amurensis) seeds regulate ARE-mediated enzyme expression via Nrf2 coupled with p38 and PI3K/Akt pathway in HepG2 cells. Int J Mol Sci. 2012;13:801–18.
100. Nazimabashir, Manoharan V, Miltonprabu S. Cadmium induced cardiac oxidative stress in rats and its attenuation by GSP through the activation of Nrf2 signaling pathway. Chem Biol Interact. 2015;242:179–93.
101. Chen S, Zhu Y, Liu Z, Gao Z, Li B, Zhang D, Zhang Z, Jiang X, Liu Z, Meng L, et al. Grape seed proanthocyanidin extract ameliorates diabetic bladder dysfunction via the activation of the Nrf2 pathway. PLoS One. 2015;10: e0126457.
102. Blazso G, Gabor M. Oedema-inhibiting effect of procyanidin. Acta Physiol Acad Sci Hung. 1980;56:235–40.
103. Li Q, Verma IM. NF-kappaB regulation in the immune system. Nat Rev Immunol. 2002;2:725–34.
104. Milenkovic D, Vanden Berghe W, Boby C, Leroux C, Declerck K, Szarc vel Szic K, Heyninck K, Laukens K, Bizet M, Defrance M, et al. Dietary flavanols modulate the transcription of genes associated with cardiovascular pathology without changes in their DNA methylation state. PLoS One. 2014;9:e95527.
105. Ruijters EJ, Haenen GR, Weseler AR, Bast A. The cocoa flavanol (-)-epicatechin protects the cortisol response. Pharmacol Res. 2014;79:28–33.

106. Ruijters EJ, Haenen GR, Willemsen M, Weseler AR, Bast A. Food-derived bioactives can protect the anti-inflammatory activity of cortisol with antioxidant-dependent and -independent mechanisms. Int J Mol Sci. 2016;17:239–48.
107. Weseler AR, Bast A. Pleiotropic-acting nutrients require integrative investigational approaches: the example of flavonoids. J Agric Food Chem. 2012;60:8941–6.
108. Dartenuc J, Marache P, Choussat H. Resistance capillaire en geriatrie: etude d'un microangioprotecteur endotelon. Bordeaux Med. 1980;13:903–7.
109. Dubos G, Durst G, Hugonot R. Evolution de la resistance capillaire, spontanement ou artificiellement diminuee par l'action d'un substance capillaro-toxique chez des personnes agees. Revue Geriatr. 1980;5:302–5.
110. Paitel D. Etude rheographique et thermographic des effets d'un endotheliotrophique sur l'hemodynamique peripherique. Vie Med. 1981;11:776–83.
111. Beylot C, Bioulac P. Essai therapeutique d'un angioprotecteur peripherique, l'Endotelon. Gaz Med (Paris). 1980;87:2919–22.
112. Elbaz C, Reinharez D, Sapin G, Brami C, Boschet P, Gounon P, Roure M, Tragit R, Vergoz L. Etude multicentrique controlee de l'endotelon dans les manifestations fonctionelles de l'insufficance veineuse chronique des membres inferieurs. Le Praticien. 1981;400:63–8.
113. Thebaut J-F, Thebaut P, Vin F. Etude de l'endotelon dans les manifestations functionelles de l'insufficisance veineuse peripherique. Resultats d'une etude en double aveugle portant sur 92 patients. Gaz Med (Paris). 1985;92:96–100.
114. Weseler AR, Ruijters EJ, Drittij-Reijnders MJ, Reesink KD, Haenen GR, Bast A. Pleiotropic benefit of monomeric and oligomeric flavanols on vascular health - a randomized controlled clinical pilot study. PLoS One. 2011;6:e28460.
115. Aragones G, Suarez M, Ardid-Ruiz A, Vinaixa M, Rodriguez MA, Correig X, Arola L, Blade C. Dietary proanthocyanidins boost hepatic NAD(+) metabolism and SIRT1 expression and activity in a dose-dependent manner in healthy rats. Sci Rep. 2016;6:24977.

Resistant starch lowers postprandial glucose and leptin in overweight adults consuming a moderate-to-high-fat diet

Mindy Patterson Maziarz[1], Sara Preisendanz[2], Shanil Juma[2], Victorine Imrhan[2], Chandan Prasad[2,3] and Parakat Vijayagopal[2*]

Abstract

Background: High-amylose maize resistant starch type 2 (HAM-RS2) stimulates gut-derived satiety peptides and reduces adiposity in animals. Human studies have not supported these findings despite improvements in glucose homeostasis and insulin sensitivity after HAM-RS2 intake which can lower adiposity-related disease risk. The primary objective of this study was to evaluate the impact of HAM-RS2 consumption on blood glucose homeostasis in overweight, healthy adults. We also examined changes in biomarkers of satiety (glucagon-like peptide-1 [GLP-1], peptide YY [PYY], and leptin) and body composition determined by anthropometrics and dual-energy x-ray absorptiometry, dietary intake, and subjective satiety measured by a visual analogue scale following HAM-RS2 consumption.

Methods: Using a randomized-controlled, parallel-arm, double-blind design, 18 overweight, healthy adults consumed either muffins enriched with 30 g HAM-RS2 (n = 11) or 0 g HAM-RS2 (control; n = 7) daily for 6 weeks. The HAM-RS2 and control muffins were similar in total calories and available carbohydrate.

Results: At baseline, total PYY concentrations were significantly higher 120 min following the consumption of study muffins in the HAM-RS2 group than control group ($P = 0.043$). Within the HAM-RS2 group, the area under the curve (AUC) glucose ($P = 0.028$), AUC leptin ($P = 0.022$), and postprandial 120-min leptin ($P = 0.028$) decreased independent of changes in body composition or overall energy intake at the end of 6 weeks. Fasting total PYY increased ($P = 0.033$) in the HAM-RS2 group, but changes in insulin or total GLP-1 were not observed. Mean overall change in subjective satiety score did not correlate with mean AUC biomarker changes suggesting the satiety peptides did not elicit a satiation response or change in overall total caloric intake. The metabolic response from HAM-RS2 occurred despite the habitual intake of a moderate-to-high-fat diet (mean range 34.5% to 39.4% of total calories).

Conclusion: Consuming 30 g HAM-RS2 daily for 6 weeks can improve glucose homeostasis, lower leptin concentrations, and increase fasting PYY in healthy overweight adults without impacting body composition and may aid in the prevention of chronic disease. However, between-group differences in biomarkers were not observed and future research is warranted before specific recommendations can be made.

Trial registration: None.

Keywords: Resistant starch, Satiety, Overweight, Gut peptides, Fiber, Leptin, PYY

* Correspondence: pvijayagopal@twu.edu
[2]Department of Nutrition and Food Sciences, Texas Woman's University, P.O Box 425888, Denton, TX 76204, USA
Full list of author information is available at the end of the article

Introduction

Epidemiological observations show that consuming a diet high in fiber can lower the risk for obesity, obesity-related comorbidities, and reduce all-cause mortality [1, 2]. One systematic review that examined the effects of dietary fiber on body weight reported that a 0.4% reduction in body weight can be achieved by consuming most dietary fibers for 4 weeks [3]. However, the amount of weight lost was dependent on the physiochemical properties (solubility, fermentability, and viscosity) of each type of fiber [3].

The purported mechanisms by which fiber contributes to weight loss such as altering gut motility, attenuating nutrient absorption, and lowering overall caloric intake are also associated with the physiochemical properties [2, 4]. Fermentable fibers are receiving attention because the metabolites produced from bacterial fermentation in the gastrointestinal (GI) tract can influence body weight. These fibers produce short chain fatty acids (SCFA; acetate, propionate, butyrate) in the distal intestine that stimulate the release of glucagon-like peptide-1 (GLP-1) and peptide YY (PYY) that act synergistically with leptin, an adipokine primarily released from adipose tissue, to induce satiety and regulate energy expenditure through central nervous system actions [5–7].

Despite increased SCFA production from fiber fermentation, the relationship between GLP-1 and PYY on satiety and food intake in humans is inconsistent. After consuming a standardized breakfast on the morning immediately following 3 days of consecutive intake of a barley kernel-based bread with resistant starch, fasting plasma GLP-1 and postprandial PYY concentrations increased in healthy middle-aged adults [8]. However, changes in appetite sensations (satiety, hunger, and desire to eat) did not occur [8]. Similarly, overweight women did not elicit a postprandial subjective satiety response despite improvements of GLP-1 and PYY after consuming an enzyme-hydrolyzed arabinoxylan from wheat or intact arabinoxylan from flax at breakfast [9]. In contrast, in healthy adults, the upregulation of GLP-1 and PYY corresponded with enhanced subjective satiety immediately after resistant maltodextrin intake [10]. However, subsequent energy intake was not suppressed despite these improvements. One recent trial found improvements in the area under the curve (AUC) PYY that corresponded with satiety and a 14% reduction in food intake in healthy adults consuming 15 g unripe banana flour rich in resistant starch for 6 weeks [11]. The different satiety peptides and satiation responses may be related to fermentability patterns, the type, amount, and duration of fiber intake, and the gut microbiota composition of individuals. Also, blood gut peptides may be too low in concentration to cross the blood brain barrier or the individuals may have hypothalamic resistance, which can occur from a high-fat diet even in lieu of obesity [12].

High-amylose maize resistant starch type 2 (HAM-RS2) is an insoluble, nonviscous fermentable fiber that has been shown to improve glucose homeostasis and/or peripheral insulin sensitivity among individuals who were healthy with normal glucose homeostasis [13] or those with metabolic syndrome [14–16]. However, many of these trials of longer duration did not report or show improvements in blood concentrations of gut peptides, satiety responses, or changes in food intake. HAM-RS2 may exert its benefits on glucose metabolism by increasing SCFA in the blood to alter free fatty acid and glycerol release from adipocytes and increased fat oxidation [17], modulate bile acid metabolism [18], or alter the gut microbiota profile [19].

Most previous trials reported the impact of HAM-RS2 on glucose homeostasis in either healthy individuals or those with metabolic syndrome [12–15]. Therefore, our primary aim was to determine the impact of the daily consumption of 30 g HAM-RS2 incorporated into muffins for 6 weeks on glucose homeostasis in normoglycemic, healthy overweight adults at risk for developing glycemic abnormalities. We also measured fasting and postprandial biomarker concentrations known to influence satiety (GLP-1, PYY, and leptin), subjective satiety, dietary intake, and body composition in these individuals.

Materials and Methods

Participants

Healthy overweight adults with a body mass index (BMI) ≥ 28 kg/m^2 between 18 and 50 years of age of any race or ethnicity were recruited from Denton, Texas and the surrounding area. Participants were sedentary (<20 min of activity no more than 2 days per week) for at least 6 months prior to enrollment in the study. Exclusion criteria included those diagnosed with or taking medication(s) for chronic conditions, such as diabetes, hypertension, cancer, diseases of the liver, kidney, or heart, or other metabolic disorders. Participants were also excluded if they gained or lost a significant amount of weight or followed a special diet ≤ 3 months prior to enrollment, consumed vitamins, minerals, or antioxidants in excess of amounts found in a daily multivitamin tablet, or dietary supplements known to alter metabolism, had an intolerance to the study foods, or smoked. Women who were pregnant, lactating, or interested in becoming pregnant were not eligible. The study was approved by the Institutional Review Board at Texas Woman's University. All participants provided written consent prior to study enrollment.

Protocol

The study was a randomized-controlled, parallel-arm, double-blind design lasting 6 weeks. Individuals who met the screening criteria and agreed to participate in the study were randomized to either the HAM-RS2 group or control group using a random numbers generator from SPSS version 19 (IBM Corporation, Armonk, NY, USA).

Prior to participant randomization, the study muffins were formulated at the University food preparation laboratory. The treatment muffins were developed to provide 50 g Hi-Maize® 260 resistant starch (~30 g HAM-RS2, ~20 g equal mixture slowly and rapidly digestible starch; Ingredion Incorporated, Westchester, IL, USA) daily. The control muffins (0 g HAM-RS2) were developed to contain similar amounts of available carbohydrate and minimal differences in total calories than the treatment muffins (Table 1). Each 60 g treatment muffin contained 16.7 g Hi-Maize® 260 resistant starch to provide 10 g HAM-RS2, therefore three muffins (180 g cooked) were required to obtain 30 g HAM-RS2 daily as indicated in the protocol. No difference in overall muffin likeability was found based on sensory evaluations of HAM-RS2 and control muffins using a 9-point hedonic scale prior to the implementation of this study [20]. All study muffins were prepared, packaged, and labeled by culinary and nutrition students twice per week to ensure freshness and quality. Two flavors of the treatment and control muffins were developed, pumpkin spice and cranberry spice. The different flavors of muffins were administered on alternating weeks to alleviate monotony and improve compliance. The two flavors of muffins were closely matched for total calories and macronutrients. The cranberry spice muffins included 4.3 g dried cranberries, but no pumpkin puree. The pumpkin spice muffins included 6.8 g pumpkin puree without dried cranberries. Different amounts of dried cranberries and pumpkin puree were added so the caloric value of each muffin type was similar.

The participants arrived for baseline data collection following an overnight fast. Anthropometric measurements were obtained in triplicate followed by the baseline blood collection (time 0). Participants consumed all three of their respective study muffins within 15 min along with 6 oz of orange juice. Immediately following muffin intake the participants completed a visual analogue scale (VAS). Four additional postprandial blood samples were collected at 15, 30, 60, and 120 min. Nutrition education and body composition analysis occurred between blood collections. Participants were instructed by a Registered Dietitian Nutritionist (RDN) to follow a balanced diet according to the Dietary Guidelines for Americans 2010 [21] adjusted for the caloric value of the study muffins and to remain sedentary during the study. Body composition was determined by whole body dual-energy x-ray absorptiometry (DXA) using the Lunar DPX NT model (GE Healthcare, Fairfield, CT, USA). Body composition analysis and blood collections were repeated using the same protocol as baseline at the end of the intervention (week 6).

Table 1 Comparison of nutrients between muffins[a]

Nutrient	HAM-RS2	Control
Energy (kcal)[b]	349.6	389.1
Available carbohydrate (g)[c]	70.5	71.6
Protein (g)	5.4	10.6
Fat (g)	5.1	6.6
Fiber (g)	30.9	11.4

[a]Nutrient analysis based on the amount consumed daily by each participant; 180 g cooked (baked) weight. Analysis conducted by Pope Labs, Irving, Texas using the following Official AOAC Methods: moisture 925.10; oil 923.03; ash 923.03; nitrogen 988.05A; total dietary fiber 991.43
[b]Energy does not include contribution from short chain fatty acids associated with fermentation
[c]Available carbohydrate excludes fiber

Dietary intake and bowel habits

Three days prior to baseline measurements, at midpoint (week 3), and the end of the study (week 6) all participants completed bowel habit logs and dietary intake journals for 3 days as instructed by a RDN. Dietary intake was analyzed using the United States Department of Agriculture National Nutrient Database for Standard Reference [22]. The bowel habit logs evaluated tolerance and potential adverse events from study muffin consumption by asking a series of questions adapted from Lewis et al. [23], such as "describe the consistency of your stools," and provided a space for comments. Participants were instructed to contact investigators immediately if abnormal changes in bowel habits, or the presence of blood or mucus, were observed. Muffin intake compliance was assessed through food intake journals.

Subjective satiety measurements

Each VAS was 100 mm in length with questions at each end to indicate feelings of subjective satiety ranging from "not at all" to "very much or a lot". The 7 questions were adapted from Flint et al. [24] and included "how hungry are you?", "how satisfied do you feel?", "how full do you feel?", "how much do you think you can eat?", "how pleasant would you find eating another mouthful of this food?" "would you like to eat something sweet?", and "would you like to eat something fatty?".

Biomarkers

A phlebotomist drew approximately 12 mL of blood at each time point into EDTA vacutainers (BD Diagnostics, Franklin Lakes, NF, USA). The tubes were centrifuged at 3,200 rpm for 12 min at 4 °C. Plasma was immediately aliquoted into 1.5 mL Eppendorf microcentrifuge tubes and stored at −80 °C until analyzed for glucose, insulin, GLP-1, PYY, and leptin. Glucose was determined using a hexokinase colorimetric method (Stanbio Laboratory, Boerne, TX, USA) with an intra-assay coefficient of variation (CV) <6%. Total insulin (CV < 8%; Alpco, Salem, NH, USA), leptin (CV < 6%; Raybiotech, Norcross, GA, USA), and total PYY ($PYY_{(1-36)}$ and PYY $_{(3-36)}$; CV < 6%; EMD Millipore, Billerica, MA, USA) were measured using an enzyme-linked immunosorbent (ELISA) technique. Total GLP-1 (GLP-$1_{(7-36)}$ and GLP-1 $_{(9-36)}$; CV < 7%; Raybiotech, Norcross, GA, USA) concentrations were determined by an enzyme immunoassay protocol.

Statistical analysis

To assess differences between and within the HAM-RS2 and control groups, change from mean baseline and final scores were calculated for anthropometric, body composition, satiety (after three questions were reverse coded), and biomarker concentrations from each individual blood collection time points (fasting, 15, 30, 60, and 120 min). Due to limited sample size and potential deviations from normality, primary analyses were conducted using nonparametric tests. The Wilcoxon Signed Ranked test compared differences within groups, while the Mann–Whitney *U* test examined between group differences. The total area under the curve (AUC) was calculated for all plasma biomarkers using the trapazoidal rule and was compared using the nonparametric tests described above. Pearson's correlation coefficient examined associations between dependent outcomes. Data are presented as mean ± standard error of the mean (SEM), unless otherwise noted. SPSS version 19 (IBM Corporation, Armonk, NY, USA) and statistical significance was achieved with a *P*-value ≤ 0.05.

Results

Participants

Twenty-five participants were enrolled in the study; however, only 18 (83% female) completed the protocol and were included in the data analysis (Fig. 1). Baseline characteristics of the participants who completed the study and were included in the data analysis did not differ between groups (Table 2).

Dietary intake and compliance

Energy and macronutrient (carbohydrate, protein, lipid) intake were similar between groups throughout the study (Table 3). Mean daily fiber intake significantly increased by 113% at midpoint in the HAM-RS2 group. At week 6, the mean fiber intake in the HAM-RS2 group increased 100% from baseline indicating fiber intake was sustained throughout the study. In contrast, the control group had a significant reduction in both fiber and carbohydrate intake from midpoint to the end of the study. Dietary fiber intake was considerably higher in the HAM-RS2 group at midpoint and the end of the study than the control. An unexplained reduction in dietary carbohydrate and fiber intake occurred from week 3 to week 6 in the control group. At baseline the HAM-RS2 group consumed a high fat diet averaging 95.8 ± 29.5 g/d (39.3% of total calories), which was non-significantly reduced to 82.1 ± 25.1 g/d (34.8% of total calories) at week 6. Based on data from the food intake journals, the HAM-RS2 and control groups consumed 94 and 98% of the study muffins, respectively, at midpoint suggesting high compliance. Compliance decreased to 85% in the HAM-RS2 group and 73% in the control group at the end of the study.

Tolerance to study muffins

In both groups, stool consistency was relatively stable throughout the study. No differences in reaching the bathroom in time, usage of toilet paper, or marks on undergarments occurred across groups at any time point. One participant in the HAM-RS2 group recorded the presence of blood or mucus in stool on two separate occasions; one prior to receiving the

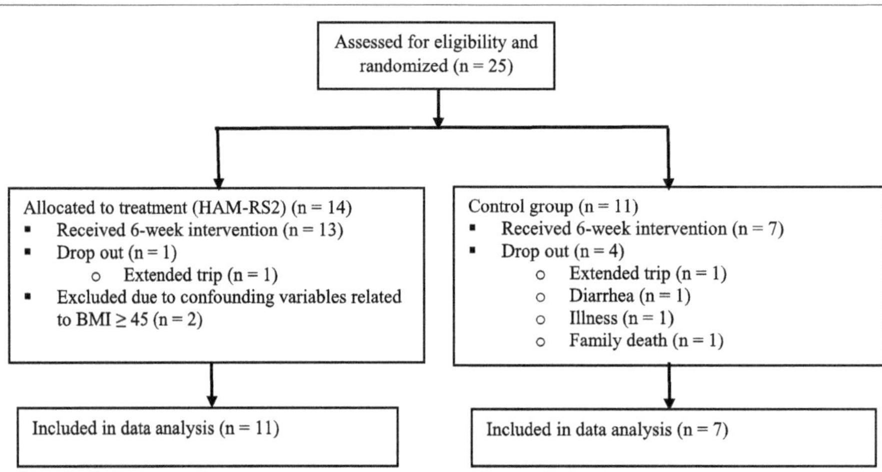

Fig. 1 Consort Diagram

Table 2 Baseline participant characteristics

Characteristic	HAM-RS2 ($n = 11$)	Control ($n = 7$)	P value[a]
Female, n (%)	9 (81.8)	6 (85.7)	
Age, years	31.0 ± 3.0	31.2 ± 4.2	0.973
Body mass index (kg/m^2)	34.8 ± 1.5	30.6 ± 1.5	0.085
Waist circumference (cm)	99.1 ± 3.7	91.6 ± 3.3	0.151
Total body fat mass (kg)[b]	42.8 ± 3.1	34.6 ± 3.0	0.085
Total body lean mass (kg)[b]	47.3 ± 1.8	43.7 ± 2.3	0.179
Trunk total mass (kg)[b]	47.1 ± 3.6	43.9 ± 6.0	0.285
Trunk fat mass (kg)[b]	22.2 ± 2.1	19.8 ± 3.0	0.285
Trunk lean mass (kg)[b]	23.8 ± 1.8	23.1 ± 2.9	0.479
Android fat (kg)[b]	50.8 ± 2.1	50.1 ± 0.8	0.791
Gynoid fat (kg)[b]	52.2 ± 2.6	49.6 ± 1.0	0.285
Visceral adipose tissue (in^3)[b]	76.8 ± 13.9	63.0 ± 18.1	0.417

Data presented as mean ± SEM except for qualitative values. All body composition measurements were obtained in triplicate after fasting for ≥8 h
[a]Between group differences determined by Mann–Whitney U test
[b]Measured by dual-energy x-ray absorptiometry (Lunar DPX NT model, GE Healthcare, Fairfield, CT, USA)

intervention and the other at midpoint. This participant was 89% compliant with muffin consumption at midpoint based on food records suggesting intake remained adequate. Overall, the HAM-RS2 and control muffins were well tolerated and few changes in bowel habit indicators were documented throughout the study.

Subjective satiety

Mean overall satiety score did not differ within or between groups ($P = 0.230$). The mean score for the question "how full do you feel?" in the HAM-RS2 group increased from baseline to the end of the study and approached significance ($P = 0.058$) (data not shown).

Body composition

Consuming muffins with HAM-RS2 did not significantly change body composition. A decrease ($P = 0.043$) in total trunk mass and a near significant decrease in lean trunk mass ($P = 0.063$) occurred in the control group (data not shown). At baseline the HAM-RS2 group had higher total leg mass ($P = 0.011$) than the control group, and the difference was sustained at the end of the intervention ($P = 0.02$) (data not shown).

Biomarkers

Changes from baseline to week 6 in the AUC for the plasma biomarkers are shown in Table 4. At the end of the 6-week treatment, the AUC change from baseline was not significantly different between HAM-RS2 and control groups for any biomarker measures. However, a significant within-group decrease in both AUC glucose ($P = 0.028$) and AUC leptin ($P = 0.022$) was observed from baseline to week 6 in the HAM-RS2 group. There were no changes from baseline to the end of the intervention in the AUC for any biomarker in the control group. Within-group comparisons for biomarkers collected at each time point at the end of the intervention are shown in Fig. 2. Only one biomarker differed between groups

Table 3 Changes in mean macronutrient intake between HAM-RS2 and control groups[1,2]

Nutrient	HAM-RS2			Control			P value**
	Baseline	Week 3	Week 6	Baseline	Week 3	Week 6	
Calories	2190 ± 564	2193 ± 397	2123 ± 424	2091.1 ± 455.3	2046. ± 1337	1910.5 ± 648.7	0.256
Carbohydrate (g)	257.5 ± 84.8	283.0 ± 73.2	268.7 ± 62.6	294.3 ± 90.4	289.4 ± 173.7[a]	261.7 ± 84.0[a]	1.000
Protein (g)	82.7 ± 15.3	78.0 ± 13.2	78.4 ± 24.7	88.0 ± 11.1	74.8 ± 48.3	67.4 ± 32.7	0.462
Lipid (g)	95.8 ± 29.5	82.5 ± 20.7	82.1 ± 25.1	75.5 ± 23.9	70.1 ± 52.4	70.8 ± 27.0	0.462
Fiber (g)	21.5 ± 13.9[a,b]	45.7 ± 8.2[1*]	43.1 ± 6.7[b]	29.5 ± 14.5	30.2 ± 18.0[a*]	23.8 ± 6.8[a]	0.001

[1]Dietary analysis software used is United States Department of Agriculture (USDA) National Nutrient Database for Standard Reference (http://ndb.nal.usda.gov)
[2]Within group values with the same letter superscript ([a,b]) in the same row are statistically different ($P < 0.05$)
*Between group values are statistically different ($P < 0.05$) by Mann–Whitney U test
**Between group comparisons at week 6 analyzed by Mann–Whitney U test

Table 4 Mean AUC biomarker comparisons within and between groups

Biomarkers	HAM-RS2		Control		*P* value[1]
	Change from baseline to week 6	*P* value[2]	Change from baseline to week 6	*P* value[2]	
Glucose	−1588 ± 545	0.028	−790 ± 706	0.310	0.285
Insulin	−908 ± 941	0.333	518 ± 1197	1.000	0.425
GLP-1	120 ± 94	0.139	208 ± 127	0.176	0.791
PYY	438 ± 719	0.285	954 ± 1465	0.866	0.085
Leptin	−664 ± 235	0.022	−191 ± 230	0.398	0.425

Data presented as mean ± SEM
[1]Between group comparisons at week 6 by Mann–Whitney *U* test
[2]Within group comparisons from baseline to week 6 by Wilcoxon Signed-Ranked test

when examining single blood collection time points. The 120 min postprandial concentration of PYY ($P = 0.043$) was higher in the HAM-RS2 group than the control group at baseline. Within-group differences in leptin and PYY were found from baseline to week 6 in the HAM-RS2 group. A decrease in postprandial leptin ($P = 0.028$) occurred at 120 min in the HAM-RS2 group. A within-group change in PYY was also observed in the HAM-RS2 group where fasting concentrations increased ($P = 0.033$) from baseline to the end of the intervention. Within the control group, no differences in the individual time points or AUC for any biomarker occurred.

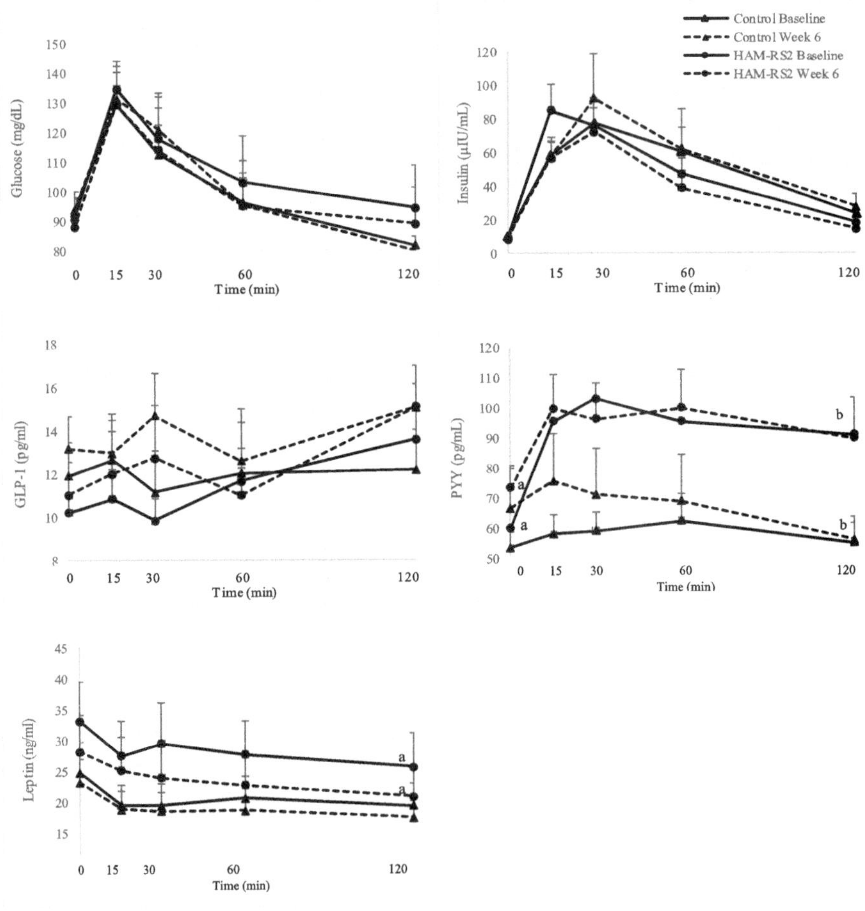

Fig. 2 Change in biomarker concentrations from baseline to week 6 in the HAM-RS2 and control groups. This figure shows within-group comparisons from Wilcoxon Signed Ranked tests and between-group comparisons from Mann–Whitney *U* tests. [a]Indicates significant within-group changes in biomarkers from baseline to week 6. Fasting PYY increased ($P = 0.033$) while leptin decreased ($P = 0.028$) 120 min after study foods were consumed in the HAM-RS2 group. A near-significant decrease ($P = 0.062$) in leptin also occurred 60 min after study foods were consumed in the HAM-RS2 group. [b]Indicates significant difference at baseline between groups in 120 min postprandial PYY concentrations ($P = 0.043$)

Relationship between subjective satiety and biomarkers of satiety

Correlations between the mean AUC for each biomarker and the mean score for each VAS question were not found in either the control or HAM-RS2 group at the end of the intervention; however, correlations between body composition measurements and the AUC for several biomarkers were found. In the HAM-RS2 group, BMI ($r = 0.655$; $P = 0.029$), percent total fat ($r = .889$; $P < 0.001$), total trunk mass ($r = 0.851$; $P = 0.001$); trunk fat ($r = 0.700$; $P = 0.017$); trunk lean ($r = 0.795$; $P = 0.003$) were associated with the AUC glucose. The percent total body fat correlated ($r = 0.652$; $P = 0.030$) with AUC leptin. In the control group AUC glucose was associated with BMI ($r = 0.814$; $P = 0.026$), total fat ($r = 0.801$; $P = 0.030$), percent fat ($r = 0.879$; $P = 0.009$), and percent trunk fat ($r = 0.772$; $P = 0.042$). Total trunk lean mass correlated with the AUC insulin ($r = 0.792$; $P = 0.034$) in the control group. The AUC glucose was associated with the AUC insulin in both the HAM-RS2 ($r = 0.710$; $P = 0.014$) and control ($r = 0.785$; $P = 0.036$) groups.

Discussion

Our primary aim was to examine changes in glucose homeostasis after consuming 30 g HAM-RS2 for 6 weeks in overweight adults. We also measured the plasma biomarkers (GLP-1, PYY, and leptin) and subjective satiety which could alter dietary intake and body composition. We found significant reductions in AUC glucose and AUC leptin in the HAM-RS2 group although differences between groups did not occur. In addition, a significant increase in fasting PYY occurred within the HAM-RS2 group after consuming the treatment muffins for 6 weeks. Interestingly, the favorable changes in biomarkers in the HAM-RS2 group did not elicit changes in overall mean subjective satiety score or body composition at the end of the intervention. Only one biomarker differed between groups throughout the duration of the study. Baseline PYY 120-min post-muffin intake was significantly higher in the HAM-RS2 group which may be attributed to initial HAM-RS2 fermentation. Increasing the duration of the. intervention or sample size may have produced additional between-group changes in biomarkers.

The decrease in AUC glucose in the HAM-RS2 group occurred under normoglycemic conditions and no change in overall mean carbohydrate intake suggesting other contributing mechanisms. One mechanism could be due to the SCFA produced from the fermentation of HAM-RS2 by bacteria in the lower GI tract. Butyrate and propionate are substrates for intestinal gluconeogenesis [25]. The newly synthesized glucose from the intestine reduces overall hepatic gluconeogenesis through portal vein sensors that contribute to overall blood glucose control [25].

Interestingly, HAM-RS2 lowered glucose AUC in the presence of a high-fat diet. At baseline habitual dietary fat intake in the HAM-RS2 group was 39.4% of total calories (~95 g per day). It is well established that diets high in fat consisting of large amounts of saturated and omega-6 polyunsaturated fatty acids and lower omega-3 polyunsaturated fatty acids contribute to chronic inflammation [26] and the development of chronic disease. Interestingly when dietary composition contains only 30.4% of calories from fat, HAM-RS2 can suppress inflammation and normalize glucose by mediating gluconeogenesis potential and altering hepatic fuel usage from lipids to carbohydrate [27]. Despite observing an improvement in AUC glucose in the HAM-RS2 group, we did not see changes in plasma insulin or insulin sensitivity (determined by Homeostasis Model Assessment estimates) that have been reported in human trials [13–15]. We did, however, observe a positive correlation between AUC glucose and AUC insulin in both groups.

A novel finding from our study is that AUC leptin significantly decreased from baseline to the end of the intervention in the HAM-RS2 group independent of changes in body composition. We also found a significant postprandial reduction at 120 min and near significant postprandial reductions at 30 ($P = 0.074$) and 60 min ($P = 0.062$) in leptin. Leptin is primarily produced by adipocytes and blood concentrations correlate with adipocyte size and percent body fat. One plausible mechanism could be enhanced fat oxidation which has been observed in healthy adults where postprandial fat oxidation increased 23% after 5.4% of dietary carbohydrate, but not 10.7%, was consumed acutely as HAM-RS2 [17]. Approximately 11% of mean daily carbohydrate intake was in the form of HAM-RS2 in our study; however, our population and study duration differed from Higgins et al. [17]. Another study found increased fat oxidation when resistant starch type 4 (RS4) plus whey protein was administered to healthy overweight and lean women [28]. Increased fat oxidation and resting energy expenditure also occurred in healthy lean males following consumption of 38 g RS4 in a mixed meal [29]. In addition, a fermentable cereal fiber reduced leptin by enhancing the gene expression of several enzymes involved in fat oxidation [30]. Similar to our findings, So et al. [31] reported lower leptin in addition to smaller adipocyte size in mice consuming HAM-RS2 compared to mice on a low resistant starch diet even though body composition did not differ between the groups. In contrast, no change in adipose leptin mRNA expression or plasma leptin concentrations occurred after a meal tolerance test in healthy males who consumed 30 g HAM-RS2 over 4 weeks [13]. The study by Robertson et al. examined healthy individuals with an average BMI of 23.7 kg/m^2 which is much lower than our mean baseline BMI of 34.8 kg/m^2, and our intervention was longer in duration. This suggests that duration of HAM-RS2 consumption and degree of adiposity may also be important in modulating leptin. Differences in adiposity (mean total body fat mass) between HAM-RS2 and control groups ($P = 0.085$) may explain why leptin did not differ between groups in our study, or that changes in leptin are more sensitive in individuals with higher fat mass.

The reduction in leptin after HAM-RS2 intake may benefit individuals with leptin resistance. Leptin resistance can develop from consuming high fat diets [12, 32] and sustained elevated leptin concentrations [33]. In our study, the HAM-RS2 group had a mean fasting leptin concentration of 33 ± 6 ng/mL. Fasting leptin concentrations of ≥15 ng/mL have been described as the cutoff value to predict insulin resistance [34]. Although we did not observe insulin resistance in the HAM-RS2 group, it is plausible that the study participants in our study were resistant to leptin due to high blood leptin concentrations and consumption of a high-fat diet at baseline. We observed significant reductions in leptin, but also a non-significant mean reduction (5.5%) in total calories from fat, but not overall total calories, in the HAM-RS2 group. This decrease in dietary fat is not likely responsible for the decrease in AUC leptin concentrations [35]. Similar to our results, leptin decreased with the addition of a fermentable soluble fiber in obese rats ingesting a high-fat diet [36]. Interestingly, the decrease in leptin in this study did not induce an orexigenic effect since overall caloric intake did not change and was similar to the control.

Our study also found an increase in total fasting PYY but not postprandial or AUC PYY in the HAM-RS2 group at the end of the study. The increase may be related to the carry-over fermentation effects of prior-day HAM-RS2 intake. Increased PYY has been observed with fermentable fiber consumption in animal studies [37]. PYY binds to the Y2 receptors of the arcuate nucleus to elicit a satiation response alongside increased energy expenditure [38]. Two isoforms of PYY exist: PYY_{1-36} and PYY_{3-36}. PYY_{1-36} predominates under fasting conditions and has a lower affinity to the Y2 receptor. This may explain why we did not see a relationship between total PYY and satiety. At baseline, PYY was significantly higher ($P = 0.043$) in the HAM-RS2 group than control 120 min after the consumption of the study muffins and may be due to the initial fermentation of HAM-RS2 following intake. A similar increase in PYY occurred in healthy adults consuming resistant starch and whey protein 180 min after intake [28]. We did not observe improvements in GLP-1, which is consistent with several human studies examining HAM-RS2 intake in overweight adults for ≥4 weeks [39, 40].

This study has several limitations. First, only inactive concentrations of GLP-1 and total PYY ($PYY_{(1-36)}$ + $PYY_{(3-36)}$) were measured. We were not able to determine the exact PYY isoform which may have explained why subjective satiety did not change. Another limitation includes the lack of adding di-peptidyl peptidase-4 inhibitors (DPP-IV) following blood collection. DPP-IV rapidly degrades GLP-1, thus we were not able to measure the physiologically active form of GLP-1 [41]. Also, the participants consumed the study muffins at any time during the day. Consuming the muffins at one meal or equally distributed throughout the day could impact metabolic response. In addition, the participants consumed the study muffins prior to postprandial blood collection instead of an isocaloric mixed meal equal in macronutrient composition. Thus, the plasma biomarker response is reflective of study muffin consumption. However, a between group 120-min improvement in PYY was observed in the HAM-RS2 group indicating fermentation can upregulate this satiety peptide. Lastly, a significant reduction in daily fiber intake from mid-point to week 6 occurred in the control group indicating the control muffins replaced other high-fiber foods in the diet.

Conclusion

In conclusion, daily consumption of 30 g of HAM-RS2 in muffins over 6 weeks can decrease leptin concentrations, assist with blood glucose homeostasis, and improve fasting PYY in healthy overweight adults. These findings occurred without changes in total caloric intake or body composition. Adding HAM-RS2 to the diet can improve fiber intake to enhance overall diet quality. However, strong conclusions cannot be made due to small sample size and between group differences in biomarkers were not observed at the end of the intervention. The mechanisms associated with biomarker changes in the HAM-RS2 group are likely related to the fermentation of HAM-RS2 by gut microbiota, but additional research is needed to determine the type, amount, and duration of resistant starch that would provide the most advantageous physiological results.

Abbreviations

AUC: Area under the curve; BMI: Body mass index; DXA: Dual-energy X-ray absorptiometry; GI: Gastrointestinal; GLP-1: Glucagon-like peptide-1; HAM-RS2: High-amylose maize resistant starch type 2; PYY: Peptide YY; RDN: Registered Dietitian Nutritionist; SCFA: Short chain fatty acids; SEM: Standard error of the mean; VAS: Visual analogue scale

Acknowledgements

None

Funding

This research was funded by the Office of Research and Sponsored Programs at Texas Woman's University through the Research Enhancement Program and Ingredion Incorporated. Ingredion Incorporated supplied the Hi-Maize® 260 resistant starch.

Availability of data and materials
Data sharing is not applicable to this article as no datasets were generated or analyzed during the current study.

Authors' contributions
PV, SJ, VI, and CP conceived and designed the experiments; MPM and SP collected data and performed the experiments; MPM and SP analyzed the data; MPM wrote the manuscript; PV, SJ, VI, and CP commented on and approved the manuscript. All authors read and approved the final manuscript.

Competing interests
The authors declare that they have no competing interests.

Consent for publication
Not applicable.

Ethics approval and consent to participate
The Institutional Review Board at Texas Woman's University approved this human research study. All participants provided informed consent prior to participating.

Author details
[1]Department of Nutrition and Food Sciences, Institute of Health Sciences, Texas Woman's University, 6700 Fannin Street, Houston, TX 77030, USA. [2]Department of Nutrition and Food Sciences, Texas Woman's University, P.O Box 425888, Denton, TX 76204, USA. [3]Department of Medicine (Endocrinology), Louisiana State University Health Science Center, New Orleans, LA 70112, USA.

References

1. Yang Y, Zhou LG, Wu QJ, Ma X, Xiang YB. Association between dietary fiber and lower risk of all-cause mortality: a meta-analysis of cohort studies. Am J Epidemiol. 2015;181(2):83–91. doi:10.1093/aje/kwu257.
2. Slavin JL. Dietary fiber and body weight. Nutrition. 2005;21(3):411–8.
3. Wanders AJ, van den Borne JJ, de Graaf C, Hulshof T, Jonathan MC, Kristensen M, Mars M, Schols HA, Feskens EJM. Effects of dietary fibre on subjective appetite, energy intake and body weight: a systematic review of randomized controlled trials. Obes Rev. 2011;12(9):724–39.
4. Lattimer JM, Haub MD. Effects of dietary fiber and its components on metabolic health. Nutrients. 2010;2(12):1266–89. doi:10.3390/nu2121266.
5. Guyenet SJ, Schwartz MW. Regulation of food intake, energy balance, and body fat mass: implications for the pathogenesis and treatment of obesity. J Clin Endocrin Metab. 2012;97(3):745–55.
6. Malijaars P, Peters H, Mela D, Masclee A. Ileal break: a sensible food target for appetite control. A review. Physiol Behav. 2008;95(3):271–81.
7. Murphy KG, Bloom SR. Gut hormones and the regulation of energy homeostasis. Nature. 2006;444(7121):854–9.
8. Nilsson AC, Johansson-Boll EV, Bjorck IME. Increased gut hormones and insulin sensitivity index following a 3-d intervention with a barley kernel-based product: a randomized cross-over study in healthy middle-aged subjects. Br J Nutr. 2015;114(6):899–907. doi:10.1017/S0007114515002524.
9. Lanfond DW, Greaves KA, Maki KC, Leidy HJ, Romsos DR. Effects of two dietary fibers as part of ready-to-eat cereal (RTEC) breakfasts on perceived appetite and gut hormones in overweight women. Nutrients. 2015;7(2): 1245–66. doi:10.3390/nu7021245.
10. Ye Z, Arumugam V, Haugabrooks E, Williamson P, Hendrich S. Soluble dietary fiber (Fibersol-2) decreased hunger and increased satiety hormones in humans when ingested with a meal. Nutr Res. 2015;35(5):393–400. doi:10.1016/j.nutres.2015.03.004.
11. Sarda FAH, Giuntini EB, Gomez ML, Lui MCY, Negrini JAE, Tadini CC, Lajolo FM, Menezes EW. Impact of resistant starch from unripe banana flour on hunger, satiety, and glucose homeostasis in healthy volunteers. J Func Foods. 2016;24:63–74.
12. Vasselli JR, Scarpace PJ, Harris RBS, Banks WA. Dietary components in the development of leptin resistance. Adv Nutr. 2013;4:164–75.
13. Robertson MD, Bickerton AS, Dennis AL, Vidal H, Frayn KN. Insulin-sensitizing effects of dietary resistant starch and effects on skeletal muscle and adipose tissue metabolism. Am J Clin Nutr. 2005;82(3):559–67.
14. Maki KC, Pelkman CL, Finocchiaro ET, Kelley KM, Lawless AL, Schild AL, Rains TM. Resistant starch from high-amylose maize increases insulin sensitivity in overweight and obese men. J Nutr. 2012;142(4):717–23.
15. Robertson MD, Wright JW, Loizon E, Debard C, Vidal H, Shojaee-Moradie F, Russell-Jones D, Umpleby AM. Insulin-sensitizing effects on muscle and adipose tissue after dietary fiber intake in men and women with metabolic syndrome. J Clin Endocrin Metabol. 2012;97(9):3326–32.
16. Johnston K, Thomas E, Bell J, Frost G, Robertson M. Resistant starch improves insulin sensitivity in metabolic syndrome. Diab Med. 2010;27(4):391–7.
17. Higgins JA, Higbee DR, Donahoo WT, Brown IL, Bell ML, Bessesen DH. Resistant starch consumption promotes lipid oxidation. Nutr Metab. 2004; 1(1):8. doi:10.1186/1743-7075-1-8.
18. Ebihara K, Shiraishi R, Okuma K. Hydroxypropyl-modified potato starch increases fecal bile acid excretion in rats. J Nutr. 1998;128:848–54.
19. Venkataraman A, Sieber JR, Schmidt AW, Waldron C, Theis KR, et al. Variable responses of human microbiomes to dietary supplementation with resistant starch. Microbiome. 2016;4:33. doi.10.1186/s40168-016-0178-x.
20. Maziarz M, Sherrard M, Juma S, Prasad C, Imrhan V, Vijayagopal P. Sensory characteristics of high-amylose maize resistant starch in three food products. Food Sci Nutr. 2012;1(2):117–24.
21. US Department of Agriculture, US Department of Health and Human Services. Dietary Guidelines for Americans. 7th ed. Washington DC: US Government Printing Office; 2010.
22. United States Department of Agriculture National Nutrient Database for Standard Reference. http://ndb.nal.usda.gov. Accessed 15 Jan 2014.
23. Lewis S, Heaton K. Stool form scale as a useful guide to intestinal transit time. Scandinav J Gastroenterol. 1997;32(9):920–4.
24. Flint A, Raben A, Blundell J, Astrup A. Reproducibility, power and validity of visual analogue scales in assessment of appetite sensations in single test meal studies. Int J Obes Rel Metab Disord. 2000;24(1):38–48.
25. De Vadder F, Kovatcheva-Datchary P, Goncalves D, Vinera J, Zitoun C, et al. Microbiota-generated metabolites promote metabolic benefits via gut-brain neural circuits. Cell. 2014;156:84–96.
26. Teng KT, Change CY, Chang LF, Nesaretnam K. Modulation of obesity-induced inflammation by dietary fats: mechanisms and clinical evidence. Nutr J. 2014;13:12. doi:10.1186/1475-2891.
27. Polakof S, Diaz-Rubio ME, Dardevet D, Martin JF, Pujos-Guillot E, Scalbert A, Sebedio JL, Mazur A, Comte B. Resistant starch intake partly restores metabolic and inflammatory alterations in the liver of high-fat-diet-fed rats. J Nutr Biochem. 2013;24:1920–30.
28. Gentile CL, Ward E, Holst JJ, Astrup A, Ormsbee MJ, Connelly S, Arciero PJ. Resistant starch and protein intake enhances fat oxidation and feelings of fullness in lean and overweight/obese women. Nutr J. 2015;14:113. doi:10.1186/s12937-015-0104-2.
29. Shimotoyodome A, Suzuki J, Kameo Y, Hase T. Dietary supplementation with hydroxypropyl-distarch phosphate from waxy maize starch increases energy expenditure by lowering the postprandial glucose-dependent insulinotropic polypeptide response in humans. Br J Nutr. 2011;106:96–104.
30. Han S, Jia J, Zhang W, Xu J, Wan Z, et al. Dietary fiber prevents obesity-related lipid toxicity by modulating sterol-regulator element binding protein pathway in C57BL/6 J mice fed a high-fat/cholesterol diet. Sci Rep. 2015;5: 15256. 10.1038/srep15256.
31. So PW, Yu WS, Kuo TU, Wasserfall C, Goldstone AP, Bell JD, Frost G. Impact of resistant starch on body fat patterning and central appetite regulation. PLosOne. 2007;2(12):e1309. 10.1371\journal.pone.0001309.
32. Enrori PJ, Evans AE, Sinnayah P, Jobst EE, Tonelli-Lemos L, Billes SK, et al. Diet-induced obesity causes severe but reversible leptin resistance in arcuate melanocortin neurons. Cell Metabol. 2007;5(3):181–94.
33. Knight AZ, Hannan KS, Greenberg ML, Friedman JM. Hyperleptinemia is required for the development of leptin resistance. PLosOne. 2010;5(6): e11376. doi:10.1371/journal.pone.0011376.
34. Askari H, Tykodi G, Liu J, Dagogo-Jack S. Fasting plasma leptin level is a surrogate measure of insulin sensitivity. J Clin Endocrinol Metab. 2010;95(8): 3836–43. doi:10.1210/jc.2010-0296.
35. Weigle DS, Duell PB, Connor WE, Steiner RA, Soules MR, Kuijper JL. Effect of fasting, refeeding, and dietary fat restriction on plasma leptin levels. J Clin Endocrin Metab. 1997;82(2):561–5.
36. Adams CL, Thomson LM, Williams PA, Ross AW. Soluble fermentable dietary fiber (pectin) decreases caloric intake, adiposity and lipidaemia in high-fat diet-induced obese rats. PLosOne. 2015;10(10):e0140392. doi:10.1371/journal.pone.0140392.

37. Zhou J, Martin RJ, Raggio AM, Shen L, McCutcheon K, Keenan MJ. The importance of GLP-1 and PYY in resistant starch's effect on body fat in mice. Mol Nutr Food Res. 2015;59:1000–3. doi:10.1002/mnfr.201400904.
38. Batterham RL, Cowley MA, Small CJ, Herzog H, Cohen MA, Dakin CL, et al. Gut hormone PYY3-36 physiologically inhibits food intake. Nature. 2002; 418(6898):650–4.
39. Bindels LB, Walter J, Ramer-Tait AE. Resistant starches for the management of metabolic disease. Curr Opin Clin Nutr Metab Care. 2015;18:559–65.
40. Keenan MJ, Zhou J, Hegsted M, Pelkman C, Durham HA, Coulon DB, Martin RJ. Role of resistant starch in improving gut health, adiposity, and insulin resistance. Adv Nutr. 2015;6:198–205. doi:10.3945/an.114.007419.
41. Holst JJ. The physiology of glucagon-like peptide-1. Physiol Rev. 2007;87:1409–39.

10

Impact of imposed exercise on energy intake in children at risk for overweight

S. Nicole Fearnbach[1*], Travis D. Masterson[1], Haley A. Schlechter[1], Amanda J. Ross[2], Michael J. Rykaczewski[2], Eric Loken[3,4], Danielle S. Downs[2], David Thivel[5,6] and Kathleen L. Keller[1,7]

Abstract

Background: Exercise not only has a direct effect on energy balance through energy expenditure (EE), but also has an indirect effect through its impact on energy intake (EI). This study examined the effects of acute exercise on daily *ad libitum* EI in children at risk for becoming overweight due to family history.

Methods: Twenty healthy-weight children (ages 9–12 years, 12 male/8 female) with at least one overweight biological parent (body mass index ≥ 25 kg/m^2) participated. Children reported to the laboratory for one baseline and two experimental visits (EX = exercise, SED = sedentary) each separated by 1 week in a randomized crossover design. Two hours into the EX day session, children exercised at 70 % estimated VO_{2max} for 30 min on a cycle ergometer. Objective EI (kcal) was measured at a standard breakfast (~285 kcal) and *ad libitum* lunch, snack and dinner. Meals were identical on the EX and SED days. Activity-related EE (kcal) was estimated with accelerometers worn on the non-dominant wrist and ankle. Relative EI (kcal) was computed as the difference between Total EI and Activity-related EE for each testing day. Paired *t*-tests were performed to test differences in Total EI, Activity-related EE and Relative EI between the EX and SED days.

Results: Across all meals, Total EI was not statistically different between the EX and SED days ($t = 1.8$, $p = 0.09$). Activity-related EE was greater on the EX day compared to the SED day ($t = 10.1$, $p < 0.001$). By design, this difference was predominantly driven by activity during the morning ($t = 20.4$, $p < 0.001$). Because children consumed a similar number of kcal on each day, but had greater Activity-related EE on the EX day, Relative EI was lower ($t = -5.15$, $p < 0.001$) for the EX day (1636 ± 456 kcal) relative to the SED day (1862 ± 426 kcal).

Conclusions: Imposed exercise was effective in reducing Relative EI compared to being sedentary. Morning exercise may help children at risk for becoming overweight to better regulate their energy balance within the course of a day.

Keywords: Children, Exercise, Energy intake, Energy expenditure, Energy balance, Obesity

Introduction

Childhood obesity rates have increased substantially over the past forty years, both in the United States and globally [1]. With increasing rates of early onset obesity, children are at the greatest risk for long-term health complications [2] because the disease is often resistant to treatment [3]. The dramatic increase in obesity prevalence has coincided with increased availability of large portions of high energy dense foods, driving a pattern of overeating [4]. In addition, levels of physical activity both in and out of the everyday school setting have decreased, reducing children's average daily energy expenditure (EE) [5]. Typical methods to reduce EI require intentional energy restriction. These methods may be difficult to sustain as a long-term lifestyle change, particularly during childhood when preferences for sweet, salty and fatty foods are high [6–8]. Therefore, alternative strategies are needed that impact EI and EE to improve obesity outcomes in children. Incorporating exercise as a regular lifestyle component may provide an alternative means to control appetite and energy balance throughout the life course.

* Correspondence: snf129@psu.edu
[1]Department of Nutritional Sciences, The Pennsylvania State University, 110 Chandlee Laboratory, University Park, PA 16802, USA
Full list of author information is available at the end of the article

The present study aims to understand the acute effects of morning exercise versus rest on daily EI in children ages 9–12 years. Exercise not only has a direct effect on energy balance through EE, but has been shown to also have an indirect effect through its impact on EI [9]. Emerging research has implicated the use of exercise as a preventative measure for overeating and subsequent development of overweight and obesity in adolescents and adults [10–31]. While exercise, relative to rest, has been shown to be effective in reducing subsequent EI and contributing to a negative energy balance in adolescents and adults [17–20, 26–29], limited research has examined this relationship in children under the age of 12 years [32]. Previous work shows that high intensity exercise can induce a state of lower 24-h energy balance by reducing subsequent EI relative to both low intensity exercise and sedentary activity in obese adolescents [27]. This is commonly referred to as the "transient anorexigenic effect" of exercise [33]. In obese adolescents, the greatest effects of high intensity exercise on EI have been seen seven hours post-exercise [27, 34]. These changes were seen without any significant differences in appetite ratings. These findings suggest the use of exercise as a possible strategy to decrease EI, at least in the short term, which could augment attempts to intentionally restrict EI.

Previous studies have focused on the impact of exercise on intake as a treatment strategy in overweight and obese adolescents, but the "anorexigenic effect" of exercise on intake has not been studied in healthy weight children who are at risk for developing obesity due to family history. From a prevention standpoint, it is vital to determine the effectiveness of exercise-related strategies to reduce overeating in children who are predisposed to genetic or environmental factors that promote positive energy balance [35, 36]. This study examined the effects of acute imposed exercise versus imposed sedentariness on daily EI in healthy-weight children with at least one overweight or obese biological parent. Based on previous research with adolescent populations [27], we hypothesized that Total EI and Relative EI (adjusted for Activity-related EE) would be lower on a day with imposed exercise compared to a day where children remained sedentary.

Methods

Study design

A within-subjects crossover design study was conducted with a community-based sample of 20 children ages 9–12 years. Children completed 1 baseline and 2 experimental visits (EX = exercise, SED = sedentary in a pre-assigned randomized order) each separated by exactly 1 week. The baseline visit was a four-hour session in the morning to familiarize children with eating in a laboratory environment (breakfast and lunch) and collect baseline measurements (described below). Outside of meal and exercise testing periods, children had access to a series of toys, books, and games and could switch freely between activities. The EX and SED days consisted of the same four-hour morning session in the laboratory, followed by five hours of free-living time at home, and then an in-laboratory dinner session (Fig. 1). Children and their parents received modest financial compensation for their time. This study was approved by the Institutional Review Board of The Pennsylvania State University.

Participants

Children were recruited using flyers posted in local schools and businesses located around the university. Interested parents completed a phone screening to determine eligibility. Children were considered eligible if by parental report they were normal weight (<85th age- and sex-specific body mass index [BMI] percentile), without food allergies, without medical conditions or contraindications to exercise testing [37], not participating in competitive sports which could skew fitness and exercise test results (year-round or > 3 practice sessions

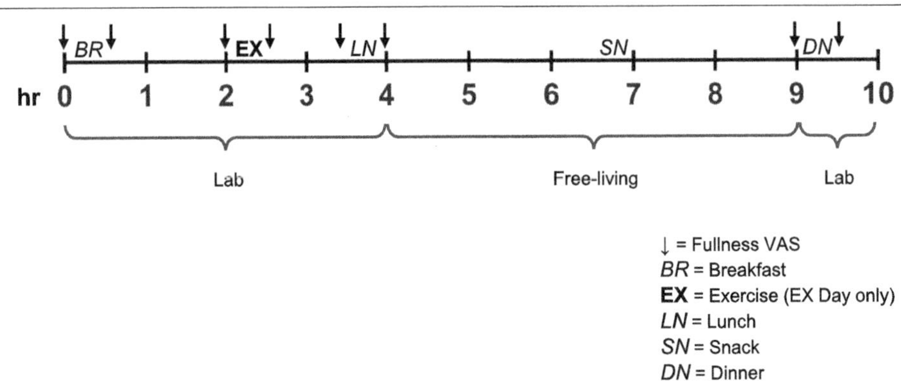

Fig. 1 Experimental day (EX or SED) timeline

per week), with at least one biological parent who was overweight or obese (BMI > 25 kg/m^2) [35, 36]. Both child and parent weight status were confirmed by measurement at the baseline visit, described below. One male child was in the overweight category (89th BMI percentile) after baseline measurements, but was retained in the study. This participant did not differ from the group mean in body composition (e.g., % body fat) or on any of the behavioral measures (e.g., food intake, physical activity, exercise test performance). On the first study visit, a parent signed informed consent for their child. Children provided written assent prior to their participation. A total of 20 children were enrolled in the study and completed all three visits. Sample characteristics for these 20 children are listed in Table 1. Sample size calculations ($n = 20$) were derived using G*Power software (version 3.1.9.2) for the primary aim to compare within-subjects differences in EI as a function of condition (EX vs. SED) using paired-sample t-tests [38].

Baseline measurements

Anthropometrics & body composition

Prior to breakfast on the baseline visit, anthropometrics (height and weight) were measured to the nearest 0.1 cm and 0.1 kg by a trained researcher. Children and their parents were each weighed and measured twice using a standard scale (Detecto model 437, Webb City, MO) and stadiometer (Seca model 202, Chino, CA) in light clothing and stocking feet. Height (m) and weight (kg) were converted to body mass index (BMI; kg/m^2) for the parent, and age- and sex-specific BMI z-score and BMI percentile for the child using the Centers for Disease Control and Prevention conversion program [39]. Percent body fat was measured using bioelectrical impedance analysis (Tanita model BF-350, Arlington Heights, IL, USA) [40].

Table 1 Participant characteristics ($n = 20$)

	Mean ± SD
Age (years)	10.3 ± 1.1
BMI percentile	41.6 ± 21.7
% body fat	15.6 ± 4.4
	N (%)
Sex	
Male	12 (60)
Female	8 (40)
Race	
White	20 (100)
Non-white	0 (0)

Abbreviations: BMI body mass index

Fitness testing

Two hours into the baseline visit, children completed the YMCA graded submaximal cycle test to estimate cardiorespiratory fitness [41]. Children were outfitted with a Polar Heart Rate Transmitter chest strap and wrist unit receiver (Polar Electro Inc. model T31-Coded, Lake Success, NY, USA). Participants remained seated for five minutes while a researcher explained the procedure and instructed the child on the use of the Borg Scale for Ratings of Perceived Exertion (RPE) [42]. At the end of the five minute period, a supervising nurse obtained resting heart rate and blood pressure measurements. Children were then familiarized with the cycle ergometer (Lode Corival V2, Lode Holding BV, Groningen, The Netherlands) and completed a three-minute warm-up, followed by the YMCA submaximal cycle test. The YMCA cycle test follows a branching, multi-stage format (Table 2) to determine the relationship between heart rate and work rate in order to estimate the individual's VO_{2max}. Children are required to pedal at a constant rate (50 ± 2 rpm) while researchers adjust the resistance (i.e., work rate) on the cycle ergometer at each stage. Heart rate values are recorded every minute, while blood pressure and RPE are measured every three minutes. The test requires that each participant completes two separate workload stages that result in steady-state heart rates between 110 and 150 beats per minute. Steady-state is achieved when two consecutive heart rate values are within ±5 beats per minute. VO_{2max} was estimated using the graph plot and extrapolation technique [41, 43]. This estimated VO_{2max} was used to determine the work rate for the 70 % intensity cycle test on the EX Day (described below).

70 % intensity exercise protocol

Two hours into the EX day session (Fig. 1), children completed the cycle ergometer exercise test. Participants were outfitted with the heart rate monitor, and resting heart rate and blood pressure measurements were taken. After a three-minute warm-up, children exercised at their individual 70 % estimated VO_{2max} for 30 min. The starting work rate (in Watts) was determined from the linear association between heart rate and work rate established during the submaximal exercise test [41]. The work rate was either confirmed or adjusted throughout the test to maintain a target heart rate between 70-80 % age-predicted maximum heart rate (e.g., 10-year-old: 147–168 beats per minute). Children could request water at any point during the test. Researchers and the attending nurse encouraged children throughout the exercise protocol with positive verbal cues, cheering and clapping. After completion of the exercise test, participants had a five-minute cool-down period on the bike, followed by ten minutes of light stretching.

Table 2 YMCA Submaximal Cycle Ergometer Test protocol; American College of Sports Medicine [36]

Stage 1	150 kg·m·min^{-1} 0.5 kg 24 W			
	HR: < 80	HR: 80–89	HR: 90–100	HR: > 100
Stage 2	750 kg·m·min^{-1} 2.5 kg 123 W	600 kg·m·min^{-1} 2.0 kg 98 W	450 kg·m·min^{-1} 1.5 kg 73 W	300 kg·m·min^{-1} 1.0 kg 49 W
Stage 3	900 kg·m·min^{-1} 3.0 kg 147 W	750 kg·m·min^{-1} 2.5 kg 123 W	600 kg·m·min^{-1} 2.0 kg 98 W	450 kg·m·min^{-1} 1.5 kg 73 W
Stage 4	1050 kg·m·min^{-1} 3.5 kg 172 W	900 kg·m·min^{-1} 3.0 kg 147 W	700 kg·m·min^{-1} 2.5 kg 114 W	600 kg·m·min^{-1} 2.0 kg 98 W

Abbreviations: HR heart rate (beats per minute), *kg* kilograms, *m* meter, *min^{-1}* per minute, *W* Watts

Accelerometer measurements

Children wore an ActiGraph GT3X-BT accelerometer on their non-dominant wrist for 10 h on each testing day (EX, SED). In addition, children wore a second accelerometer on their non-dominant ankle for the YMCA submaximal cycle test and the 30-min exercise test (70 % individual estimated aerobic capacity) to more accurately measure activity in the seated position on the cycle ergometer. We used this hybrid measure to estimate Activity-related EE [44]. The 4 h during the morning session were considered in-laboratory time, while the 6 h in the afternoon were considered free-living time. Activity-related EE was extracted for each child for the entire 10-h period, and then separately for the morning (in-lab) versus the afternoon (free-living). All data were validated and scored in ActiLife 6 software (ActiGraph, LLC, Pensacola, FL, USA) using Freedson Combination (1998) to calculate Activity-related EE.

Food intake measurement

Test-meal procedures

Children arrived to the laboratory after an overnight fast on all three testing days. Objective EI (kcal) was measured at a standard breakfast and lunch, snack and dinner test-meals. Meals were identical on the EX and SED days. Fullness ratings were completed before and after each laboratory meal on a vertical 150 mm visual analog scale (VAS) referred to as "Freddy Fullness" (data not shown) [45]. On the first visit, children conducted taste tests to report liking and wanting for each breakfast, lunch and snack food on VAS. On the second visit, children tasted and rated liking and wanting on VAS for each dinner food (data not shown). Timing for the meals and VAS ratings is depicted in Fig. 1.

Breakfast All children were required to consume a standardized breakfast on all three test days consisting of an English muffin toasted with one tablespoon butter, banana and orange juice (285 kcal total) (Table 3). Children's liking for and willingness to eat the breakfast foods were confirmed at screening, prior to the first visit. Children were considered to have finished the meal if they consumed ≥ 95 % of each individual food item within 30 min (average duration = 11 ± 5 min). All 20 children met these requirements at each of the three breakfast meals.

Lunch Prior to the first visit, children were given the opportunity to select from a pre-set menu of available items for lunch. Children chose a sandwich (peanut butter & jelly or deli meat & cheese), vegetable (carrots or tomatoes) with ranch dip, fruit (apple slices or grapes), and salty snack (pretzels or baked chips). All children also received brownies and a bottle of water with their lunch. All serving sizes were controlled to ensure that any combination of food items provided approximately the same number of total calories (997–1014 kcal), which provided > 50 % of children's caloric needs for the day. Possible food choices and serving sizes are reported in Table 3. Children were instructed that they had up to 30 min to eat freely from the food items provided. If they were finished before the 30 min had elapsed, they notified a researcher (average duration = 19 ± 6 min).

Snack The snack consisted of a granola bar, fruit cocktail and juice (~302 kcal) (Table 3). All foods were pre-weighed and packed for children to take home during free-living time on the EX and SED days. Parents were given written and verbal instructions to provide the snack at a set time and to return any packaging and uneaten food items to researchers upon arrival for dinner. Additional written and verbal instructions were given to not eat or drink anything except water before the snack, or for the 2 h prior to dinner. Compliance was checked by sending text message reminders to parents at snack time and requesting a response. These messages asked parents to remind children that they could eat as much

Table 3 Food items, serving sizes and calorie contents for each meal. Abbreviations: g, grams; fl oz., fluid ounces; kcal, kilocalories

Breakfast Food Item	Serving Size	Kcal per Serving
English muffin (with butter)	1 muffin + 1 tablespoon butter	151
Banana (without peel)	60 g	51
Orange juice	178 g (6 fl oz.)	83
Total		285
Lunch Food Item	Serving Size	Kcal per Serving
Wheat bread	2 slices	170
Deli meat (pick one)		
Ham	114 g	100
Turkey	95 g	100
+ Cheese (pick one)		
Cheddar	42 g	157
Provolone	38 g	140
American	53 g	151
OR		
Peanut butter	30 g	190
+ Jelly	36 g	60
Pretzels	42 g	165
OR		
Baked chips	39 g	65
Apple slices	102 g	53
OR		
Grapes	77 g	53
Carrots	100 g	41
OR		
Tomatoes	140 g	41
Ranch dip	30 g	140
Brownies (3)	43 g	188
Total		997–1014
Snack Food Item	Serving Size	Kcal per Serving
Chocolate chip granola bar	1 bar	104
Mixed fruit cocktail	117 g	62
Apple juice	250 g (8 fl oz.)	136
Total		302
Dinner Food Item	Serving Size (multiple servings available)	Kcal per Serving
Macaroni & cheese	400 g	551
Garlic bread	75 g	270
Broccoli (with butter)	120 g	53
Applesauce	128 g	110
Cookies (3)	46 g	243
Total		1,227

as they wanted of any of the snack foods. Upon return, packaging was re-weighed to measure snack intake.

Dinner On the EX and SED days, children reported to the laboratory at least 2 h fasted for an *ad libitum* dinner test-meal consisting of macaroni and cheese, garlic bread, broccoli, applesauce and cookies (~1227+ kcal) (Table 3). Children were instructed that they had up to 30 min to eat as much as they wanted from the available foods. They were also able to request additional servings of the foods at this meal. A researcher was available in the room during the meal and prompted the child if they finished a serving of a particular food. Children could also notify the researcher if they finished eating before the 30 min had elapsed (average duration = 19 ± 5 min).

Nutrient analysis

Pre- and post-meal weights for each food item were measured to the nearest 0.1 g, and used to calculate intake in grams. This was later converted to EI (kcal) by meal (Breakfast, Lunch, Snack and Dinner) and in SPSS Statistics (Version 22; IBM Corporation, Armonk, NY, USA) using nutrition label information. Total EI (kcal) was computed as the sum of EI from each of the individual meals (Breakfast, Lunch, Snack and Dinner EI). Macronutrient intake (kcal) was also calculated for each day using nutrition label information for each food item, summed across each testing day. Relative EI (kcal) was computed as the difference between Total EI and Activity-related EE for each testing day.

Statistical analysis

Descriptive statistics for participant characteristics (i.e., means and standard deviations on continuous variables and frequencies on categorical variables) were calculated on the full sample. Pearson's correlations were computed to determine the association between Total EI on the EX and SED days. Paired *t*-tests were performed to test differences in Total EI, EI by meal (standard breakfast, lunch, snack and dinner EI), macronutrient intake, Activity-related EE (total, morning, afternoon) and Relative EI between the EX and SED days. Effect sizes (Cohen's *d*) were calculated for all paired *t*-test results. Data were analyzed using SPSS. Test results were considered significant at $p < 0.05$.

Results

Across all meals, Total EI was not statistically different between the EX and SED days ($t = 1.8$, $p = 0.09$). Total intake on the two days was highly correlated ($r = 0.93$, $p < 0.01$). By design, EI at the standard breakfast was not different between the two days ($t = 0.2$, $p = 0.87$). In addition, EI at the lunch ($t = 2.0$, $p = 0.06$), snack ($t = -1.9$, $p = 0.08$), or dinner ($t = 1.2$, $p = 0.24$) did not differ on the EX day versus the SED day. In regards to macronutrient intake, energy intake from protein ($t = 2.1$, $p < 0.05$) and fat ($t = 2.3$, $p < 0.05$) were higher on the EX day compared to the SED day, with no differences in carbohydrate intake ($t = 1.2$, $p = 0.24$). However, this did not result in a significant difference in the proportion of calories from each macronutrient (all $p > 0.05$, data not shown) between the two testing days.

Activity-related EE was greater on the EX day compared to the SED day ($t = 10.1$, $p < 0.001$). This difference was predominantly driven by in-laboratory activity during the morning ($t = 20.4$, $p < 0.001$). Afternoon free-living Activity-related EE was not different between the two days ($t = 1.8$, $p = 0.09$).

Because children ate a similar number of kcal on each day, but had greater Activity-related EE on the EX day, Relative EI was lower ($t = -5.15$, $p < 0.001$) for the EX day (1636 ± 456 kcal) compared to the SED day (1862 ± 426 kcal) (Fig. 2). In other words, Total EI adjusted for Activity-related EE was 226 kcal lower on the EX Day than the SED day. Paired t-test results for EI and EE variables and effect sizes for these results are summarized in Table 4.

Discussion

The purpose of this pilot study was to examine the effects of acute exercise on daily EI in healthy-weight 9–12 year-old children who were at risk for becoming overweight due to family history. Based on previous research on adolescents with obesity [27], we hypothesized that Total EI and Relative EI (Total EI adjusted for Activity-related EE) would be lower on the EX day compared to the SED day. In line with our hypothesis, we did find that Relative EI was 226 kcal lower on the EX day compared to the SED day, indicating a beneficial effect of imposed exercise on children's energy balance over the course of a day. This finding was a result of the fact that children did not significantly adjust their daily EI to fully compensate for differences in activity-related EE between the two days. Participants consumed essentially the same number of calories (within 85 kcal) on the EX day and the SED day, but had greater Activity-related EE (~310 kcal) on the EX day than the SED day. There were small but statistically significant increases in calories consumed from protein (11 kcal) and fat (39 kcal) on the EX day relative to the SED day. In sum, we found that imposed exercise had a beneficial impact on daily energy balance in children who are at risk for becoming overweight by increasing Activity-related EE without a significant increase in subsequent EI.

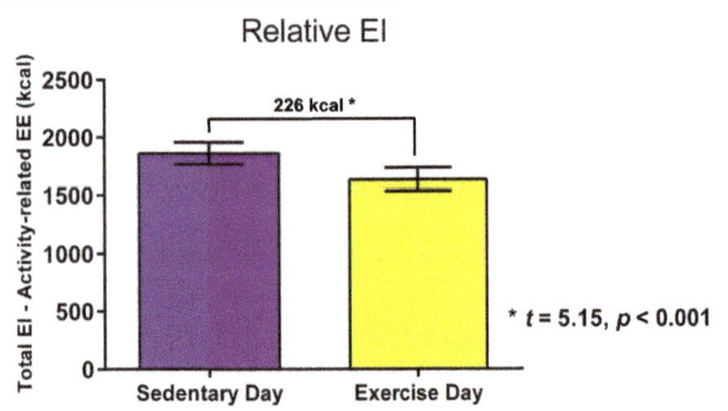

Fig. 2 Relative EI (kcal) was 226 kcal lower on the EX Day (1636 ± 456 kcal) compared to the SED Day (1862 ± 426 kcal); $t = 5.15$, $p < 0.001$

In the current study, we looked to extend previous findings in adolescents with obesity regarding the "anorexigenic effect" of exercise on subsequent food intake [27]. We used a similar design to previous studies to examine the effects of exercise in a younger age group of pre-adolescent children who were at risk for becoming overweight. We found that imposed exercise was effective in reducing Relative EI when compared to the SED day. We did not find evidence of a compensatory response to the exercise bout in regards to children's EI at subsequent meals. Children consumed approximately the same number of calories on both days, demonstrating that they did not adjust their EI to match differences in Activity-related EE between the EX day and the SED day. In other words, the short-term benefits of exercise on EE were not immediately offset by compensatory EI in our sample of healthy weight children. Previous studies in adolescents and adults have shown mixed results for acute post-exercise EI [33, 46], which can be attributed to differences in participant characteristics (e.g., lean versus obese) or exercise methodologies (e.g., intensity, modality). Generally, subsequent EI is not greater after exercise relative to rest in healthy populations, whether at a single meal or over the course of a day [30, 46]. Once differences in EE from exercise are accounted for, Relative EI is typically lower after exercise versus a control condition [23, 27, 31]. These results, together with ours, suggest that morning moderate-to-vigorous intensity exercise may be an effective strategy to prevent positive energy balance in children at risk for becoming overweight, at least in the short term. Additional longer-term studies are needed to assess the effectiveness of structured morning exercise for childhood obesity prevention.

It is important to note that the timing of the exercise bout relative to the meals can affect subsequent EI, but previous studies disagree regarding the most effective time interval to reduce EI. A recent study in healthy weight adolescent males demonstrated that exercise immediately prior to lunch was more effective in reducing lunch EI when compared to an identical exercise bout approximately 2 h prior to lunch [11]. There are several proposed mechanisms for the effects of acute exercise

Table 4 Results of paired *t*-tests for mean comparisons of energy intake (EI) and energy expenditure (EE) variables between the Exercise (EX) and Sedentary (SED) Days

	EX Day	SED Day	Paired Diff. (± SD)	*t*	*p*	*Effect size (d)*
Total EI (kcal)	2171 ± 566	2088 ± 497	83 ± 204	1.8	0.09	0.41
Breakfast EI (kcal)	287 ± 8.2	286 ± 8.5	0 ± 9	0.2	0.87	0.04
Lunch EI (kcal)	683 ± 186	639 ± 193	45 ± 100	2.0	0.06	0.45
Snack EI (kcal)	245 ± 72	256 ± 61	−12 ± 28	−1.9	0.08	0.43
Dinner EI (kcal)	956 ± 362	907 ± 310	50 ± 182	1.2	0.24	0.27
EI from Macronutrients (kcal)						
Carbohydrate (kcal)	1269 ± 337	1235 ± 295	33 ± 122	1.2	0.24	0.85
Protein (kcal)	207 ± 68	196 ± 67	11 ± 23	2.1	0.04 *	1.48
Fat (kcal)	694 ± 181	655 ± 155	39 ± 76	2.3	0.03 *	1.61
Total Activity-related EE (kcal)	534 ± 263	226 ± 146	308 ± 137	10.1	0.001*	2.25
Morning Activity-related EE (kcal)	394 ± 123	116 ± 77	278 ± 61	20.4	0.001*	4.56
Afternoon Activity-related EE (kcal)	144 ± 147	110 ± 74	33 ± 86	1.8	0.09	0.40
Relative EI (kcal)	1636 ± 456	1862 ± 426	−226 ± 196	−5.15	0.001 *	1.15

*Significance at $p < 0.05$

on appetite and EI regulation. Exercise can act indirectly on energy balance through influences on body composition (e.g., fat and lean mass), gut peptide signaling (e.g., polypeptide YY 3–36, glucagon-like peptide-1) and brain responses to food-related cues [9, 47]. These signals, in theory, impact appetite and subsequent food intake [9, 47]. Given the short half-life of many appetite-regulating hormones, it may be expected that a shorter delay between an exercise bout and a meal is more effective in reducing EI than a longer interval. In the current study, the delay between the exercise bout and the lunch test-meal was approximately 45 min. We did not find a significant difference in lunch EI between the EX and SED days. Other studies have found lasting effects of acute morning exercise on EI later in the day. For example, Thivel and colleagues found that high intensity exercise was effective in reducing intake at a dinner test-meal 7 h post-exercise [27]. The mechanism for these more sustained effects is unclear, but important to investigate given that obesity prevention requires chronic regulation of energy balance.

One major methodological difference in our study, versus previous studies [27], is that EE was not matched across the two days (EX versus SED). Activity-related EE was controlled during the four hours of in-laboratory time in the morning, but we also allowed children free-living time in the afternoon. This allowed us to test whether children would compensate for the morning exercise by increasing sedentary time later in the day. We did not find any differences in afternoon Activity-related EE between the EX and SED days. In other words, children were not less active following the exercise bout than they were following imposed sedentary time. The lack of a compensatory response in our sample is suggestive of one promising behavioral attribute that could help children maintain a healthy weight. A recent study in overweight boys found that after a vigorous exercise session, the participants spontaneously decreased their physical activity EE during the following 24 h [48]. Participation in structured exercise may be a more effective strategy in healthy weight populations with fewer negative consequences on subsequent leisure-time physical activity. A systematic review in healthy adults found minimal evidence that prescribed exercise affects non-exercise physical activity and EE [49]. Further research in children is warranted to determine which characteristics make an individual more or less likely to compensate for imposed exercise.

This preliminary study represents a novel application of the working model of energy balance in a sample of children at risk for becoming overweight. There are several strengths of this study. First, we have objective measures of daily EI across multiple test-meals during which we were able to assess children's energy intake. Objective intake measures are advantageous compared to self-reported EI, a method which introduces misreporting biases [50]. In addition, identical meals across the two experimental days allowed us to look specifically at the within-subjects effect of the exercise bout on Total EI. Another strength is the inclusion of objective measures of Activity-related EE, both in the laboratory and free-living. Our study was designed to facilitate acclimation to the laboratory environment (research personnel, exercise testing and test-meals) at the baseline visit. This helped to reduce the novelty effect on our outcome variables on the experimental days. Finally, we had a 100 % retention rate and full reported and/or observed compliance with instructions and protocols across the three testing days.

Some limitations of the current study should be noted. We were not able to assess intake outside of the 10-h experimental day and are unsure whether children's EI differed in the late evening (e.g., dessert) or the following day. While there were no reports of additional food or beverage intake during the free-living period between lunch and dinner, we acknowledge that our compliance rates with food-related study procedures are subject to the biases of self-report. In addition, a few of the differences in intake between the two days were non-significant trends ($p < 0.10$), including lunch EI ($p = 0.06$). Post-hoc analyses demonstrated we were underpowered (Power < 0.30) to detect differences in intake of individual meals/snack between the two days. It is possible that these differences would be significant with a larger sample size. Our sample was homogenous in demographic characteristics, which limits the generalizability of our findings. In addition, our classification of "at risk for becoming overweight" was solely based on parent weight status [35, 36], and not inclusive of additional genetic, family or environmental-level factors that can impact energy balance-related behaviors [51]. Future studies may be able to identify more specific phenotypes of obesity risk in the recruitment phase. Finally, this study did not include measures of resting metabolic rate or thermic effect of food. Therefore, we cannot evaluate effects of exercise on total daily EE or overall energy balance.

Conclusions

Children in this study did not adjust their EI to match differences in Activity-related EE, resulting in relative positive energy balance on the SED compared to the EX day. Imposed exercise may help children at risk for becoming overweight better regulate their food intake within the course of a day. In order to allow for more personalized prevention strategies, future research is necessary to determine the individual-level child characteristics that are likely to impact the effect of exercise on energy intake in this population.

Abbreviations

ad lib: *ad libitum*; BMI: Body mass index; EE: Energy expenditure; EI: Energy intake; EX: Exercise; kcal: Kilocalories; RPE: Ratings of perceived exertion; SED: Sedentary; VAS: Visual analog scale; VO_{2max}: Maximal aerobic capacity

Acknowledgements

The project described was also supported by the National Center for Advancing Translational Sciences, National Institutes of Health, through Grant UL1 TR000127. The content is solely the responsibility of the authors and does not necessarily represent the official views of the NIH. We would like to thank the Penn State Clinical and Translational Science Institute, including the Clinical Research Center and the Biostatistics, Epidemiology and Research Design services. Finally, we would like to acknowledge the Metabolic Kitchen and Children's Eating Behavior Laboratory at Penn State.

Funding

This project was supported by Agriculture and Food Research Initiative Grant #2011-67001-30117 from the USDA National Institute of Food and Agriculture, Childhood Obesity Prevention: Transdisciplinary Graduate Education and Training in Nutrition and Family Sciences, Program A2121.

Availability of data and materials

Data from this project will not be shared because additional results from the study are yet to be published.

Authors' contributions

SNF, DSD, DT & KLK conceptualized and designed the study. SNF, TDM, HAS, AJR & MJR developed study materials and completed data collection. SNF analyzed the data. SNF, EL, DSD, TD & KLK were involved in interpretation the results. SNF was primarily responsible for drafting the manuscript, and all authors gave critical feedback and approval prior to submission of the final manuscript.

Competing interests

The authors declare that they have no competing interests.

Consent for publication

Not applicable.

Ethics approval and consent to participate

This study was approved by the Institutional Review Board of The Pennsylvania State University (#00578). A parent signed informed consent for their child. Children provided written assent prior to their participation.

Author details

[1]Department of Nutritional Sciences, The Pennsylvania State University, 110 Chandlee Laboratory, University Park, PA 16802, USA. [2]Department of Kinesiology, The Pennsylvania State University, 276 Recreation Building, University Park, PA 16802, USA. [3]Department of Human Development and Family Studies, The Pennsylvania State University, 119 Health and Human Development Building, University Park, PA 16802, USA. [4]Department of Educational Psychology, University of Connecticut, 328 Charles B. Gentry Building, Storrs, CT 06269, USA. [5]Laboratory of the Metabolic Adaptations to Exercise under Physiological and Pathological Conditions (AME2P), Clermont Auvergne University, EA 3533 Clermont-Ferrand, France. [6]CRNH-Auvergne, 58 Rue Montalembert, 63009 Clermont-Ferrand, France. [7]Department of Food Science, The Pennsylvania State University, 202 Rodney A. Erickson Food Science Building, University Park, PA 16802, USA.

References

1. Finucane MM, et al. National, regional, and global trends in body-mass index since 1980: systematic analysis of health examination surveys and epidemiological studies with 960 country-years and 9.1 million participants. Lancet. 2011;377(9765):557–67.
2. Must A, Strauss RS. Risks and consequences of childhood and adolescent obesity. Int J Obes Relat Metab Disord. 1999;23 Suppl 2:S2–S11.
3. Jeffery RW, et al. Long-term maintenance of weight loss: current status. Health Psychol. 2000;19(1 Suppl):5–16.
4. Rolls BJ, Morris EL, Roe LS. Portion size of food affects energy intake in normal-weight and overweight men and women. Am J Clin Nutr. 2002; 76(6):1207 13.
5. Page A, et al. Physical activity patterns in nonobese and obese children assessed using minute-by-minute accelerometry. Int J Obes (Lond). 2005; 29(9):1070–6.
6. Berman EM. Factors influencing motivations in dieting. J Nutr Educ. 1975; 7(4):155–9.
7. Lanfer A, et al. Taste preferences in association with dietary habits and weight status in European children: results from the IDEFICS study. Int J Obes (Lond). 2012;36(1):27–34.
8. Mennella JA, et al. Preferences for salty and sweet tastes are elevated and related to each other during childhood. PLoS One. 2014;9(3):e92201.

9. Blundell JE, et al. Role of resting metabolic rate and energy expenditure in hunger and appetite control: a new formulation. Dis Model Mech. 2012;5(5):608–13.
10. Alajmi N, et al. Appetite and Energy Intake Responses to Acute Energy Deficits in Females versus Males. Med Sci Sports Exerc. 2016;48(3):412–20.
11. Albert MH, Drapeau V, Mathieu ME. Timing of moderate-to-vigorous exercise and its impact on subsequent energy intake in young males. Physiol Behav. 2015;151:557–62.
12. Blundell JE, King NA. Physical activity and regulation of food intake: current evidence. Med Sci Sports Exerc. 1999;31(11 Suppl):S573–83.
13. Blundell JE, et al. Cross talk between physical activity and appetite control: does physical activity stimulate appetite? Proc Nutr Soc. 2003;62(3):651–61.
14. Chaput JP, et al. Modern sedentary activities promote overconsumption of food in our current obesogenic environment. Obes Rev. 2011;12(5):e12–20.
15. Chaput JP, Sharma AM. Is physical activity in weight management more about 'calories in' than 'calories out'? Br J Nutr. 2011;106(11):1768–9.
16. Finlayson G, et al. Acute compensatory eating following exercise is associated with implicit hedonic wanting for food. Physiol Behav. 2009; 97(1):62–7.
17. Hagobian TA, et al. Effects of acute exercise on appetite hormones and ad libitum energy intake in men and women. Appl Physiol Nutr Metab. 2013; 38(1):66–72.
18. Hopkins M, King NA, Blundell JE. Acute and long-term effects of exercise on appetite control: is there any benefit for weight control? Curr Opin Clin Nutr Metab Care. 2010;13(6):635–40.
19. Hubert P, King NA, Blundell JE. Uncoupling the effects of energy expenditure and energy intake: appetite response to short-term energy deficit induced by meal omission and physical activity. Appetite. 1998;31(1):9–19.
20. Imbeault P, et al. Acute effects of exercise on energy intake and feeding behaviour. Br J Nutr. 1997;77(4):511–21.
21. King NA, Hester J, Gately PJ. The effect of a medium-term activity- and diet-induced energy deficit on subjective appetite sensations in obese children. Int J Obes (Lond). 2007;31(2):334–9.
22. King NA, et al. Individual variability following 12 weeks of supervised exercise: identification and characterization of compensation for exercise-induced weight loss. Int J Obes (Lond). 2008;32(1):177–84.
23. King NA, Tremblay A, Blundell JE. Effects of exercise on appetite control: implications for energy balance. Med Sci Sports Exerc. 1997;29(8):1076–89.
24. Kriemler S, et al. Impact of a single exercise bout on energy expenditure and spontaneous physical activity of obese boys. Pediatr Res. 1999;46(1):40–4.
25. Schubert MM, et al. Acute exercise and subsequent energy intake. A meta-analysis. Appetite. 2013;63:92–104.
26. Thivel D, Duché P, Morio B. Energy intake and appetite response to acute short duration exercise in obese youths. Appl Physiol Nutr Metab. 2012; 37(5):1014–5.
27. Thivel D, et al. The 24-h energy intake of obese adolescents is spontaneously reduced after intensive exercise: a randomized controlled trial in calorimetric chambers. PLoS One. 2012;7(1):e29840.
28. Thivel D, et al. Gender effect on exercise-induced energy intake modification among obese adolescents. Appetite. 2011;56(3):658–61.
29. Thivel D, Saunders TJ, Chaput JP. Physical activity in children and youth may have greater impact on energy intake than energy expenditure. J Nutr Educ Behav. 2013;45(1):e1.
30. Thompson DA, Wolfe LA, Eikelboom R. Acute effects of exercise intensity on appetite in young men. Med Sci Sports Exerc. 1988;20(3):222–7.
31. Cameron JD, et al. Energy depletion by diet or aerobic exercise alone: impact of energy deficit modality on appetite parameters. Am J Clin Nutr. 2016;103(4):1008–16.
32. Moore MS, et al. Short-term appetite and energy intake following imposed exercise in 9- to 10-year-old girls. Appetite. 2004;43(2):127–34.
33. Thivel D, et al. Acute post-exercise energy and macronutrient intake in lean and obese youth: A systematic review and meta-analysis. It J Obes (Lond). 2016. doi:10.1038/ijo.2016.122.
34. Thivel D, et al. Intensive exercise: a remedy for childhood obesity? Physiol Behav. 2011;102(2):132–6.
35. Danielzik S, et al. Parental overweight, socioeconomic status and high birth weight are the major determinants of overweight and obesity in 5–7 y-old children: baseline data of the Kiel Obesity Prevention Study (KOPS). Int J Obes Relat Metab Disord. 2004;28(11):1494–502.
36. Reilly JJ, et al. Early life risk factors for obesity in childhood: cohort study. BMJ. 2005;330(7504):1357.
37. Pescatello LS, American College of Sports Medicine. ACSM's guidelines for exercise testing and prescription. 9th ed. Philadelphia: Wolters Kluwer/ Lippincott Williams & Wilkins Health; 2014. p. 456. xxiv.
38. Faul F, et al. G*Power 3: a flexible statistical power analysis program for the social, behavioral, and biomedical sciences. Behav Res Methods. 2007;39(2):175–91.
39. Cole TJ, et al. Establishing a standard definition for child overweight and obesity worldwide: international survey. BMJ. 2000;320(7244):1240–3.
40. Tyrrell VJ, et al. Foot-to-foot bioelectrical impedance analysis: a valuable tool for the measurement of body composition in children. Int J Obes Relat Metab Disord. 2001;25(2):273–8.
41. Kaminsky LA, American College of Sports Medicine. ACSM's health-related physical fitness assessment manual. 3rd ed. Philadelphia: Wolters Kluwer Health/Lippincott Williams & Wilkins Health; 2010. p. 172. xiii.
42. Borg GA. Psychophysical bases of perceived exertion. Med Sci Sports Exerc. 1982;14(5):377–81.
43. Quinart S, et al. Evaluation of cardiorespiratory fitness using three field tests in obese adolescents: validity, sensitivity and prediction of peak VO2. J Sci Med Sport. 2014;17(5):521–5.
44. Mannini A, et al. Activity recognition using a single accelerometer placed at the wrist or ankle. Med Sci Sports Exerc. 2013;45(11):2193–203.
45. Keller KL, et al. Potential of an analog scaling device for measuring fullness in children: development and preliminary testing. Appetite. 2006;47(2):233–43.
46. Donnelly JE, et al. Does increased exercise or physical activity alter ad-libitum daily energy intake or macronutrient composition in healthy adults? A systematic review. PLoS One. 2014;9(1):e83498.
47. Cornier MA, et al. The effects of exercise on the neuronal response to food cues. Physiol Behav. 2012;105(4):1028–34.
48. Paravidino VB, et al. Effect of Exercise Intensity on Spontaneous Physical Activity Energy Expenditure in Overweight Boys: A Crossover Study. PLoS One. 2016;11(1):e0147141.
49. Washburn RA, et al. Does increased prescribed exercise alter non-exercise physical activity/energy expenditure in healthy adults? A systematic review. Clin Obes. 2014;4(1):1–20.
50. Champagne CM, et al. Assessment of energy intake underreporting by doubly labeled water and observations on reported nutrient intakes in children. J Am Diet Assoc. 1998;98(4):426–33.
51. Xu S, Xue Y. Pediatric obesity: Causes, symptoms, prevention and treatment. Exp Ther Med. 2016;11(1):15–20.

11

A dietary cholesterol challenge study to assess *Chlorella* supplementation in maintaining healthy lipid levels in adults: a double-blinded, randomized, placebo-controlled study

Sangmi Kim[1†], Joohee Kim[1†], Yeni Lim[1], You Jin Kim[1], Ji Yeon Kim[2] and Oran Kwon[1*]

Abstract

Background: Previous animal studies suggested that *Chlorella*, a unicellular green alga, has a preventive role in maintaining serum cholesterol levels against excess dietary cholesterol intake. This study aimed to conduct a pioneering investigation to clarify this issue in healthy subjects by adopting a dietary cholesterol challenge, which has not been used previously in similar studies of *Chlorella* in hypercholesterolemia.

Methods: In this double blind, randomized, placebo-controlled study, 34 participants ingested 510 mg of dietary cholesterol from three eggs concomitantly with a usual dose of *Chlorella* (5 g/d) or a matched placebo for 4 weeks.

Results: The dietary cholesterol challenge induced consistently higher concentrations of serum total cholesterol (TC, $P < 0.001$), LDL-C ($P = 0.004$), and HDL-C ($P = 0.010$) compared with baseline values, suggesting that the challenge was reliable. Thus, we observed a preventive action of *Chlorella* in maintaining serum TC versus placebo levels (3.5 % versus 9.8 %, respectively; $P = 0.037$) and LDL-C versus placebo levels (1.7 % versus 14.3 %, respectively; $P = 0.012$) against excessive dietary cholesterol intake and in augmenting HDL-C versus placebo levels (8.3 % versus 3.8 %, respectively). Furthermore, serum α-carotene showed the best separation between the placebo and *Chlorella* groups (R^2X and $R^2Y > 0.5$; $Q^2 > 0.4$).

Conclusion: The results suggest that a fully replicated dietary cholesterol challenge may be useful in assessing the effectiveness of dietary supplements in maintaining the serum lipid profiles of adults whose habitual diets are high in cholesterol.

Trial registration: WHO International Clinical Trials Registry Platform (KCT0000258)

Keywords: Carotenoids, *Chlorella*, Dietary cholesterol challenge, Healthy adult

Background

Cardiovascular disease (CVD) is the leading cause of mortality worldwide as a result of the aging population and increased urbanization. A high serum cholesterol level is thought to be a major risk factor for CVD [1]. Each 1 % increase in the serum cholesterol is predicted to increase the risk of coronary disease by approximately 2 % [2]. An impressive body of evidence has accumulated regarding the hypocholesterolemic effects associated with several plant-based foods compared with the placebo group in at risk subjects such as those with mild to severe hypercholesterolemia [3] or compared before and after administration in healthy subjects [4]. In animal models, a preventive effect of a food or food ingredient against hypercholesterolemia could be shown by the co-administration of excess dietary cholesterol in normal animals [5]. However, no successful

* Correspondence: orank@ewha.ac.kr
[†]Equal contributors
[1]Department of Nutritional Science and Food Management, Ewha Womans University, Seoul 03760, Republic of Korea
Full list of author information is available at the end of the article

placebo-controlled clinical trial has yet been explored to validate this concept in human subjects.

Chlorella is a unicellular green alga that contains a wide array of nutrients, including carotenoids, chlorophyll, minerals, vitamins and long-chain polyunsaturated fatty acids [5]. Animal experiments have shown that *Chlorella* inhibited the intestinal absorption of excess cholesterol from the diet and enhanced fecal steroid excretion, thereby preventing hypercholesterolemia [6]. However, several previous human clinical trials, including our own, have attempted only to determine only whether *Chlorella* supplementation is useful to reduce the high cholesterol levels of hypercholesterolemic subjects [7].

Here, we performed a double-blinded, randomized, placebo-controlled trial to investigate the hypothesis that a dietary cholesterol challenge might be useful to evaluate the effectiveness of *Chlorella* supplementation in maintaining healthy serum cholesterol concentration in adults consuming a high cholesterol meal. This approach is based on the previous findings of other investigations, which indicated that consuming three eggs daily could increase serum cholesterol levels in healthy subjects [8, 9]. Furthermore, we examined whether carotenoids derived from the eggs may have hampered the prediction of the responses of serum lipids to *Chlorella* carotenoids by using partial least squares (PLS) regression.

Methods

Test samples

Tablets containing 416 mg of dried *Chlorella* (*Chlorella vulgaris*) or a color-matched placebo (lactose) were kindly provided by Daesang Corp. (Seoul, Korea). *Chlorella* is a unicellular green alga and listed as a functional ingredient in the Korean Health/Functional Food Code with the following specifications: total chlorophyll content > 10 mg/g for identification; and lead < 3.0 mg/kg, cadmium < 1.0 mg/kg, total mercury < 0.5 mg/kg, total pheophorbide < 1,000 mg/kg, and coliform bacteria negative for purity. Daily *Chlorella* supplementation (12 tablets/d) provides 5 g of *Chlorella* containing the following nutrients: 3 g of protein, 180 mg of total carbohydrates, 640 mg of total lipids, 650 mg of dietary fiber, 225 mg of ash, 2,945 IU of vitamin A, 3.7 mg of vitamin C, and 1.1 mg of vitamin E [6]. The dietary source of the cholesterol challenge were pasteurized whole eggs were purchased from a retail market in Seoul, Korea. Daily egg consumption (3 eggs/d) provides 540 μg of lutein, 330 μg of zeaxanthin, 10 μg of β-carotene and trace amount of α-carotene, and 510 mg cholesterol.

Study design

The double blind, randomized, and placebo-controlled study was performed in two phases, a 4-week lead-in phase and a 4-week intervention phase. The length of the intervention phase was determined based on a meta-analysis of plant sterols as cholesterol lowering agents [10]. To detect the postulated difference with 80 % power using a two-sided 5 %, and a 20 % dropout rate, the sample size was estimated to be 34 subjects. The study protocol was approved by the Institutional Review Boards of Ewha Womans University (Seoul, Korea) and registered at the WHO International Clinical Trials Registry Platform as KCT0000258. The study was conducted in accordance with the Declaration of Helsinki, and the results are reported according to the Consolidated Standards of Reporting Trials guidelines [11].

Subjects

After the initial screening, 34 eligible subjects were entered at baseline. For study inclusion, a serum total cholesterol (TC) levels of < 5.18 mmol/L (desirable level) [12] was required of the subjects at the screening visit. The following exclusion criteria were applied: the regular use of medications or dietary supplements; presence of CVD, hypertension, type 2 diabetes, liver disease, renal failure, thyroid disease, or malignant tumors; a family history of hypercholesterolemia; known hypersensitivity to the study products; and pregnancy or lactation. All of the participants provided written informed consent before participation.

Study procedures

Following the 4 week lead in period, the participants were randomly assigned to either the placebo or *Chlorella* group. At the beginning of the study, the participants received one bottle of the test sample and 21 eggs (packaged in threes for a daily supply), enough for seven days, thus allowing for weekly visits. They were asked to take four tablets of the test sample and one egg with each meal, for a total of 5 g of *Chlorella* powder and 510 mg of cholesterol daily. Cooking methods for the eggs were provided to thereby minimize influences on carotenoid absorption. To determine a compliance status, the subjects were asked to answer whether they had followed the dietary instruction and the remaining pills were counted at each visit. The subjects were also required to report any possible adverse events. To assess nutrient intake and monitor dietary compliance, three-day dietary records were analyzed using a computer aided nutritional analysis program (Can-Pro 3.0, the Korean Nutrition Society, Seoul, Korea).

Outcome measurements

At the beginning of the study and 4 weeks after the intervention, overnight fasting blood was collected in serum separator tubes (Becton Dickinson, Franklin Lakes, NJ, USA). The samples were then centrifuged, and the supernatants were stored at -80 °C before analysis. The serum TC, triglycerides (TG), and high-density lipoprotein cholesterol (HDL-C) concentrations were assessed using commercially available kits (Daiichi Pure Chemicals, Tokyo, Japan). The low-density lipoprotein cholesterol (LDL-C) level was calculated using the Friedewald equation (LDL-C = TC−HDL-C−TG/2.2). Serum carotenoid concentrations were measured by HPLC (Shiseido SP 3023, Tokyo, Japan) with a reverse-phase C18 column (Shiseido Capcell Pak, MG type, 5 μm, 4.6 × 250 mm) and UV detector.

Statistical analysis

Data analyses were performed on the intention-to-treat (ITT) population, which included all randomized subjects. Additionally, per protocol (PP) analysis was performed on participants who completed the study. The results of the ITT and PP analyses were comparable, thus only those of the ITT analysis are shown. Variables were tested for normal distribution using the Shapiro-Wilk *W*-test and log transformation was performed on skewed variables. A Student's *t*-test or Fisher's exact test was used to compare the baseline characteristics between groups. An analysis of variance (ANOVA) mixed-effects model was applied to compare changes in nutrient intake, serum lipids, and serum carotenoids with group and time as fixed effects factors and subject as random effect factor. A two-tailed value of $P < 0.05$ was considered to be significantly different. PLS regression was used to correlate measured values of serum carotenoids for serum lipids and identify predictors for responses to *Chlorella* during the dietary cholesterol challenge. PLS regression with 5-fold cross-validation leads to the calculation of the R^2X, R^2Y, and Q^2 factors, representing the explanation, fitness, and prediction power, respectively. $R^2 > 0.5$ and $Q^2 > 0.4$ [13] were considered acceptable for PLS regression. The data were analyzed using the SAS 9.3 statistical software (SAS Institute, Cary, NC, USA) or TANAGRA (version1.4.50, University of Lyon, France).

Results

Subject characteristics and dietary monitoring

The CONSORT flow chart of the study is shown in Fig. 1. Following the 4-week lead-in period, 34 eligible subjects were randomized into two groups. Five subjects were withdrawn from the study due to lack of interest ($n = 1$) or loss of contact ($n = 4$). The compliance was excellent (mean compliance ratio for all subjects = 97.5 %) with no subjects were excluded due to insufficient compliance. No participant reported any significant subjective symptoms or serious events.

The participant characteristics at baseline are shown in Table 1. All subjects were in good health, as determined by physical examination and routine blood and urine biochemical screening. Randomization was successful, and no significant differences were observed in the baseline findings between the groups. The daily intakes of calories and some selected nutrients at baseline and week 4 are listed in Table 2. Within each group, cholesterol intake increased by approximately 3-fold by adding three eggs to the usual diet ($P < 0.001$ for time effect). No significant between-group differences were observed for any nutrient, however, β-carotene intake was significantly increased in the *Chlorella* group compared to the placebo group ($P = 0.010$ for interaction). Unexpectedly, carbohydrate intake was decreased in both groups ($P = 0.033$ for time effect).

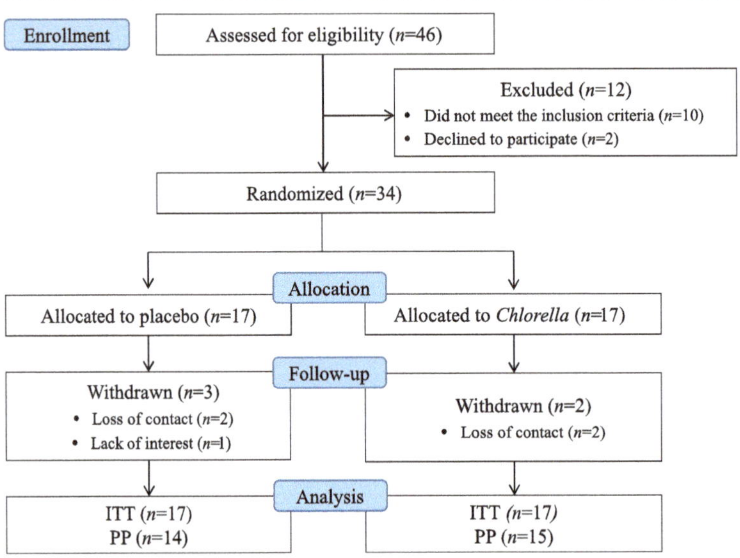

Fig. 1 CONSORT diagram for the flow of subjects through the study. ITT, intention-to-treat; PP, per protocol

Table 1 Characteristics of the participants at baseline

	Placebo group ($n = 17$)	*Chlorella* group ($n = 17$)	*P*-value
Age, y	23.7 ± 0.8	23.2 ± 0.6	0.639
Female/Male, *n*	15/2	15/2	1.000
BMI, kg/m^2	19.7 ± 0.5	20.7 ± 0.4	0.130
SBP, mmHg	106.4 ± 2.4	104.4 ± 2.3	0.557
DBP, mmHg	63.8 ± 1.9	64.6 ± 1.7	0.737
Fasting serum levels, mmol/L			
TC	4.24 ± 0.16	4.38 ± 0.12	0.495
TG	0.76 ± 0.07	0.83 ± 0.08	0.678
LDL-C	2.28 ± 0.11	2.49 ± 0.11	0.186
HDL-C	1.58 ± 0.08	1.55 ± 0.06	0.737

Values are the means ± SEMs (all such values). *P*-values are for Student's *t*-test or Fisher's exact test used to compare the between-group differences. *BMI* body mass index, *SBP* systolic blood pressure, *DBP* diastolic blood pressure, *TC* total cholesterol, *TG* triglycerides, *LDL-C* low-density lipoprotein cholesterol, *HDL-C* high-density lipoprotein cholesterol

The role of Chlorella in maintaining health serum lipid profiles following a dietary cholesterol challenge

No difference in baseline concentrations of serum lipids was observed between the two groups. After 4 weeks, the 3-egg dietary cholesterol challenge induced significant increases in serum TC ($P < 0.001$ for time effect), LDL-C ($P = 0.004$ for time effect), and HDL-C ($P = 0.010$ for time effect) in the placebo group. In contrast, concomitant ingestion of 5 g *Chlorella* significantly suppressed the increases of TC (9.8 % versus 3.5 %; $P = 0.037$ for interaction) and LDL-C (14.3 % versus 1.7 %; $P = 0.012$ for interaction), but accelerated the increase of HDL-C (3.8 % versus 8.3 %), a finding that lacked statistical significance (Table 3, upper part).

Serum carotenoids as a predictor of serum lipid responses to Chlorella supplementation

The daily ingestion of three eggs resulted in significant increases in the serum lutein, α-carotene and β-carotene levels ($P < 0.001$ for time effect for all) in the placebo group. Concomitant intake of *Chlorella* supplementation led to a significant enhancement of lutein (76 % versus 123 %; $P = 0.006$ for interaction) and α-carotene (31.2 % versus 228 %, $P < 0.001$ for interaction) levels. However, serum β-carotene concentration remained unchanged between the two groups (Table 3, lower part).

PLS regressions for each combination of serum carotenoids and lipids showed that data points from β-carotene (Fig. 2a) and lutein (Fig. 2b) were randomly dispersed in the plane and did not show clear discrimination between groups. In contrast, α-carotene showed better separations between the placebo and *Chlorella* groups (R^2X and $R^2Y > 0.5$; $Q^2 > 0.4$) (Fig. 2c). The finding suggests that α-carotene may serve an important parameter for predicting the maintenance effect of *Chlorella* on healthy cholesterol concentrations.

Discussion

The data obtained in this study validated the hypothesis that a dietary cholesterol challenge permitted the determination of a beneficial impact of *Chlorella* on modifying serum cholesterol concentration in subjects whose habitual diets are high in cholesterol. Early changes in metabolic markers may not be easily identified due to the robustness of homeostatic vigor of healthy subjects [14]. The administration of additional dietary cholesterol from three eggs daily created a temporary perturbation in serum cholesterol levels, thus providing a unique opportunity to evaluate the intervention effect of *Chlorella* on the earliest changes in

Table 2 Mean daily intakes of selected nutrients at baseline and during the 4-week intervention

Nutrients	Placebo group ($n = 17$)		*Chlorella* group ($n = 17$)		*P*-value[a]		
	Week 0	Week 4	Week 0	Week 4	Group	Time	Group x time
Energy, kcal/d	1558 ± 124	1505 ± 92	1511 ± 111	1485 ± 81	0.800	0.642	0.860
Carbohydrate, g/d	204.0 ± 16.6	185.6 ± 13.7	214.7 ± 15.3	186.0 ± 11.7	0.734	0.033	0.680
Protein, g/d	63.0 ± 5.5	65.3 ± 3.2	56.2 ± 7.3	64.9 ± 3.8	0.400	0.065	0.394
Fat, g/d	52.7 ± 5.1	55.3 ± 3.3	46.2 ± 3.5	50.5 ± 2.5	0.189	0.338	0.815
SFA, *g/d*	8.2 ± 1.1	9.5 ± 1.1	7.4 ± 1.2	9.6 ± 0.8	0.723	0.071	0.643
PUFA, *g/d*	5.8 ± 0.7	6.5 ± 0.8	6.4 ± 0.9	6.4 ± 0.5	0.664	0.194	0.810
Cholesterol, mg/d	323.5 ± 54.5	725.9 ± 17.5	219.1 ± 32.2	754.1 ± 25.7	0.312	< 0.001	0.220
Dietary fibers, g/d	12.7 ± 1.3	12.6 ± 1.1	11.3 ± 1.1	11.9 ± 0.6	0.665	0.316	0.568
β-carotene, mg/d	2.2 ± 0.4	1.7 ± 0.3	1.9 ± 0.4	2.6 ± 0.2	0.266	0.302	0.010

Values are the means ± SEMs. Intakes were estimated from 3-day dietary records using CAN-pro (Korean Nutrition Society, Seoul, Korea). Egg, *Chlorella* and placebo intakes were included in the analysis. *SFA* saturated fatty acids, *PUFA* polyunsaturated fatty acids

[a]Mixed-effects ANOVA model, with group and time as fixed effects factors and subject as random effect factor

Table 3 Serum lipid and carotenoid responses to the 4-week intervention with *Chlorella* supplementation with three eggs daily

Fasting serum levels (mmol/L)	Placebo group (*n* = 17)		*Chlorella* group (*n* = 17)		*P*-value[a]		
	Week 0	Week 4	Week 0	Week 4	*Group*	*Time*	*Group x Time*
Serum lipids							
TC	4.24 ± 0.16	4.71 ± 0.15	4.38 ± 0.12	4.47 ± 0.12	0.962	< 0.001	0.037
LDL-C	2.28 ± 0.11	2.59 ± 0.11	2.49 ± 0.11	2.51 ± 0.12	0.619	0.004	0.012
HDL-C	1.58 ± 0.08	1.67 ± 0.10	1.55 ± 0.06	1.62 ± 0.05	0.917	0.010	0.404
Serum carotenoids							
Lutein	0.54 ± 0.05	0.89 ± 0.08	0.65 ± 0.03	1.39 ± 0.12	0.001	< 0.001	0.006
α-carotene	0.06 ± 0.01	0.07 ± 0.01	0.08 ± 0.01	0.24 ± 0.02	< 0.001	< 0.001	< 0.001
β-carotene	0.19 ± 0.02	0.27 ± 0.05	0.22 ± 0.02	0.29 ± 0.03	0.292	< 0.001	0.753

Values are the means ± SEMs. *TC* total cholesterol, *LDL-C* low-density lipoprotein cholesterol, *HDL-C* high-density lipoprotein cholesterol
[a]Mixed-effects ANOVA model with group and time as fixed effects factors and subject as random effect factor

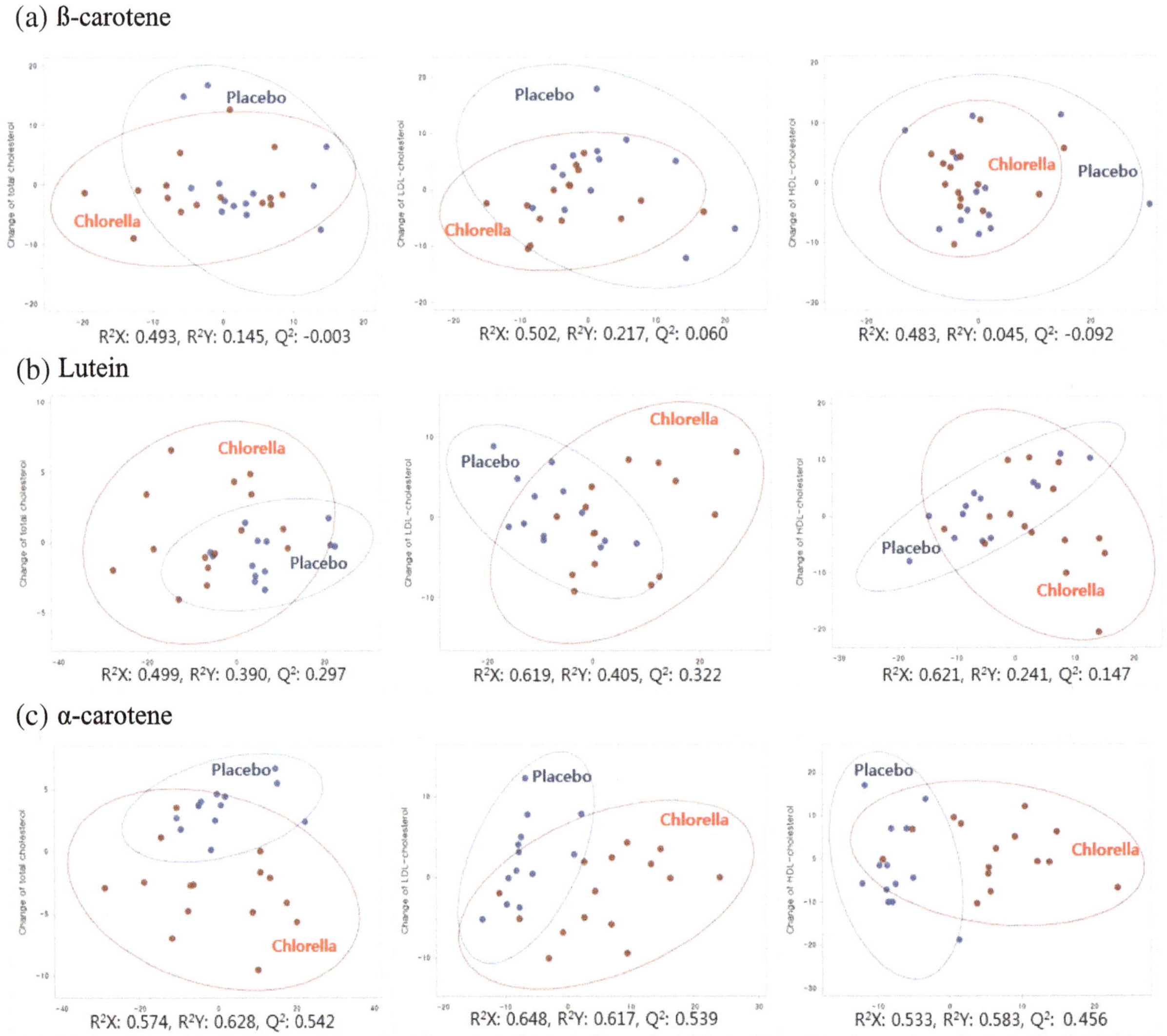

Fig. 2 PLS-regression score plots of each serum lipid and carotenoid obtained from the placebo and *Chlorella* group. R^2X, modeled variation of X; R^2Y, predicted variation of Y; Q^2, cross-validated prediction of Y. (**a**) β-carotene, (**b**) Lutein, (**c**) α-carotene

serum lipid profiles. To the best of our knowledge, this is the first attempt to use a dietary cholesterol challenge to investigate the modifying effect of a food or food component on serum lipid profile in healthy subjects.

Notably, the serum lipid profile changes that ensued from the three egg consumption were modest; (1) the alterations were quantitatively within the normal ranges and the LDL particle subclass was identified as the larger LDL particle [15], which is believed to have a reduced susceptibility to oxidation and endothelial penetration [16]. Furthermore, the 0.40 mmol/L increase in the serum cholesterol we observed in this study in response to the ingestion of 510 mg of additional cholesterol from three eggs was in agreement with previous studies that estimated a 0.05 ~ 0.12 mmol/L increase in the serum TC for each additional 100 mg of dietary cholesterol [17, 18]. Together, these results suggest that the 4-week dietary cholesterol challenge from three eggs each day was fully replicated in magnitude the expected changes in serum cholesterol.

Chlorella contains a wide range of bioactive substances that may act to optimize lipid metabolism. In our previous study, we observed that *Chlorella* carotenoids are highly bioavailable [7, 19]. In this study, we examined whether serum carotenoids derived from *Chlorella* may be used to predict serum lipid responses to *Chlorella* consumption during a dietary cholesterol challenge. Because the eggs also contain high level of carotenoids, we first compared the serum carotenoid levels for each group. In the case of lutein, the daily lutein consumption from three eggs (540 μg/d) increased mean serum lutein levels by 58 % at 4 weeks compared to the baseline value. When *Chlorella* lutein (7,450 μg/d) was added, the mean serum lutein levels increased 2-fold compared to egg consumption only. In regard to α-carotene, *Chlorella* provided high levels (500 μg/d), whereas eggs provided trace amounts. The mean serum α-carotene level was increased 8-fold following *Chlorella* supplementation compared to egg consumption only. However, the additional β-carotene consumption from *Chlorella* (900 μg/d) was not associated with a significant increase of serum β-carotene level compared to egg consumption only, likely because of the rapid conversion of β-carotene to vitamin A [20].

Then, PLS regression analysis was performed to identify the carotenoids that contributed to predicting the effectiveness of *Chlorella* on serum lipid profile during the dietary cholesterol challenge. Consistent with our previous study in subjects with hypercholesterolemia, the data points from α-carotene showed a better separation by PLS regression analysis. Taken together, the cumulative data suggested that serum α-carotene concentration might be useful, at least in part, to predict *Chlorella* effects on serum lipid concentrations during the dietary cholesterol challenge. However, it is a limitation of this study that we did not determine the underlying mechanism that could explain how the results obtained may have been due to the high concentration of serum α-carotene. Future studies will be needed to confirm the concomitant effects of carotenoids on cholesterol absorption and to understand the pathways and responses initiated by *Chlorella* supplementation following a high dietary cholesterol challenge in laboratory animals and human subjects.

Conclusions

Given the modest nature of the serum lipid response to dietary cholesterol challenge from three eggs daily for 4 weeks, our findings provide an essential foundation for applying a dietary cholesterol challenge can be applied to evaluate candidate foods or food components with hypocholesterolemic properties in healthy subjects. Thereby it is plausible to implicate that *Chlorella* as playing a useful role in maintaining healthy serum cholesterol levels in the environment of free access to high-lipid foods, thus preventing or delaying the risk for CVD.

Abbreviations

CVD: cardiovascular disease; HDL-C: high-density lipoprotein cholesterol; HPLC: high performance liquid chromatography; ITT: intention-to-treat; LDL-C: low-density lipoprotein cholesterol; PP: per protocol; TC: total cholesterol; TG: triglycerides.

Competing interests

The authors declare that they have no competing interests.

Authors' contribution

OK, JK, and JYK were responsible for the study conception and study design; OK and JK were responsible for the supervision of the human study, sample handling, conduction of the analyses, and statistical analysis; SMK and YL conducted the study and performed analyses of the data; JK and YK performed the statistical analysis; OK and JK prepared the manuscript. All authors read and approved the final manuscript.

Acknowledgments

We wish to thank the study participants. This study was supported by an unrestricted grant from Daesang Corp. (Seoul, Korea) and the Ministry of Science, ICT & Future Planning (NRF 2012M3A9C4048761). The funding sources had no involvement in the collection, analysis, and interpretation of the data, the writing of this report, or the decision to submit this manuscript for publication.

Author details

[1]Department of Nutritional Science and Food Management, Ewha Womans University, Seoul 03760, Republic of Korea. [2]Department of Food Science and Technology, Seoul National University of Science and Technology, Seoul 01811, Republic of Korea.

References

1. Wu T, Trevisan M, Genco RJ, Falkner KL, Dorn JP, Sempos CT. Examination of the relation between periodontal health status and cardiovascular risk factors: serum total and high density lipoprotein cholesterol, C-reactive protein, and plasma fibrinogen. Am J Epidemiol. 2000;151:273–82.
2. The Lipid Research Clinics Coronary Primary Prevention Trial results. II. The relationship of reduction in incidence of coronary heart disease to cholesterol lowering. JAMA 1984; 251:365-374.

3. Lu TM, Chiu HF, Shen YC, Chung CC, Venkatakrishnan K, Wang CK. Hypocholesterolemic efficacy of quercetin rich onion juice in healthy mild hypercholesterolemic adults: a pilot study. Plant Foods Hum Nutr. 2015;70: 395–400.
4. Alvarez-Suarez JM, Giampieri F, Tulipani S, Casoli T, Di Stefano G, Gonzalez-Paramas AM, Santos-Buelga C, Busco F, Quiles JL, Cordero MD, et al. One-month strawberry-rich anthocyanin supplementation ameliorates cardiovascular risk, oxidative stress markers and platelet activation in humans. J Nutr Biochem. 2014;25:289–94.
5. Bocanegra A, Bastida S, Benedí J, Ródenas S, Sánchez-Muniz FJ. Characteristics and nutritional and cardiovascular-health properties of seaweeds. J Med Food. 2009;12:236–58.
6. Lee HS, Park HJ, Kim MK. Effect of Chlorella vulgaris on lipid metabolism in Wistar rats fed high fat diet. Nutr Res Pract. 2008;2:204–10.
7. Ryu NH, Lim Y, Park JE, Kim J, Kim JY, Kwon SW, Kwon O. Impact of daily Chlorella consumption on serum lipid and carotenoid profiles in mildly hypercholesterolemic adults: a double-blinded, randomized, placebo-controlled study. Nutr J. 2014;13:57–64.
8. Weggemans RM, Zock PL, Katan MB. Dietary cholesterol from eggs increases the ratio of total cholesterol to high-density lipoprotein cholesterol in humans: a meta-analysis. Am J Clin Nutr. 2001;73:885–91.
9. Fernandez ML. Dietary cholesterol provided by eggs and plasma lipoproteins in healthy populations. Curr Opin Clin Nutr Metab Care. 2006;9:8–12.
10. Abumweis SS, Barake R, Jones PJ: Plant sterols/stanols as cholesterol lowering agents: A meta-analysis of randomized controlled trials. Food Nutr Res 2008, 52 doi: 10.3402/fnr.v52i0.1811
11. Moher D, Hopewell S, Schulz KF, Montori V, Gøtzsche PC, Devereaux PJ, Elbourne D, Egger M, Altman DG, CONSORT. CONSORT 2010 explanation and elaboration: updated guidelines for reporting parallel group randomised trials. Int J Surg. 2012;10:28–55.
12. National Cholesterol Education Program (NCEP) Expert Panel on Detection, Evaluation, and Treatment of High Blood Cholesterol in Adults (Adult Treatment Panel III). Third report of the National Cholesterol Education Program (NCEP) expert panel on detection, evaluation, and treatment of high blood cholesterol in adults (adult treatment panel III) final report. Circulation. 2002;106:3143–421.
13. Paban V, Fauvelle F, Alescio-Lautier B. Age-related changes in metabolic profiles of rat hippocampus and cortices. Eur J Neurosci. 2010;31:1063–73.
14. Wopereis S, Rubingh CM, van Erk MJ, Verheij ER, van Vliet T, Cnubben NH, Smilde AK, van der Greef J, van Ommen B, Hendriks HF. Metabolic profiling of the response to an oral glucose tolerance test detects subtle metabolic changes. PLoS One. 2009;4:e4525.
15. Greene CM, Zern TL, Wood RJ, Shrestha S, Aggarwal D, Sharman MJ, Volek JS, Fernandez ML. Maintenance of the LDL cholesterol: HDL cholesterol ratio in an elderly population given a dietary cholesterol challenge. J Nutr. 2005;135:2793–8.
16. Aiyer AN, Kip KE, Marroquin OC, Mulukutla SR, Edmundowicz D, Reis SE. Racial differences in coronary artery calcification are not attributed to differences in lipoprotein particle sizes: the Heart Strategies Concentrating on Risk Evaluation (Heart SCORE) study. Am Heart J. 2007;153:328–34.
17. Hegsted DM. Serum-cholesterol response to dietary cholesterol: a re-evaluation. Am J Clin Nutr. 1986;44:299–305.
18. Hopkins PN. Effects of dietary cholesterol on serum cholesterol: a meta-analysis and review. Am J Clin Nutr. 1992;55:1060–70.
19. Jung HY, Ok HM, Park MY, Kim JY, Kwon O. Bioavailability of carotenoids from chlorella powder in healthy subjects: A comparison with marigold petal extract. J Funct Foods. 2016;21:27–35.
20. Yeum KJ, Russell RM. Carotenoid bioavailability and bioconversion. Annu Rev Nutr. 2002;22:483–504.

Replacing American snacks with tree nuts increases consumption of key nutrients among US children and adults: results of an NHANES modeling study

Colin D. Rehm* and Adam Drewnowski

Abstract

Background: Replacing typical American snacks with tree nuts may be an effective way to improve diet quality and compliance with the 2015–2020 Dietary Guidelines for Americans (DGAs).

Objective: To assess and quantify the impact of replacing typical snacks with composite tree nuts or almonds on diet metrics, including empty calories (i.e., added sugars and solid fats), individual fatty acids, macronutrients, nutrients of public health concern, including sodium, fiber and potassium, and summary measures of diet quality.

Methods: Food pattern modeling was implemented in the nationally representative 2009–2012 National Health and Examination Survey (NHANES) in a population of 17,444 children and adults. All between-meal snacks, excluding beverages, were replaced on a per calorie basis with a weighted tree nut composite, reflecting consumption patterns in the population. Model 1 replaced all snacks with tree nuts, while Model 2 exempted whole fruits, non-starchy vegetables, and whole grains (>50% of total grain content). Additional analyses were conducted using almonds only. Outcomes of interest were empty calories (i.e., solid fats and added sugars), saturated and mono- and polyunsaturated fatty acids, fiber, protein, sodium, potassium and magnesium. The Healthy Eating Index-2010, which measures adherence to the 2010 Dietary Guidelines for Americans, was used as a summary measure of diet quality.

Results: Compared to observed diets, modeled food patterns were significantly lower in empty calories (−20.1% and −18.7% in Model 1 and Model 2, respectively), added sugars (−17.8% and −16.9%), solid fats (−21.0% and −19.3%), saturated fat (−6.6% and −7.1%)., and sodium (−12.3% and −11.2%). Modeled patterns were higher in oils (65.3% and 55.2%), monounsaturated (35.4% and 26.9%) and polyunsaturated fats (42.0% and 35.7%), plant omega 3 s (53.1% and 44.7%), dietary fiber (11.1% and 14.8%), and magnesium (29.9% and 27.0%), and were modestly higher in potassium (1.5% and 2.9%). HEI-2010 scores were significantly higher in Model 1 (67.8) and in Model 2 (69.7) compared to observed diets (58.5). Replacing snacks with almonds only produced similar results; the decrease in sodium was more modest and no increase in plant omega-3 fats was observed.

Conclusion: Replacing between-meal snacks with tree nuts or almonds led to more nutrient-rich diets that were lower in empty calories and sodium and had more favorable fatty acid profiles. Food pattern modeling using NHANES data can be used to assess the likely nutritional impact of dietary guidance.

Keywords: Nuts, Diet quality, Snacks

* Correspondence: crehm@uw.edu
Center for Public Health Nutrition, University of Washington, Seattle, WA 98195-3410, USA

Introduction

Between-meal snacks represent an important source of solid fats, added sugars, and sodium in the American diet [1–6]. The USDA has identified solid fats and added sugars (SoFAs) as the main sources of "empty" calories, contributing ample energy but few nutrients [7, 8]. Snacking between meals is consistently listed among potential causes of obesity and weight gain [9–11] and is an issue of public health concern.

Healthier snacking patterns could improve diet quality by reducing empty calories and sodium, and increasing intakes of some insufficiently consumed nutrients [12, 13], including fiber and potassium [14]. Healthier snack patterns may also shift the fatty acid ratio away from solid fats towards oils, by increasing mono- and polyunsaturated fats (MUFAs and PUFAs), and plant-based omega-3 fatty acids, and reducing saturated and *trans* fat consumption [15, 16]. In the United States, consumption of added empty calories (e.g., added sugars and solid fats) and sodium is much higher than recommended, while consumption of some food groups, including whole grains, plant and seafood protein, whole fruits and vegetables lags well below recommended levels [17–19].

Tree nuts, including almonds, walnuts, and cashews, have been featured prominently in multiple dietary recommendations and guidelines [14], as well as consumer-facing recommendations regarding healthy snacking from numerous profesional and advocacy groups, including the American Heart Association, the American Diabetes Association and Academy of Nutrition and Dietetics [20–22]. In the nationally representative cross-sectional National Health and Nutrition Examination Surveys (NHANES), tree nut consumption was associated with better nutrient adequacy, higher diet quality, and improved health risk markers [15, 16, 23]. Prospective cohorts have also observed that consumption of tree nuts reduces the risk of all-cause mortality, deaths due to heart disease, cancer and respiratory disease, the incidence of heart disease, and may reduce the likelihood of weight gain [24–28]. Analyses of dietary trends suggest that the consumption of nuts/seeds among US adults has risen from 0.43 to 0.69 oz-equivalents per day from 1999–2000 to 2011–2012. In 2011–2012, just over 30% of adults consumed ≥5 servings of nuts/seeds per week, the recommended amount per 2000 kcal/d from the 2015–2020 Dietary Guidelines for Americans [14]. While no specific recommendation exists for tree nuts, the trend in their consumption has been particularly strong, increasing 145% from 0.11 to 0.27 oz-equivalents per day from 1999–2000 to 2011–2012 [17]. Among the reasons for the substantial growth in tree nut consumption may be their well-documented health benefits as well as the certification of a qualified health claim for nuts and heart disease in 2003 [29].

Following earlier studies on food pattern modeling [30, 31], we sought to quantify the nutritional impact of replacing between-meal snacks with tree nuts or almonds. First, a tree nut composite was created based on the relative frequency of consumption within the population (e.g., a weighted average of almonds, walnuts, pecans and other tree nuts). In substitution models, between-meal snacks (excluding beverages) were replaced, on a per calorie basis, with this weighted tree nut composite. One model replaced all solid snack foods and a second model replaced all solid snacks, with the exception of whole fruits, non-starchy vegetables and whole grain foods. Based on the well-documented high nutrient density of tree nuts [32], we expected to observe measurable improvements in the quality of food patterns generated. The primary goal was to quantify the impact of such a replacement on key dietary constituents of public health interest, including added sugars, solid fats, empty calories, fatty acids, sodium, potassium and magnesium.

Methods

Study population & dietary data

Dietary data were drawn from two cycles of the nationally representative National Health and Nutrition Examination Survey (NHANES) for 2009–2010 and 2011–2012. Data were available for 17,444 children, adolescents and adults age ≥ 1y. Any children who consumed breast milk were excluded. The sample included 6,881 children and adolescents (age 1–19y) and 10,563 adults (age ≥ 20y). At the time of study initiation (late Summer 2015), these were the latest NHANES dietary data available.

Data from two non-consecutive 24-h recalls were used. The first 24-h recall was completed in-person at the Mobile Examination Center with a trained interview. The second recall was completed over the telephone many days later. The 24-h recall queries all foods/beverages consumed by participants from midnight-to-midnight on the previous day [33]. Eighty-five percent of respondents completed two dietary recalls and the remaining 15% completed a single dietary recall.

Nutrient data was obtained from the Food and Nutrient Database for Dietary Studies (FNDDS); FNDDS 5.0 for 2009–2010 data and FNDDS 2011–2012 for 2011–2012 data were used [34]. Data on consumption of food groups of interest (e.g., nuts/seeds), added sugars, solid fats, and oils were obtained from the Food Patterns Equivalent Database (FPED); the cycle-specific version of FPED was used for each NHANES cycle (e.g., FPED 2009–2010 for 2009–2010 data) [35].

Modeling strategy

Two models were developed. Model 1 replaced all between-meal solid snacks with tree nuts on a calorie-per-calorie basis. Model 2 exempted between meal snacks consisting of whole fruit, non-starchy vegetables, or grain products containing more than 50% whole grains. The models were applied to solid snacks only and did not replace between-meal beverages, whether fruit juices, soft drinks, cola, or alcohol. Between-meal beverages were not included in the substitution models for two reasons. First, we wanted the substitution models to be a like-for-like comparison, where solid foods were replaced with other solid foods. Second, we wanted to keep the amount of energy being replaced to levels that could feasibly be replaced with tree nuts, by including beverages in the substitution models the amount of energy being replaced would lead to infeasible intakes of tree nuts. Beverage additions (i.e., sugar added to coffee) were not replaced. Diets of individuals already consuming tree nuts as exclusive snacks were not modified. Foods were replaced on a calorie-per-calorie basis to observe the impact on diet quality within an isocaloric context.

A composite tree nut was created based on current consumption patterns. First, a list of all tree nuts consumed by NHANES participants from 2009 to 2012 was made (n = 21). Second, the weighted frequency of consumption was estimated and a weight was assigned to each tree nut corresponding to its frequency of consumption. For example, "almonds, not formally specified" were identified as the most frequently consumed tree nut and contributed a weight of 0.268 to the composite tree nut. Other important components of the composite tree nut were walnuts (weight = 0.208), pecans (0.088), dry roasted almonds (0.086), cashews (0.076), dry roasted almonds without salt (0.071), and pistachio nuts (0.069) (see Fig. 1). The nutrient profile for the composite tree nut (per 100 kcal) was then estimated based on these weights. The nutrient profile of the composite tree nut was then used in the models based on the amount of snack energy eligible for substitution. Because almonds were the most frequently consumed tree nut (~44% of all tree nuts), secondary analyses were conducted with a composite almond alone.

The primary outcome measures were dietary outcomes based on nutrients of interest, selected based on their overall importance to current dietary recommendations [14, 36]. Nutrients of interest included dietary fiber, potassium and magnesium; each of which are underconsumed per the 2015–2020 Dietary Guidelines for Americans and the first two are nutrients of public health concern [14]. Furthermore, the 2010 Healthy Eating Index (HEI-2010) was examined as a summary measure of diet quality to measure the global impact of the models on diet quality. The HEI-2010 is an energy-adjusted measure of diet quality based on 12 components, including 9 components to encourage, including total fruit, whole fruit, total vegetables, greens and beans, whole grains, dairy, total protein, protein from plant and seafood sources and the fatty acid ratio (favoring higher ratio of mono- and polyunsaturated fatty acids to saturated fatty acids); and 3 components to discourage, including refined grains, energy from solid fat and added sugars, and sodium. Details on the HEI-2010 algorithm have been previously described [37]. A version of the Healthy Eating Index corresponding to the 2015–2020 Dietary Guidelines for

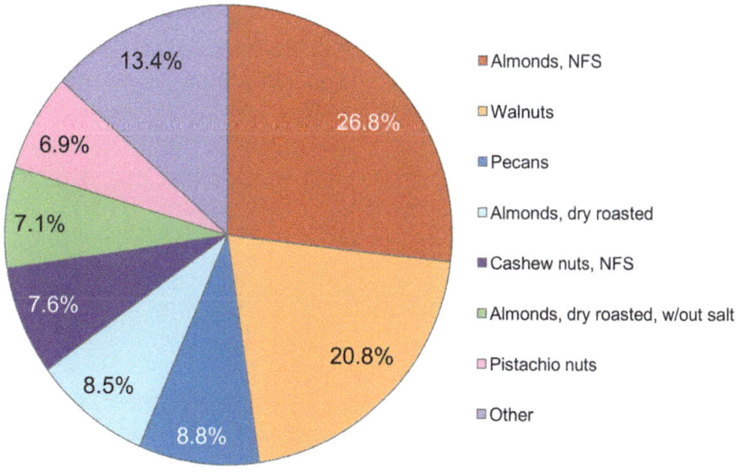

Fig. 1 Breakdown of composite tree nut. Value indicates the relative weight of each tree nut type. For example, "almonds, not formally specified" contributed 26.8% to the composite tree nut. Graph shows all tree nuts contributing more than 5%. Other nuts contributing between 1-5% include, cashews (dry roasted), almonds (unroasted), cashews (dry roasted, no salt), and almonds roasted

Americans is not yet available, but the 2010 and 2015–2020 Dietary Guidelines are generally in alignment regarding nutrients/food groups whose consumption should be encouraged and/or limited [14, 38].

Analyses

The National Cancer Institute (NCI) method was used to characterize the usual intake of nutrients and food groups of interest as observed and for each of the two substitution models [39, 40]. This method can be used to estimate the usual intake of nutrients and food groups, including the population-distribution of intakes. Two models were fit using this method; one for ubiquitously consumed nutrients (i.e., foods/nutrients consumed by most individuals on all days, such as fiber) and another, which incorporates both the mean and probability of consumption for episodically consumed foods/nutrients (i.e., not consumed by most individuals on all days, such as whole grains). Additional covariates were included in the model to account for whether the recall data were from a weekday or weekend and whether it was the first or second recall, which accounted for mode (e.g., telephone vs. in-person) and order effects. Estimates of the population mean and standard error and distribution of intakes were conducted for observed diets and each modeling scenario for the entire population and by age group. The NCI method makes uses of both the first and second recall, and includes all individuals regardless of whether they completed a second recall. To estimate population means for the HEI-2010, the population ratio method was used, which uses a single recall [37, 41]. Code developed by the United States Department of Agriculture was used to estimate the population average HEI-2010 and HEI-2010 component values for the observed diet and two models [42].

In order to account for the complex survey design of NHANES data, balanced repeated replication (BRR) weights were constructed using WesVar software (Westat, Rockville, MD, 2012) and a Fay's adjustment of 0.7. A total of 32 BRR runs were repeated for each analysis, making the results representative of the US population. To determine if mean intakes differed for the different models as compared to the observed we conducted survey-weighted t-tests with an unequal variance, comparing the results of each model to baseline intakes. To place the results in context, we defined a relative change of less than 5% to be "marginal" if the difference was statistically significant ($p < 0.05$). Statistically significant differences ($p < 0.05$), for which the relative change was between 5% and less than 10% (or between −5% and greater than −10%), are described as "modest" or "moderate" changes, while statistically significant changes greater than 10% (or less than −10%), are described as "strong" or "dramatic". Ten percent was selected as the cut-off for "strong" effects as it corresponds to the definition of a "good source" of nutrients or minerals according to the US Food and Drug Administration [43]. A reference line corresponding to the Daily Value (DV) for nutrients with a daily value in units consistent with our analysis are included in all graphics [44]. All output for this paper was generated using SAS software, Version 9.3 and are representative of the US population (SAS Institute Inc. Cary, NC, USA).

Data availability and ethical approval

The necessary IRB approval for NHANES had been obtained by the National Center for Health Statistics (NCHS) [45]. For adult participants, written informed consent was obtained directly from the participating adult. For child participants, parental/guardian written informed consent was obtained and children/adolescents ≥ 12y provided additional written consent. All data used here are publicly available on the NCHS and USDA websites [46]. Publicly available data, such as those used here per University of Washington policies, do not involve "human subjects" and their use requires neither IRB review nor an exempt determination. According to University of Washington policies, these data may be used without any involvement of the Human Subjects Division or the University of Washington Institutional Review Board.

Results

Among the 17,444 study participants, 76.9% consumed a snack on their first recall day (defined as any energy from any food or beverage identified as a snack). Overall, mean energy from all snacks was 303 kcal/d, whereas the median was 204 kcal/d. Among snack-consumers, mean energy from snacks was 394 kcal/d, whereas the median was 293 kcal/d. Mean energy from solid snacks eligible for substitution was 252 kcal/d and the median was 148 kcal/d. For Model 1, the amount of solid snack energy in kcal/d that was eligible for substitution depended on age: 250 (ages 1–3y), 341(4–8y), 374 (9–13y), 350 (14–19y), 316 (20–30y), 309 (31–50y), 285 (51–70y), and 206 (71 + y). Median energy from snacks (293 kcal/d) corresponds to 51 g of almonds or 45 g of walnuts.

The distribution of calories from solid food snacks is presented in Table 1 for snacks eligible for replacement under Model 1 and Model 2, respectively. Under both substitution scenarios, cookies and brownies, ice cream and frozen dairy desserts, cakes and pies and candy containing chocolate were the primary sources of snack calories from solid food. Popcorn, apples, bananas and other fruits and fruit salads each contributed more than 1% of snack calories from solid foods.

Table 1 Summary of snack calories by food category, NHANES 2009-2012

	% of solid food snack calories from each food group under Modeling scenarios	
Food Category[a]	Model 1[b]	Model 2[b]
Cookies and brownies	11.2%	13.5%
Ice cream and frozen dairy desserts	9.1%	10.9%
Cakes and pies	7.2%	8.6%
Candy containing chocolate	5.9%	7.1%
Tortilla, corn, other chips	4.9%	4.8%
Candy not containing chocolate	4.1%	4.9%
Crackers, excludes saltines	3.9%	4.2%
Potato chips	3.6%	4.3%
Doughnuts, sweet rolls, pastries	3.6%	4.3%
Popcorn	3.5%	-
Cheese	3.3%	4.0%
Yeast breads	2.6%	2.6%
Apples	2.0%	-
Pretzels/snack mix	1.9%	2.3%
Bananas	1.8%	-
Pizza	1.7%	2.0%
Ready-to-eat cereal, higher sugar (>21.2 g/100 g)	1.5%	0.8%
Cereal bars	1.4%	0.4%
Yogurt, lowfat and nonfat	1.3%	1.6%
Biscuits, muffins, quick breads	1.3%	1.5%
Cold cuts and cured meats	1.1%	1.3%
Other fruits and fruit salads	1.1%	-
Burritos and tacos	0.9%	1.1%
Other foods	21.0%	19.7%

[a]Food categories from USDA What We Eat in America Food Groups
[b]Snacks eligible for replacement in Model 1 include all solid foods; snacks eligible for replacement in Model 2 include all solid foods, with the exception of non-starchy vegetables, whole fruit, and foods where more than 50% of the grain content comes from whole grains. The USDA considers popcorn to be a whole grain

Results of primary models

The nutrient content of modeled food patterns is presented in Figs. 2, 3, 4 and 5 for the entire population and by age group. Model 1 and Model 2 showed significant declines in consumption of empty calories (–20.1% and –18.7%), and a significant drop in solid fats (–21.0% and –19.3%) and in added sugars (–17.8% and –16.9%). Consistent with the decline in solid fats, consumption of saturated fatty acids (SFA) declined modestly in both models (–6.6% and –7.1%). By contrast, the consumption of oils (+65.3% and +55.2%), total polyunsaturated fatty acid (PUFA, +42.0% and +35.7%), alpha-linolenic acid (ALA, +53.1% and +44.7%) and monounsaturated fatty acid (MUFA, 35.4% and 29.6%) all increased. The significant increase in total fat (+20.5% and +16.8%) was accompanied by a greatly improved mono- and polyunsaturated to saturated fat ratio. Dietary carbohydrates dropped significantly (–13% and –10%), whereas a small but statistically significant increase was observed for protein (+2.6% and +1.7%).

Sodium declined from 3,518 mg/d in observed diets to 3,086 mg/d (–12.3%) and 3,124 mg/d (–11.2%) in Model 1 and 2, respectively. For dietary fiber, an 11.1% and 14.8% increase was observed compared to observed diets. Small changes were observed for potassium (not shown, +1.5% and +2.9%) and strong increases were observed for magnesium (+29.9% and +27.0%).

Change in percent of population meeting recommendations

A change in the proportion of individuals meeting prespecified dietary recommendations is an alternative way of assessing diet quality. For sodium, the percent of the population consuming less than 2300 mg/d nearly doubled from 11.7% as observed to 21.6% and 20.4% in Models 1 and 2, respectively. For dietary fiber, the percent of the population consuming more than 25 g/d increased from 10.7 to 15.9% and 18.8% in Models 1 and 2, respectively.

Age-specific results

Figures 2, 3, 4 and 5 also show the nutrient quality of modeled food patterns for specific age groups. Age-specific effects were impacted by a number of factors, including the frequency of snacking within that age group and the types of snacks typically consumed within that age group. For example, children 4–8y and 9–13y were most likely to consume candy/confectionary as snacks, so their models had a more dramatic impact in reducing sugars. By contrast, older adults were least likely to consume between meal snacks, so the results of snack substitution tended to be weaker in this population as compared to younger adults. Significant declines in empty calories, solid fats and added sugars were observed for all groups, but were most profound among children 4–8y and 9–13y.

Results of almond-only modeling

Sensitivity analyses evaluated the impact of a snack substitution model using almonds only. Almonds were the most frequently consumed type of tree nut during the NHANES 2009–2012 data collection period (see Fig. 1). Substitution modeling using the tree nut composite and almonds-alone produced very similar results (see Table 2). Significant declines in empty calories, added sugars, and solid fats were observed for modeled food

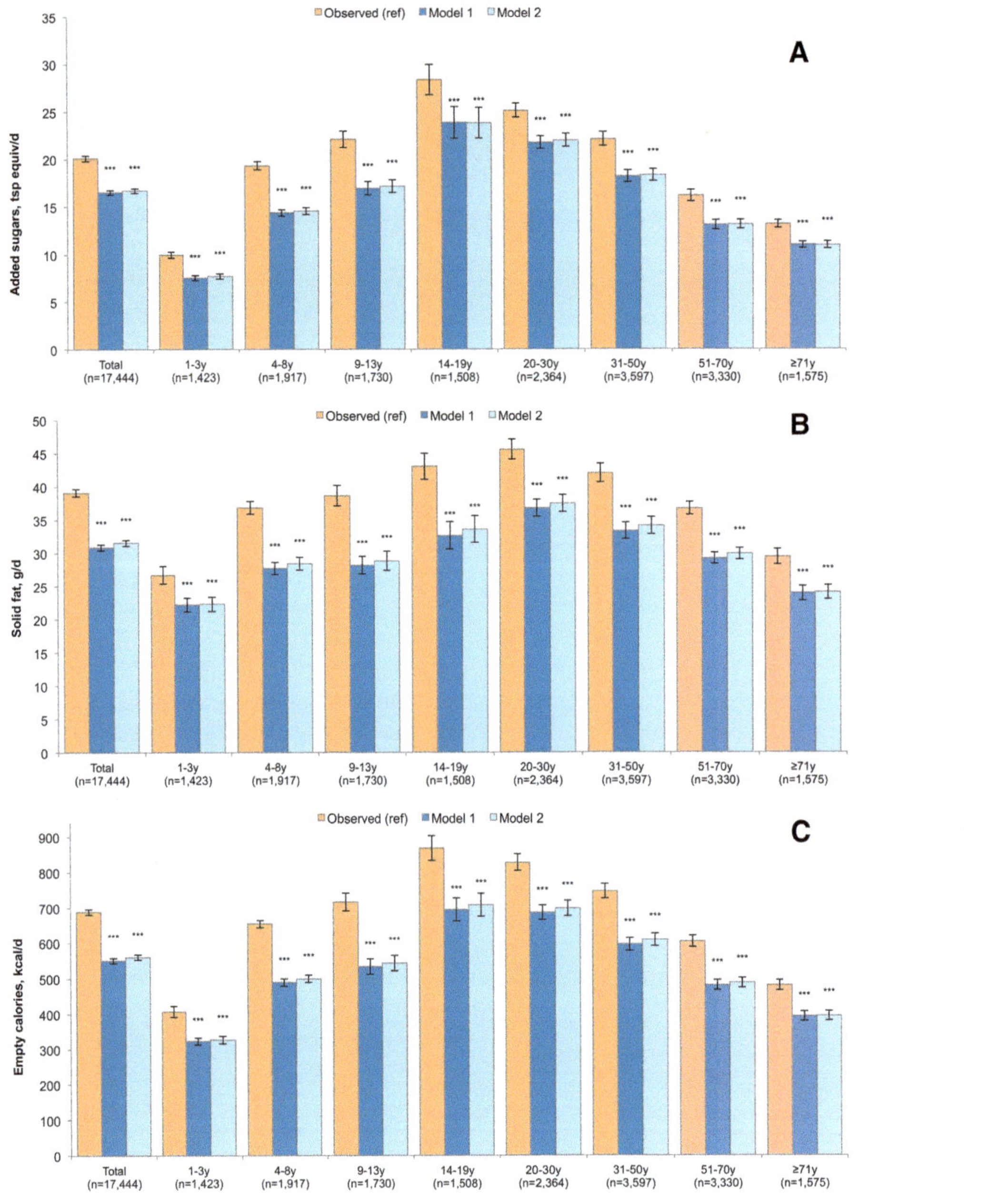

Fig. 2 Added sugars (Panel **a**), solid fats (Panel **b**) and energy from empty calories (Panel **c**) in observed and modeled diets, overall and by age group. Error bars are 95% confidence intervals. Model 1 is substitution of all solid snack foods with the composite tree nut and Model 2 is substitution of all solid foods except for whole fruit, non-starchy vegetables and foods where more than 50% of the total grain comes from whole grains. *P*-value of difference comparing each model to observed value is indicated by asterisk (***$p < 0.001$; **$0.001 < p$-value < 0.01; *$0.05 < p < 0.01$). Hypothesis testing comparing Model 1 to Model 2 was not conducted

patters in both models. A drop in sodium in the almond-only model was weaker but statistically significant. The only difference was a decrease in dietary alpha-linolenic acid (plant based omega 3 essential fatty acid) in the almond-only model as compared to the composite model. This is likely due to the fact that walnuts contain high levels of alpha-linolenic acid whereas almonds do not.

Impact of models on healthy eating index-2010

To measure the total impact of the substitution models on diet quality, the HEI-2010 was examined (see Fig. 6). Based on observed diets, the population mean HEI-2010 value was 58.5 (95% CI 57.4, 59.7). For both models, the HEI-2010 values were significantly higher, 67.8 for Model 1 and 69.7 for Model 2 ($p < 0.001$ for each). For all age groups, the HEI-2010 score was significantly

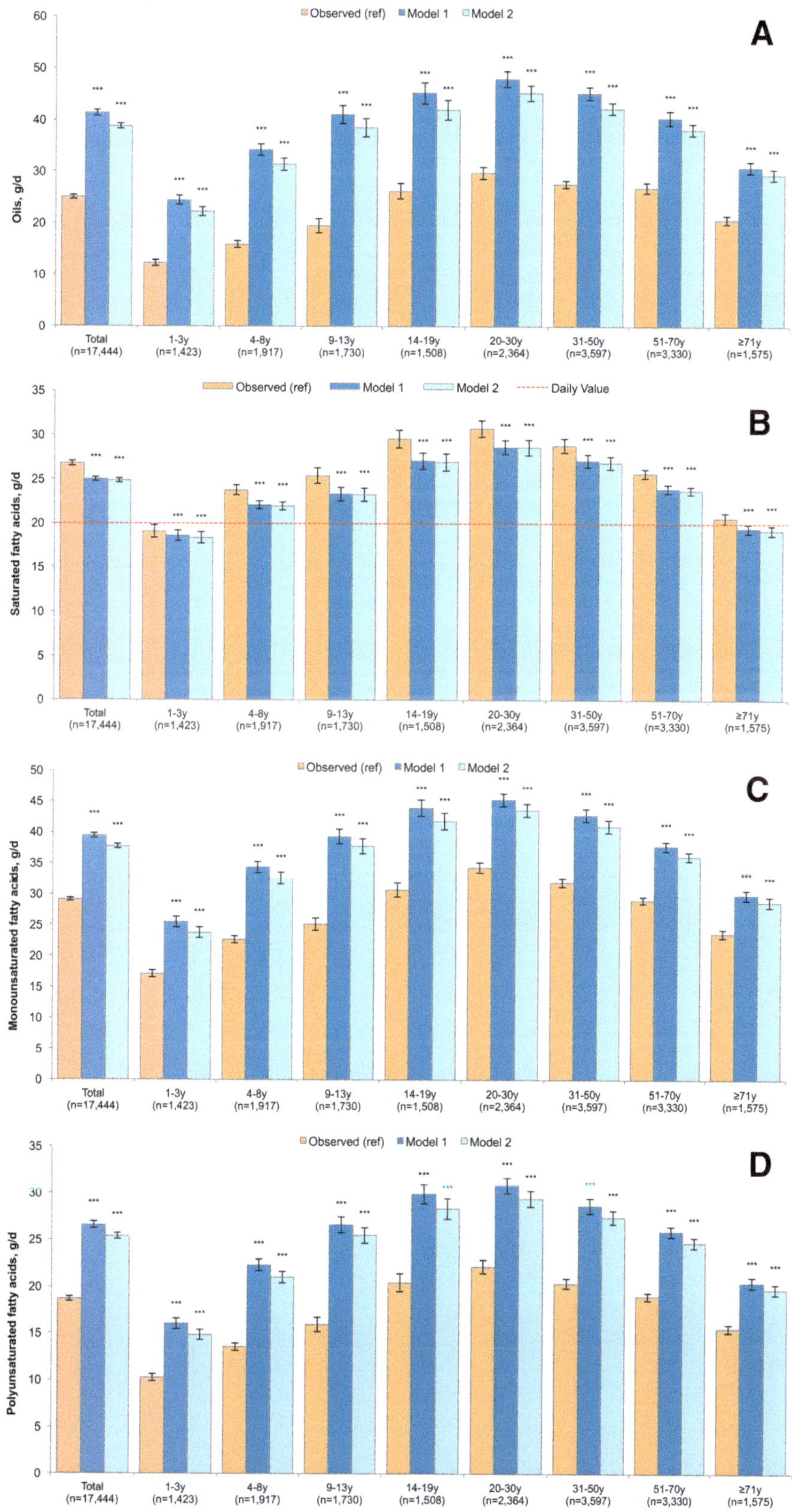

Fig. 3 (See legend on next page.)

(See figure on previous page.)
Fig. 3 Oils (Panel **a**), saturated fatty acids (Panel **b**), monounsaturated fatty acids (Panel **c**), and polyunsaturated fatty acids (Panel **d**) in observed and modeled diets, overall and by age group. Error bars are 95% confidence intervals. Model 1 is substitution of all solid snack foods with the composite tree nut and Model 2 is substitution of all solid foods except for whole fruit, non-starchy vegetables and foods where more than 50% of the total grain comes from whole grains. *P*-value of difference comparing each model to observed value is indicated by asterisk (***$p < 0.001$; **$0.001 < p\text{-value} < 0.01$; *$0.05 < p < 0.01$). Hypothesis testing comparing Model 1 to Model 2 was not conducted. A reference line is provided for saturated fatty acids, which corresponds to the Daily Value, commonly used on food labels. The Daily Value may not apply to children less than 4y and for pregnant or lactating women

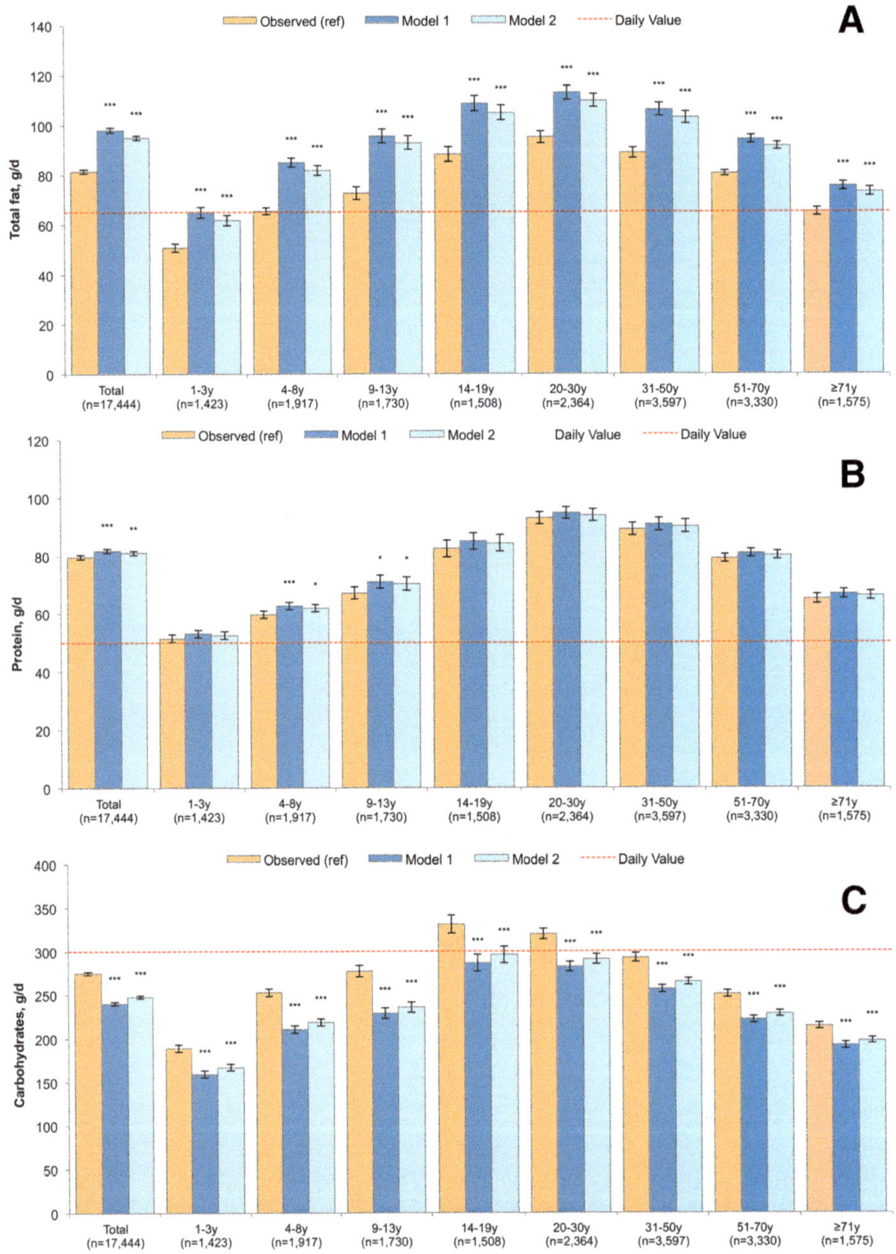

Fig. 4 Total fat (Panel **a**), protein (Panel **b**), total carbohydrates (Panel **c**) in modeled and observed diets, overall and by age group. Error bars are 95% confidence intervals. Model 1 is substitution of all solid snack foods with the composite tree nut and Model 2 is substitution of all solid foods except for whole fruit, non-starchy vegetables and foods where more than 50% of the total grain comes from whole grains. *P*-value of difference comparing each model to observed value is indicated by asterisk (***$p < 0.001$; **$0.001 < p\text{-value} < 0.01$; *$0.05 < p < 0.01$). Hypothesis testing comparing Model 1 to Model 2 was not conducted. A reference line is provided which corresponds to the Daily Value, commonly used on food labels. The Daily Value may not apply to children less than 4y and for pregnant or lactating women

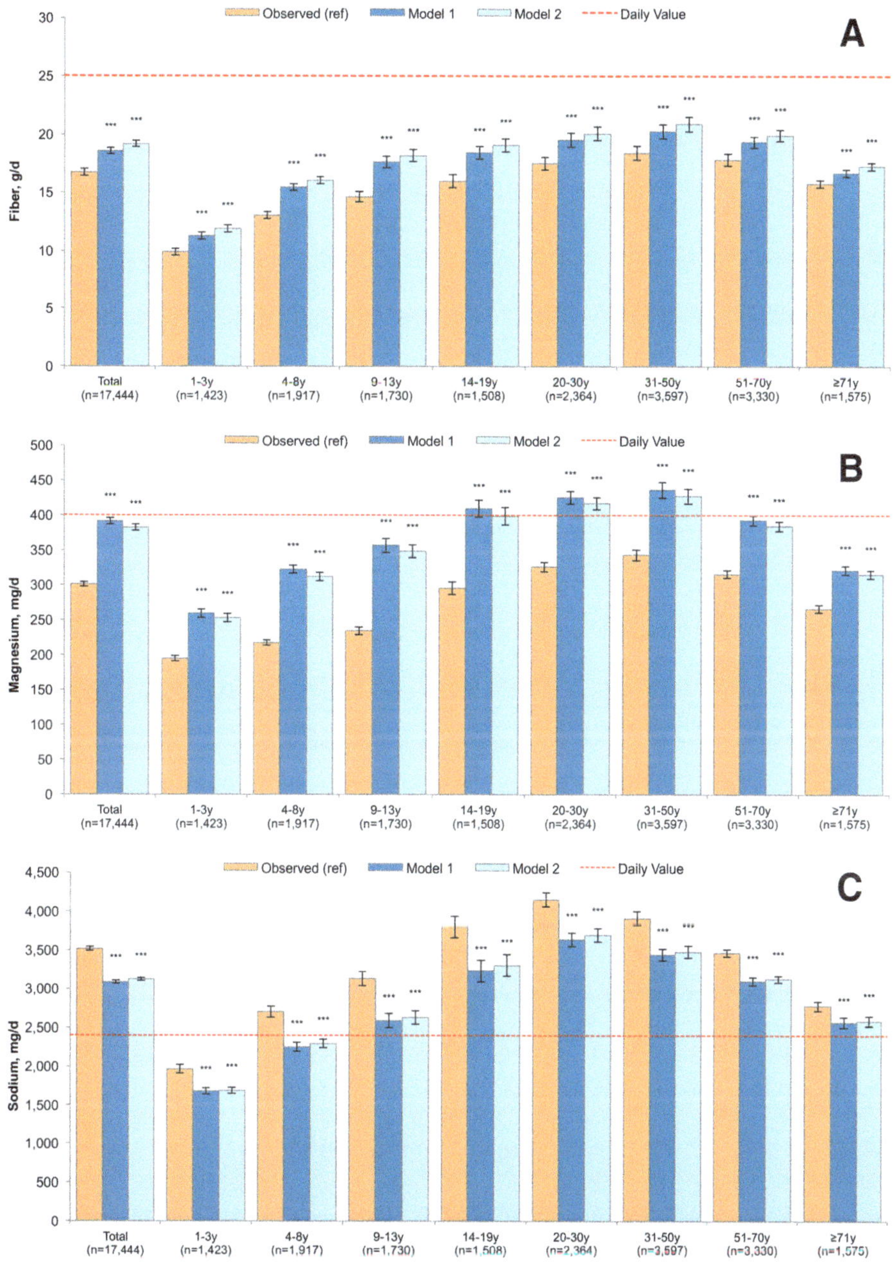

Fig. 5 Dietary fiber (Panel **a**), magnesium (Panel **b**), and sodium (Panel **c**) in modeled and observed diets, overall and by age group. Error bars are 95% confidence intervals. Model 1 is substitution of all solid snack foods with the composite tree nut and Model 2 is substitution of all solid foods except for whole fruit, non-starchy vegetables and foods where more than 50% of the total grain comes from whole grains. *P*-value of difference comparing each model to observed value is indicated by asterisk (***$p < 0.001$; **$0.001 < p\text{-value} < 0.01$; *$0.05 < p < 0.01$). Hypothesis testing comparing Model 1 to Model 2 was not conducted. A reference line is provided which corresponds to the Daily Value, commonly used on food labels. The Daily Value may not apply to children less than 4y and for pregnant or lactating women

higher in both Model 1 and Model 2 as compared to observed diets. The effect was particularly profound among children and adolescents due to low HEI-2010 baseline values and higher frequency of consuming lower quality snacks. As expected, the results of Model 2 tended to be stronger than for Model 1. When evaluating individual HEI-2010 components (see Fig. 7), modest but statistically significant declines were observed for total vegetables, total fruit, whole fruit, whole grains and dairy comparing observed diets to Model 1. However, component values for seafood and plant protein, fatty acid ratio, sodium, refined grains, and energy from solid fat and added sugars all significantly improved. Similar results by component were observed for Model 2, but with no

Table 2 Results of almond-only substitution models, NHANES 2009-2012

	Population mean (95% CI)		
	Observed	Model 1[a]	Model 2[b]
Macronutrients			
Total fat (g/d)	81.5 (80.7, 82.2)	97.2 (96.3, 98.1)***	94.1 (93.2, 95)***
Saturated fat (g/d)	26.8 (26.5, 27.1)	24.2 (24, 24.5)***	24.2 (24, 24.5)***
Monounsaturated fat (g/d)	29.1 (28.9, 29.4)	42.9 (42.4, 43.4)***	40.6 (40.2, 41.1)***
Polyunsaturated fat (g/d)	18.7 (18.4, 19)	22.9 (22.6, 23.2)***	22.2 (21.9, 22.5)***
Alpha-linolenic acid (mg/d)	1651 (1626, 1675)	1420 (1399, 1441)***	1442 (1420, 1463)***
Protein (g/d)	79.8 (79.1, 80.5)	83.8 (83.0, 84.5)***	82.9 (82.2, 83.5)***
Oils (g/d)	25.0 (24.6, 25.5)	40 (39.5, 40.6)***	37.6 (37.1, 38.1)***
Solid fats (g/d)	39.1 (38.6, 39.6)	31 (30.5, 31.4)***	31.6 (31.1, 32.1)***
Carbohydrates (g/d)	275 (273, 277)	240 (239, 242)***	248 (246, 250)***
Added sugars (tsp/d)	20.1 (19.8, 20.4)	16.6 (16.4, 16.9)***	16.8 (16.5, 17)***
Empty calories (kcal/d)	689 (681, 696)	553 (546, 560)***	563 (556, 570)***
Vitamins & Minerals			
Fiber (g/d)	16.7 (16.4, 17)	19.9 (19.6, 20.2)***	20.4 (20.1, 20.7)***
Magnesium (mg/d)	301 (298, 305)	424 (419, 429)***	410 (405, 415)***
Potassium (mg/d)	2683 (2655, 2710)	2777 (2751, 2803)***	2814 (2786, 2841)***
Sodium (mg/d)	3518 (3493, 3543)	3220 (3200, 3240)***	3410 (3387, 3433)***

***Indicates that population mean values between the Model and Observed diets were highly statistically significant ($p < 0.001$)
[a]Model 1 replaced all snack foods
[b]Model 2 replaced all snack foods with the exception of non-starchy vegetables, fruits and foods where more than 50% of the grain comes from whole grains

change in whole fruit, total fruit and whole grains, and modest declines in dairy and total vegetables.

Discussion

Faced with the need to improve US diets, the 2015–2020 Dietary Guidelines for Americans stressed that making small shifts in eating patterns can make a big difference in diet quality overall [14]. One recommendation was to improve the nutrient quality of between-meal snacks, replacing high-calorie snacks with more nutrient-rich options [14]. In a parallel effort to improve diets of children, new federal rules require healthier snacks in schools [47]. Quantifying the impact of replacing typically consumed solid food snacks with tree nuts was the primary purpose of the present study. For the same amount of calories the modeled food patterns replacing

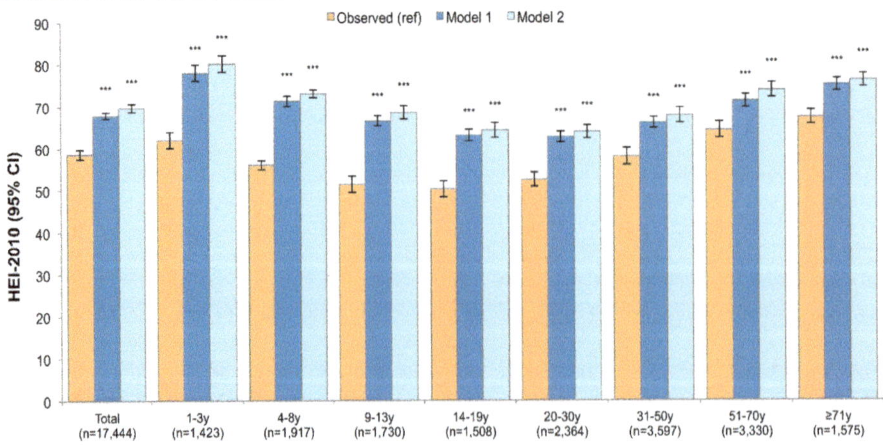

Fig. 6 Healthy Eating Index-2010 in modeled and observed diets, overall and by age group. Error bars are 95% confidence intervals. Model 1 is substitution of all solid snack foods with the composite tree nut and Model 2 is substitution of all solid foods except for whole fruit, non-starchy vegetables and foods where more than 50% of the total grain comes from whole grains. P-value of difference comparing each model to observed value is indicated by asterisk (***$p < 0.001$; **$0.001 < p$-value < 0.01; *$0.05 < p < 0.01$). Hypothesis testing comparing Model 1 to Model 2 was not conducted

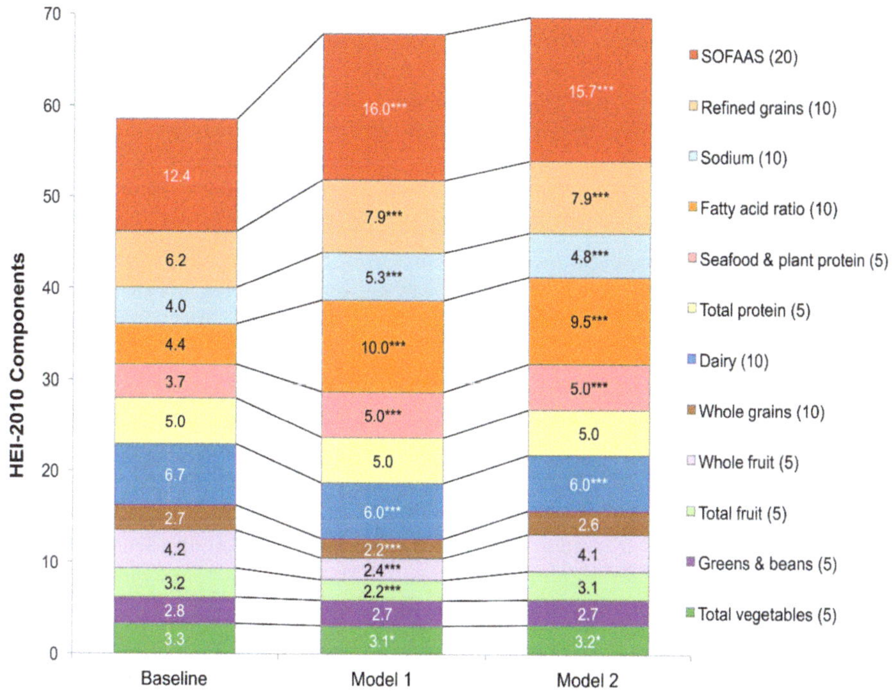

Fig. 7 Healthy Eating Index-2010 components in modeled and observed diets. Model 1 is substitution of all solid snack foods with the composite tree nut and Model 2 is substitution of all solid foods except for whole fruit, non-starchy vegetables and foods where more than 50% of the total grain comes from whole grains. *P*-value of difference comparing each model to observed value is indicated by asterisk (***$p < 0.001$; **$0.001 < p$-value < 0.01; *$0.05 < p < 0.01$). Hypothesis testing comparing Model 1 to Model 2 was not conducted

currently consumed solid food snacks with tree nuts were more nutrient dense. First, there was a significant reduction in empty calorics. Second, there was a shift in dietary fat profiles. The modeled diets had much less saturated fat and a more favorable fatty acid profile, characterized by more oils, more MUFAs and PUFAs, and more plant omega-3 s (alpha-linolenic acid). The ratio of PUFA and MUFA to saturated fatty acids was much more favorable than in observed diets. Total fat content was higher, as might be expected after replacing many refined grains or sugar-sweetened grains with nuts containing fat, fiber, and protein. Overall, Healthy Eating Index-2010 scores improved in the modeled compared to observed diets.

Frequent between-meal snacking has long been an issue of public health concern [48, 49]. In several past studies, increased snacking frequency has been linked to rising obesity rates [9, 10]. First, more frequent snacking has been associated with consuming more calories overall [8]. Second, some of the commonly eaten snacks were of low, if not minimal, nutritional value [8]. Foods and beverages consumed as snacks provided higher proportions of alcohol, carbohydrates, and total sugars relative to calories, while providing lower proportions of many other nutrients. On average, US adults consumed 24% of daily calories as snacks [49]. Consistent with prior reports [3, 50, 51], the most commonly eaten snacks in the US were sweet desserts high in carbohydrates, sugars, and saturated fats. The top items in the 2009–2012 NHANES were cookies, brownies, cakes and pies, ice cream and frozen dairy desserts, chocolate candy and doughnuts, pastries and sweet rolls. Also on the list were corn chips, crackers and potato chips. Between-meal snacks consisting of apples, bananas, yogurts and other fruit were eaten less often.

Substitution modeling of dietary patterns offers a compelling way to test the nutritional impact of dietary guidance [30]. When based on nationally representative dietary data, such models can provide insight into the impact of federal dietary guidelines on the diet of the entire population or specific population sub-groups [30, 31]. The modeled food patterns can be used to evaluate, compare, and rank the impact of following dietary advice on measures of diet quality at the population level. Results of modeling studies can be used to inform effective nutrition communications and the sub-populations that may benefit most from such efforts. For example, we observed the greatest impact of replacing snacks with tree nuts among children and adolescents, as they tended to consume proportionally more nutrient sparse and less healthful snacks as compared to adults. In addition, children/adolescents are less likely to consume nuts/seeds both overall and as a snack [14].

With that said, such models also have limitations. First, for any substitution model, the units of the substitution model are critical (e.g., whether foods are replaced on per-calorie or per-serving). Given the diverse number of foods in the present study and the arbitrary nature of serving sizes, we opted for an isocaloric substitution model. In simple terms, such a model would result in no change in energy intakes, and therefore no change in body weight. However, if applied in practice, given the relatively high satiety of nuts compared to commonly consumed solid snacks, we might expect fewer calories to be consumed [52, 53]. However, this assumption is not verifiable, so relying on an isocaloric model seems most appropriate. Beyond impacts on weight, substantial improvements to the diet independent of energy changes is likely to have considerable population health benefits. Second, as evidenced by the impact of the models on Healthy Eating Index-2010 component scores, replacement of all solid snacks with tree nuts resulted in modest declines in whole fruit, vegetable, whole grain and dairy intakes. Model 1 was agnostic as to the foods being replaced; both less healthful and more healthful snacks were replaced. As expected Model 2, which did not replace whole fruits, non-starchy vegetables or whole grain snacks with tree nuts, resulted in better improvements and no significant declines in HEI-2010 component scores, with the exception of total dairy. However, because it is important to quantify both the positive and potentially negative impact of any model, we opted to use two models, one that universally replaced solid snack foods and another, which more judiciously replaced snack foods. Despite major improvements observed for many of the modeled dietary constituents evaluated, in many cases population mean intakes remained well below recommended levels (e.g., for sodium, fiber and potassium), suggesting that multiple other changes would need to be implemented simultaneously. For example, increasing whole grain, whole fruit or vegetable consumption, specifically through replacing refined grains and foods high in empty calories would also have tremendous population health impact. As such, these models should be viewed as an approach for quantifying and comparing the impact of various strategies, not as a prescription for specific changes an individual should make.

Substitution modeling complements and builds upon past studies comparing the diets of tree nut consumers and non-consumers. In past studies, based on 2005–2010 NHANES data, usual diets of tree nut consumers were also determined using two 24-h dietary recalls and the NCI Method [16]. That study assessed diet quality based on percentages of tree nut consumers below the estimated average requirement (EAR) or above the adequate intakes (AI) relative to non-consumers. Diets of tree nut consumers showed more favorable intakes for vitamins A and C, folate, calcium, iron, magnesium and zinc as well as potassium and fiber. The Healthy Eating Index 2005 score (HEI 2005) was higher for tree nut consumers as compared to non-consumers.

In cross-sectional studies, tree nut consumers and non-consumers were of necessity different people, who may differ by both observed (e.g., age) and unobserved or difficult to measure factors (e.g., health-seeking behavior). By contrast, substitution modeling offers some insight into how diets of individual consumers can be improved by making some small changes in food choices that are based, in part, on the existing eating patterns of the broader population as the tree nut composite was tailored based on population consumption patterns.

Past studies of tree nut consumers and non-consumers found that the two groups did not differ in their usual sodium intakes and both exceeded recommended adequate intake [16]. Given that tree nuts are generally very low in sodium, nut consumers, typical of the American diet consumed excessive amounts of sodium from other sources. In some past studies, tree nut consumers had lower sodium intakes than did non-consumers [15, 54]. Consistent with those data, the present modeling study showed that the sodium content in modeled diets was much lower than in observed diets. Given that a small increase was observed for potassium, there was a decline in the dietary sodium to potassium ratio, another index of diet quality. Comparable patterns were observed for almonds only modeling. These modeled data counter the perceptions that tree nut snacks may act as a vehicle for increasing dietary sodium.

The present study quantifies the impact of replacement of solid food snacks with tree nuts, suggesting that such a replacement may have a profound effect on population diet quality. However, the critical question moving forward is what policies and interventions may be most effective at increasing consumption of tree nuts at the population-level. Schools and childcare settings may be one environment where tree nut consumption could be increased. A number of tools were recently made available online by the US Department of Agriculture to help schools identify those food items that meet Smart Snacks Standards, which were implemented in 2014–15 [55]. Based on these Standards, almonds, dry roasted without salt in 1 oz packages (167 kcal) are compliant with the school guidelines, providing <200 kcal per serving [56], as nuts/seeds are exempt from the total fat threshold. Products consisting of only dried fruit with nuts and/or seeds with no added sugars or fats are also exempt from the saturated fat standard [57]. Additional policies that may promote nut consumption include the adoption of healthy vending policies, though the contribution of vending machines to snack intake at the population-level remains limited. Additional strategies to increase nut consumption may include social marketing and/or mass communication efforts to increase awareness regarding the health benefits of nuts or address potential misconceptions (e.g., that nuts consumption may lead to weight gain) [58]. In addition, targeted subsidies to reduce their cost in comparison to less healthful snacks might be an additional approach to increase their intake [59]. The efficacy of these approaches specific to increasing nut consumption has not yet been established.

The present study had a number of strengths. First, the data are nationally representative and we used the NCI method to estimate usual intake distributions for the entire population and by age group. Second, same-person replacement modeling complements past studies based on consumers and non-consumers of a specific food. Third, we used a composite tree nut, based on existing nut consumption patterns, which allows for a more precise assessment of the potential nutritional effects of behavioral changes. Further, the tree nut composite included both salted and unsalted nuts, weighted by consumption frequency. Therefore, the modeled results are representative of what would be observed if current consumption patterns continued.

Numerous limitations are also worth noting. First, all NHANES data were based on self-reports. Proxy reports were used for young children [60] and some foods may be under-reported, either through omission or error in recording portion sizes [61]. It is also possible that some participants reported tree nuts, while eating peanuts [15]. In addition, the results presented here are based on models and do not reflect actual behavior of individuals. Nonetheless, substitution modeling in the context of a specific meal or eating occasion, offers one way to test the potential nutritional impact of dietary guidance.

Conclusion

Based on present modeling analyses, widespread replacement of solid food snacks with tree nuts or almonds would improve the quality of the diet. Even a partial replacement, exempting already nutrient rich snacks, had a significant positive effect on diet quality. Substitution modeling can provide added insight into the likely impact of following 2015–2020 DGAs on diet quality in the US.

Acknowledgements
Not Applicable.

Funding
Funding for secondary analyses of publicly available federal datasets was provided to the University of Washington Center for Public Health Nutrition from the Almond Board of California. The funder approved the study proposal, but played no role in the data analysis, interpretation, or decision to submit this research for publication.

Availability of data and materials
The datasets supporting the conclusions of this article are available in publicly repository as described below. The authors do not own the data.
National Health and Nutrition Examination Survey data are available from the National Center for Health Statistics (http://www.cdc.gov/nchs/nhanes/nhanes_questionnaires.htm).
The Food Patterns Equivalent Database is available from the United States Department of Agriculture (http://www.ars.usda.gov/Services/docs.htm?docid=23869).

Author contributions
CR and AD conceptualized and designed the study. CR carried out the analyses, reviewed and revised the manuscript, and approved the final manuscript as submitted. AD drafted the initial manuscript, reviewed and revised the manuscript, and approved the final manuscript as submitted.

Competing interest
AD has received grants, contracts, honoraria, and consulting fees from numerous food and beverage companies and other commercial and nonprofit entities with interests in diet quality and health. The University of Washington has received grants, donations, and contracts from both the public and the private sectors. CDR has no financial relationships relevant to this article to disclose.

Consent for publication
Not applicable.

Ethics approval and consent to participate
The necessary IRB approval for NHANES had been obtained by the National Center for Health Statistics (NCHS). For adult participants, written informed consent was obtained directly from the participating adult. For child participants, parental/guardian written informed consent was obtained and children/adolescents ≥ 12y provided additional written consent. Publicly available data, such as those used here per University of Washington policies, do not involve "human subjects" and their use requires neither IRB review nor an exempt determination. According to University of Washington policies, these data may be used without any involvement of the Human Subjects Division or the University of Washington Institutional Review Board.

References

1. Nicklas TA, O'Neil CE, Fulgoni VL 3rd. Snacking patterns, diet quality, and cardiovascular risk factors in adults. BMC Public Health. 2014;14:388.
2. Hess J, Slavin J. Snacking for a cause: nutritional insufficiencies and excesses of U.S. children, a critical review of food consumption patterns and macronutrient and micronutrient intake of U.S. children. Nutrients. 2014;6:4750–9.
3. Piernas C, Popkin BM. Trends in snacking among U.S. children. Health Aff (Millwood). 2010;29:398–404.
4. Evans EW, Jacques PF, Dallal GE, Sacheck J, Must A. The role of eating frequency on total energy intake and diet quality in a low-income, racially diverse sample of schoolchildren. Public Health Nutr. 2015;18:474–81.
5. Hickson DA, Diez Roux AV, Smith AE, Tucker KL, Gore LD, Zhang L, et al. Associations of fast food restaurant availability with dietary intake and weight among African americans in the Jackson heart study, 2000–2004. Am J Public Health. 2011;101(Sppl 1):S301–309.
6. Leung CW, Laraia BA, Kelly M, Nickleach D, Adler NE, Kushi LH, et al. The influence of neighborhood food stores on change in young girls' body mass index. Am J Prev Med. 2011;41:43–51.
7. Choose MyPlate.gov. What are empty calories? Available at: http://www.choosemyplate.gov/weight-management-calories/calories/empty-calories.html. Accessed 16 May 2016.
8. Huth PJ, Fulgoni VL, Keast DR, Park K, Auestad N. Major food sources of calories, added sugars, and saturated fat and their contribution to essential nutrient intakes in the U.S. diet: data from the national health and nutrition examination survey (2003–2006). Nutr J. 2013;12:116.
9. Whybrow S, Mayer C, Kirk TR, Mazlan N, Stubbs RJ. Effects of two weeks' mandatory snack consumption on energy intake and energy balance. Obesity. 2007;15:673–85.
10. Rolls BJ, Roe LS, Kral TV, Meengs JS, Wall DE. Increasing the portion size of a packaged snack increases energy intake in men and women. Appetite. 2004;42:63–9.

11. Mazlan N, Horgan G, Whybrow S, Stubbs J. Effects of increasing increments of fat- and sugar-rich snacks in the diet on energy and macronutrient intake in lean and overweight men. Br J Nutr. 2006;96:596–606.
12. Zizza CA, Xu B. Snacking is associated with overall diet quality among adults. J Acad Nutr Diet. 2012;112:291–6.
13. Leidy HJ, Todd CB, Zino AZ, Immel JE, Mukherjea R, Shafer RS, et al. Consuming high-protein soy snacks affects appetite control, satiety, and diet quality in young people and influences select aspects of mood and cognition. J Nutr. 2015;145:1614–22.
14. U.S. Department of Health and Human Services and U.S. Department of Agriculture. 2015 – 2020 Dietary guidelines for americans. 8th ed. 2015.
15. O'Neil CE, Keast DR, Nicklas TA, Fulgoni 3rd VL. Out-of-hand nut consumption is associated with improved nutrient intake and health risk markers in US children and adults: national health and nutrition examination survey 1999–2004. Nutr Res. 2012;32:185–94.
16. O'Neil CE, Nicklas TA, Fulgoni 3rd VL. Tree nut consumption is associated with better nutrient adequacy and diet quality in adults: national health and nutrition examination survey 2005–2010. Nutrients. 2015;7:595–607.
17. Rehm CD, Penalvo JL, Afshin A, Mozaffarian D. Dietary intake among US adults, 1999–2012. JAMA. 2016;315:2542–53.
18. Powell ES, Smith-Taillie LP, Popkin BM. Added sugars intake across the distribution of US children and adult consumers: 1977–2012. J Acad Nutr Diet. 2016;116(10):1543–50.
19. Banfield EC, Liu Y, Davis JS, Chang S, Frazier-Wood AC. Poor adherence to US dietary guidelines for children and adolescents in the national health and nutrition examination survey population. J Acad Nutr Diet. 2016;116(1):21–7.
20. American Heart Association. Healthy Snacking. Available at: https://health.gov/dietaryguidelines/2015-scientific-report/pdfs/scientific-report-of-the-2015-dietary-guidelines-advisory-committee.pdf. Accessed 15 Nov 2016.
21. American Diabetes Association. Snacks. http://www.diabetes.org/food-and-fitness/food/what-can-i-eat/food-tips/snacks.html? Accessed 15 Nov 2016.
22. Academy of Nutrition and Dietetics. Smart Snacking for Adults and Teens. http://www.eatright.org/~/media/eatright%20files/nationalnutritionmonth/handoutsandtipsheets/nutritiontipsheets/smartsnackingforadultsandteens.ashx. Accessed 15 Nov 2016.
23. O'Neil CE, Nicklas TA, III VLF. Almond consumption is associated with better nutrient intake, nutrient adequacy, and diet quality in adults: national health and nutrition examination survey 2001–2010. Food Nutr Sciences. 2016;7(7):12.
24. Bao Y, Han J, Hu FB, Giovannucci EL, Stampfer MJ, Willett WC, et al. Association of nut consumption with total and cause-specific mortality. N Engl J Med. 2013;369:2001–11.
25. Afshin A, Micha R, Khatibzadeh S, Mozaffarian D. Consumption of nuts and legumes and risk of incident ischemic heart disease, stroke, and diabetes: a systematic review and meta-analysis. Am J Clin Nutr. 2014;100:278–88.
26. Hu FB, Stampfer MJ, Manson JE, Rimm EB, Colditz GA, Rosner BA, et al. Frequent nut consumption and risk of coronary heart disease in women: prospective cohort study. BMJ. 1998;317(7169):1341–5.
27. Mozaffarian D, Hao T, Rimm EB, Willett WC, Hu FB. Changes in diet and lifestyle and long-term weight gain in women and men. N Engl J Med. 2011;364(25):2392–404.
28. Bes-Rastrollo M, Sabaté J, Gómez-Gracia E, Alonso A, Martínez JA, Martínez-González MA. Nut consumption and weight gain in a Mediterranean cohort: The SUN study. Obesity (Silver Spring). 2007;15(1):107–16.
29. Qualified health claims: letter of enforcement discretion—nuts and coronary heart disease. (Docket 02P-0505). pp. 1–4. US Food and Drug Administration. US Department of Health and Human Services; 2003. Available at: http://www.fda.gov/Food/IngredientsPackagingLabeling/LabelingNutrition/ucm072926.htm. Accessed on 16 May 2016.
30. Monsivais P, Rehm CD. Potential nutritional and economic effects of replacing juice with fruit in the diets of children in the United States. Arch Pediatr Adolesc Med. 2012;166:459–64.
31. Rehm CD, Drewnowski A, Monsivais P. Potential population-level nutritional impact of replacing whole and reduced-fat milk with low-fat and skim milk among US children aged 2–19 years. J Nutr Educ Behav. 2015;47:61–8. e61.
32. Salas-Salvado J, Casas-Agustench P, Salas-Huetos A. Cultural and historical aspects of Mediterranean nuts with emphasis on their attributed healthy and nutritional properties. Nutr Metab Cardiovasc Dis. 2011;21 Suppl 1:S1–6.
33. US Department of Health and Human Services: Centers for Disease Control and Prevention (CDC), National Center for Health Statistics. About the National Health and Nutrition Exmaination Survey (NHANES). Hyattsville; 2013.
34. USDA Food and Nutrient Database for Dietary Studies 2011–2012. Food Surveys Research Group Home Page, http://www.ars.usda.gov/ba/bhnrc/fsrg U.S. Department of Agriculture, Agricultural Research Service, 2014.
35. Food Patterns Equivalents Database. United States Department of Agriculture (USDA), Agricultural Research Service, 2014. Available at: http://www.ars.usda.gov/Services/docs.htm?docid=23871. Accessed 15 May 2016.
36. U.S. Department of Agriculture. Scientific report of the 2015 Dietary Guidelines Advisory Committee 2015. 2015. https://health.gov/dietaryguidelines/2015-scientific-report/. Accessed 16 May 2016.
37. Guenther PM, Casavale KO, Reedy J, Kirkpatrick SI, Hiza HA, Kuczynski KJ, et al. Update of the healthy eating index: HEI-2010. J Acad Nutr Diet. 2013;113:569–80.
38. U.S. Department of Health and Human Services and U.S. Department of Agriculture. 2010 Dietary guidelines for Americans. 7th ed. 2010.
39. Tooze JA, Midthune D, Dodd KW, Freedman LS, Krebs-Smith SM, Subar AF, et al. A new statistical method for estimating the usual intake of episodically consumed foods with application to their distribution. J Am Diet Assoc. 2006;106(10):1575–87.
40. Tooze JA, Kipnis V, Buckman DW, Carroll RJ, Freedman LS, Guenther PM, et al. A mixed-effects model approach for estimating the distribution of usual intake of nutrients: The NCI method. Stat Med. 2010;29:2857–68.
41. Freedman LS, Guenther PM, Krebs-Smith SM, Kott PS. A population's mean Healthy Eating Index-2005 scores are best estimated by the score of the population ratio when one 24-h recall is available. J Nutr. 2008;138:1725–9.
42. HEI Tools for Researchers. Available at: http://epi.grants.cancer.gov/hei/tools.html. Accessed 15 May 2016.
43. Guidance for Industry. A Food Labeling Guide (10. Appendix B: Additional Requirements for Nutrient Content Claims). US Department of Health and Human Services. January, 2013. Available at: http://www.fda.gov/Food/GuidanceRegulation/GuidanceDocumentsRegulatoryInformation/LabelingNutrition/ucm064916.htm. Accessed 15 May 2016.
44. Food and Drug Administration. Guidance for Industry: A Food Labeling Guide (14. Appendix F: Calculate the Percent Daily Value for the Appropriate Nutrients). https://www.fda.gov/Food/GuidanceRegulation/GuidanceDocumentsRegulatoryInformation/LabelingNutrition/ucm064928.htm. Accessed 5 Nov 2016.
45. National Center for Health Statistics. National Health and Nutrition Examination Survey. NCHS Research Ethics Review Board (ERB) Approval. Available at: http://www.cdc.gov/nchs/nhanes/irba98.htm. Accessed 15 May 2016.
46. National Center for Health Statistics. National Health and Nutrition Examination Survey. Questionnaires, Datasets, and Related Documentation. https://www.cdc.gov/nchs/nhanes/nhanes_questionnaires.htm. Accessed 15 May 2016.
47. National School Lunch Program and School Breakfast Program. Nutrition standards for all foods sold in school as required by the healthy, hunger-free kids Act of 2010. Fed Regist. 2013;78:39068–120.
48. Piernas C, Popkin BM. Snacking Increased among U.S. Adults between 1977 and 2006. J Nutrition. 2010;140:325–32.
49. Sebastian RS, Wilkinson Enns C, Goldman JD. Snacking patterns of U.S. adults: What we eat in America, NHANES 2007–2008. Food Surveys Research Group Dietary Data Brief No. 4 June, 2011.
50. Jacquier EF, Eldridge AL. Eating dessert foods: behavioral patterns in American children. FASEB J. 2016;30:677.611.
51. Gobbling Up Snacks: Cause or potential cure for childhood obesity? Available at: https://www.ers.usda.gov/amber-waves/2012/december/gobbling-up-snacks-cause-or-potential-cure-for-childhood-obesity/. Accessed 15 May 2016.
52. Mattes RD, Dreher ML. Nuts and healthy body weight maintenance mechanisms. Asia Pac J Clin Nutr. 2010;19(1):137–41.
53. Hull S, Re R, Chambers L, Echaniz A, Wickham MS. A mid-morning snack of almonds generates satiety and appropriate adjustment of subsequent food intake in healthy women. Eur J Nutr. 2015;54(5):803–10.
54. O'Neil CE, Keast DR, Fulgoni 3rd VL, Nicklas TA. Tree nut consumption improves nutrient intake and diet quality in US adults: an analysis of National Health and Nutrition Examination Survey (NHANES) 1999–2004. Asia Pac J Clin Nutr. 2010;19:142–50.

55. Healthier school day. Tools for schools: Focusing on smart snacks. Available at: http://www.fns.usda.gov/healthierschoolday/tools-schools-focusing-smart-snacks. Accessed 15 May 2016.
56. Alliance for a Healthier Generation. Alliance Product Calculator. Available at: https://www.healthiergeneration.org/take_action/schools/snacks_and_beverages/smart_snacks/alliance_product_calculator/. Accessed 16 May 2016.
57. U.S. Department of Agriculture, Food and Nutrition Service. National School Lunch Program and School Breakfast Program: Nutrition Standards for All Foods Sold in School as Required by the Healthy, Hunger-Free Kids Act of 2010: Proposed Rules. Federal Register. 2013;78(27):50132–51.
58 Pawlak R, Colby S, Herring J. Beliefs, benefits, barriers, attitude, intake and knowledge about peanuts and tree nuts among WIC participants in eastern North Carolina. Nutr Res Pract. 2009;3(3):220–5.
59 Afshin A, Penalvo J, Del Gobbo L, Kashaf M, Micha R, Morrish K, Pearson-Stuttard J, Rehm C, Shangguan S, Smith JD. Mozaffarian D1 CVD prevention through policy: a review of mass media, food/menu labeling, taxation/subsidies, built environment, school procurement, worksite wellness, and marketing standards to improve diet. Curr Cardiol Rep. 2015;17(11):98.
60 Troiano RP, Briefel RR, Carroll MD, Bialostosky K. Energy and fat intakes of children and adolescents in the United States: data from the national health and nutrition examination surveys. Am J Clin Nutr. 2000;72:1343s–53s.
61 Lafay L, Mennen L, Basdevant A, Charles MA, Borys JM, Eschwège E, Romon M. Does energy intake underreporting involve all kinds of food or only specific food items? Results from the Fleurbaix Laventie Ville Santé (FLVS) study. Int J Obes Relat Metab Disord. 2000;24(11):1500–6.

Two ghrelin receptor agonists for adults with malnutrition

Jianhua Su[1,2†], Jin Geng[3†], Jisheng Bao[2], Yin Tang[2], Menglan Liu[2], Haibin Yu[2], Yi Han[1], Wei Huang[2*] and Suming Zhou[1*]

Abstract

Background: Ghrelin receptor agonists have been established to be important in ameliorating the nutritional conditions in patients with malnutrition. However, some studies have reported inconsistent results. We aimed to coalesce the available evidence on the efficacy of ghrelin receptor agonists for the treatment of malnutrition.

Methods: We searched PubMed, the Cochrane Central Register of Controlled Trials, and EMBASE for relevant articles published through March 2016. Studies comparing the efficacy of ghrelin receptor agonists versus placebo in malnourished patients were eligible for inclusion.

Results: A total of 12 studies involving 1377 patients were included. Compared with placebo, ghrelin receptor agonists could increase the energy intake (standard mean difference [SMD] 2.67, 95% confidence interval [CI] 1.48 to 3.85, $P < 0.001$), lean body mass (weighted mean difference [WMD] 0.25 kg, 95% CI 0.07 to 0.42, $P = 0.006$), fat mass (WMD 0.92 kg, 95% CI 0.05 to 1.8, $P = 0.038$), and grip strength (WMD 0.31 kg, 95% CI 0.207 to 0.414, $P < 0.001$) of patients with malnutrition.

Conclusion: Our analysis indicated that ghrelin receptor agonists could improve the poor nutritional state of malnourished patients by increasing their energy intake, ameliorating their irregular body composition and improving their grip strength. However, these results might be less conclusive due to the limited sample sizes and one potential publication that has not been released.

Keywords: Ghrelin, Ghrelin receptor agonist, Anamorelin, Malnutrition, Anorexia, Cachexia

Introduction

Malnutrition, a condition that is strongly associated with poor prognosis, is a state of nutrition in which a deficiency of energy, protein and micronutrients causes measurable adverse effects on the body composition, function, and clinical outcomes as well as unintentional weight loss [1]. Malnutrition is a common complication of many diseases, such as chronic heart failure [2], chronic obstructive pulmonary disease(COPD) [3], chronic renal failure(CRF) [4], and cancer cachexia [5]. It may also result from other causes of anorexia, sarcopenia or emaciation, including anorexia nervosa [6], functional dyspepsia [7], and ageing [8]. Thus, a single approach can not reverse all aspects of these complicated syndromes and expect to provide prominent benefits. A comprehensive intervention requires the combination of nutritional support, pharmacotherapeutic methods, and exercise [9].

Ghrelin, a compound predominantly secreted by gastric endocrine cells, is an endogenous ligand for the growth hormone secretagogue receptor and has been shown to increase growth hormone(GH) secretion from the pituitary gland [10]. Ghrelin stimulates appetite and food intake and triggers a positive energy balance through GH-dependent mechanisms [11]. However, because the half-life of ghrelin is short and it must be

* Correspondence: huanwei2212@medmail.com; zhousuming1113@hotmail.com
†Equal contributors
[2]Department of Geriatric Medicine, Wuxi NO.2 People's Hospital, Nanjing Medical University, Zhongshan road 68, Wuxi 214002, China
[1]Department of Geriatric Intensive Care Unit, The First Affiliated Hospital, Nanjing Medical University, Guangzhou road 300, Nanjing 210029, China
Full list of author information is available at the end of the article

administered by either intravenous or subcutaneous injection [12], the clinical applications of ghrelin are restricted. Several orally active, and selective ghrelin receptor agonists that have a longer half-life than ghrelin were consequently developed, including anamorelin [13], ibutamoren(MK-677) [14], ulimorelin(TZP-101) [15], ipamorelin [16], relamorelin [17], and macimorelin [18]. A number of studies revealed that ghrelin receptor agonists could stimulate appetite and food intake, improve body composition and muscle wasting, and ameliorate the disregulated nutritional condition in malnourished patients. However, some studies have reported inconsistent results [19–23]. In a recent report, Temel et al. demonstrated that anamorelin could significantly increase lean body mass (LBM) but could not significantly enhance the grip strength of patients with cancer cachexia. Additionally, they did not report caloric intake [24].

Therefore, we performed this meta-analysis to confirm the superiority of ghrelin receptor agonist administration compared with placebo in malnourished patients. Our primary outcome was energy intake(EI), and the secondary outcomes were LBM, fat mass(FM), and grip strength(GS).

Methods

We conducted this meta-analysis in accordance with PRISMA guidelines [25] and the Cochrane Handbook for Systematic Reviews of Interventions [26] following a registered protocol from the PROSPERO database(CRD42016037466).

Searching strategy

PubMed, the Cochrane Central Register of Controlled Trials (CENTRAL), and EMBASE were electronically searched by independent investigators(JS and JG) to identify any randomized controlled trial (RCT) published through March 2016 that investigated the comparative effects of ghrelin and its analogues versus placebo in patients with malnutrition. We used following search terms embedded in specific files involving the title, keywords, and abstract: "ghrelin", "ghrelin receptor agonists", "malnutrition", "under-nutrition", "anorexia", "cachexia", "weight loss", and relevant variants of these items. The search strings were constructed with a Boolean operator. We also manually detected any eligible studies among the references of identified papers and several corresponding reviews to include any potential studies, which would guarantee the precision and recall ratio. No language or publication restrictions were imposed. We did not assess the grey literature.

Identification of studies

The inclusion criteria were described according to the PICOS acronym (participant, intervention, comparison, outcomes of interest, and study design). For population (P), all of the malnourished patients who were treated with ghrelin receptor agonists were included in this study. For intervention(I) and comparison (C), the studies investigated the comparative effects of ghrelin receptor agonists versus placebo. For outcome of interests (O), we accessed the following outcomes: EI, LBM, FM and GS. Regarding the study design (S), only RCT with or without blind methodology were considered.

The exclusion criteria were as follows: healthy volunteers; subjects under 18 years old; patients with either normal nutrition or obesity; a lack of essential information; animal studies; a review, letter or specialist comment; and non-RCT.

Data extraction

Two independent investigators (JS and YT) extracted the baseline information and essential data of the expected outcomes from each study, including the last name of the first author, publication year, country, sample size of each group, average age and body mass index(BMI) of participants, disease status of the included patients, interventional protocol, follow-up, and reported outcomes of interest. We contacted the authors to acquire any missing data when necessary. Any divergence was resolved by either consensus or consultation with a third author (JB).

Accessing the quality of methodology

Two independent investigators (HY and ML) were assigned to critically appraise the methodological quality of all eligible studies in accordance with the Cochrane Handbook of Systematic Review of Interventions. Seven indexes were independently assessed, and the following results were crosschecked: randomization sequence generation, allocation concealment, blinding of participants and study personnel, blinding of outcome assessors, incomplete outcome data, selective reporting, and other biases. The risk of each incorporated study was rated as " high bias risk " ," unclear bias risk " or " low bias risk " according to the extracted information. A third investigator (JB) was assigned to resolve any disagreement.

Statistical analysis

Stata 12.0 software (Stata Corp, College Station, Texas, USA) was employed to analyse the pooled effect of EI with the SMD and 95% CI, and of the LBM, FM, and GS with WMD and 95% CIs. Heterogeneity was assessed using the $\chi 2$-base Q test with a $p < 0.10$ and the I^2 test with $I^2 > 50\%$ suggesting significant heterogeneity [27]. We preferentially used the fixed effects model (Mantel-Haenszel method) for pooled analysis [28]; if high heterogeneity was identified, we used the random effects model (DerSimonian and Larid method) [29]. Given the considerable heterogeneity, we also performed sensitivity analyses by excluding each study to evaluate the contribution of the inclusion of studies for heterogeneity. Publication bias was estimated using Egger's test and funnel plots with the trim and fill method [30, 31], which were also utilized to adjust for publication bias from potential unpublished studies. Statistical significance was considered when a 2-tailed P value was less than 0.05.

Results

Figure 1 shows the flow diagram for study selection. We identified 785 potentially relevant studies based on above search strategy at the initial search stage. After screening the title and abstract, 20 studies were selected for the full-text assessment, and eight trials were excluded due to several reasons such as lack of interested outcomes, ineligible control regimens, and non-RCTs. All selection procedures were performed independently by two investigators. Finally, 12 eligible studies [13, 20, 24, 32–39] were incorporated into this meta-analysis.

Studies characteristics

The 12 included RCTs comprised 1377 patients, including 1008 male subjects and 369 females. Among the total cohort, 854(62%) patients were assigned to the ghrelin receptor agonists group, and 523(38%) to the control group. The sample size ranged from 14 to 495 subjects, and the follow-up ranged from one day to 12 weeks. All of the included studies compared the efficacy of ghrelin receptor agonists with a corresponding placebo. Nine studies enrolled patients with cancer, while the other three studies did not. Seven studies administered ghrelin, whereas the remaining five trials used anamorelin. The basic characteristics of included studies are shown in Table 1.

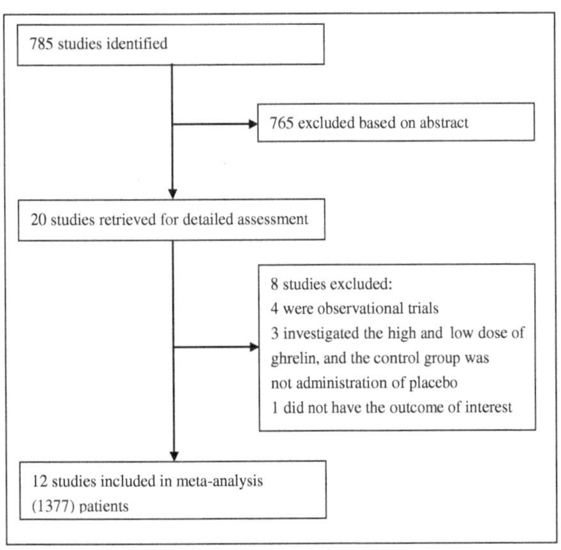

Fig. 1 Flow diagram of the retrieval and selection of qualifying literature

Risk of bias in the included studies

We carefully appraised the methodological quality of the included studies according to the Cochrane Collaboration's Risk of Bias Tool. Four studies provided detailed information regarding the seven total indexes. In the remaining studies, varying degrees of methodological bias were identified. All of the included trials were rated as low bias risk regarding incomplete outcome data because the authors described the drop-out reasons in detail and used the intent-to-treat method to analyse the data. No other bias sources were identified. The graphical results of the methodological quality are shown in Figs. 2 and 3.

Energy intake

Eight studies reported the EI data: seven measured the total calories of ingested food, whereas the eighth estimated the total calories by using a calorie count. In total, 201 participants were included for the pooled analysis, which showed a significantly increased EI after administration of ghrelin receptor agonists (SMD 2.67, 95%CI 1.48 to 3.85, $P < 0.001$, Fig. 4). There was significant heterogeneity among the studies ($I^2 = 89.3\%$, $P < 0.001$). Subgroup analyses showed that the increased EI after the administration of ghrelin receptor agonists remained evident irrespective of the different areas, diseases, therapeutic drug, and follow-up.

Sensitivity analyses showed no alterations of the main outcome after eliminating each study. However, we found no significant heterogeneity when we excluded the studies that did not include cancer patients($I^2 = 0\%$, $P = 0.99$) with a new pooled SMD of 1.12 (95%CI 0.74 to 1.50, $P < 0.001$).

Egger's test was statistically significant ($P = 0.037$) and visual inspection of the funnel plot seemed to be asymmetric. The trim and fill method suggested that there might be one unpublished studies (Fig. 5). Using trim and fill method, we found that our finding remained significant after adjusting for one unpublished study(SMD 2.18, 95%CI 0.913 to 3.448, $P = 0.001$).

Lean body mass

A total of six studies comprising 1178 participants reported LBM data as measured by dual energy x-ray absorptiometry(DEXA). The meta-analysis showed that administration of ghrelin receptor agonists could increase the LBM in malnourished patients (WMD 0.25 kg, 95%CI 0.07 to 0.42, $P = 0.006$, Fig. 6). There was also significant heterogeneity among the studies regarding LBM ($I^2 = 95.2\%$, $P = 0.000$). The subgroup analyses showed that increased LBM after administration of

Table 1 Basic Characteristics of the Included Studies Comparing Ghrelin Receptor Agonists versus Placebo

Study ID	Country	Sample size	Age of participants (Mean ± SD)	Disease	Primary BMI (kg/m^2, Mean ± SD)	Regimen for the interventional group	Control regimen	Follow up	Reported outcomes
Neary 2004 [36]	UK	7/7	54.3 ± 8.4/ 54.3 ± 8.4	cancer	22.6 ± 4.1/22.6 ± 4.1	Grelin(5 pmol/kg.min), IVP, single dose	placebo	1 day	EI
Wynne 2005 [38]	UK	9/9	49.8 ± 5.2/ 49.8 ± 5.2	CRF	24.7 ± 4.4/24.7 ± 4.4	Ghrelin(3.6 nmol/kg), HD, single dose	placebo	3 days	EI
Ashby 2009 [33]	UK	12/12	49.4 ± 14.6/ 49.4 ± 14.6	CRF	24.3 ± 4.1/24.3 ± 4.1	Ghrelin(12 μg/kg), HD, qd, 7 days	placebo	7 days	EI
Yamamoto 2010 [39]	Japan	10/10	63 ± 6/ 65 ± 6	cancer	20 ± 2/22 ± 4	Ghrelin(3 μg/kg), IVP, bid, 10 days	placebo	10 days	EI
Shinichi 2010 [32]	Japan	10/10	64.8 ± 10.4/ 61.6 ± 8.4	cancer	23.1 ± 3.1/24.5 ± 3.8	Ghrelin(3 μg/kg), IVP, bid, 10 days	placebo	10 days	EI, LBM, FM
Miki 2012 [20]	Japan	18/15	70.5 ± 6.2/ 73.9 ± 6.0	COPD	18.6 ± 2.1/18.0 ± 2.1	Ghrelin(2 μg/kg) , IVP, bid, 3 weeks	placebo	3 week	EI, LBM, FM, GS
Hiura 2012 [35]	Japan	20/20	65.8 ± 5.2/ 61.8 ± 10.9	cancer	21.6 ± 3/21.0 ± 2.7	Ghrelin(3 μg/kg), IVP, bid, 7 days	placebo	7 days	EI
Garcia 2012 [13]	USA	16/16	61.9 ± 10.29/ 62.9 ± 8.43	cancer	22.1 ± 3.51/21.6 ± 3.93	Anamorelin, 50 mg, PO, qd, 3 days	placebo	3 days	EI
Garcia 2015 [34]	USA	44/38	65.5 ± NR/ 65 ± NR	cancer	21.5 ± NR/21.1 ± NR	Anamorelin, 50 mg, PO, qd, 12 weeks	placebo	12 weeks	LBM, FM, GS
Takayama 2016 [37]	Japan	55/60	65.7 ± 8.8/ 66 ± 9.4	cancer	20.23 ± 3.21/19.80 ± 2.86	Anamorelin, 100 mg, PO, qd, 12 weeks	placebo	12 weeks	LBM, GS
Temel 2016(1) [24]	USA	323/161	63 ± NR/ 63 ± NR	cancer	23.2 ± 3.6/23.3 ± 3.7	Anamorelin, 100 mg, PO, qd, 12 weeks	placebo	12 weeks	LBM, FM, GS
Temel 2016(2) [24]	USA	330/165	63 ± NR/ 62 ± NR	cancer	22.5 ± 3.7/22.1 ± 3.7	Anamorelin, 100 mg, PO, qd, 12 weeks	placebo	12 weeks	LBM, FM, GS

Abbreviations: *SD* standard deviation, *NR* not reported

ghrelin receptor agonists remained evident irrespective of the different regions, diseases, or therapeutic drug. Sensitivity analyses showed no alterations of the main outcome after eliminating each study. However, we found no significant heterogeneity when excluded the study by Miki (I^2 = 43%, P = 0.14) with a pooled WMD of 1.64 kg (95%CI 1.31 to 1.97, P < 0.001). Egger's test revealed no statistical significance (P = 0.054), indicating that there is no publication bias.

Fat mass

There were four studies(923 subjects) that reported FM data, which was also measured by DEXA. The meta-analysis revealed that administration of either ghrelin or anamorelin to malnourished patients could increase the FM (WMD 0.92 kg, 95%CI 0.05 to 1.8, P = 0.038) with no evidence for heterogeneity across the studies (I^2 = 0%, P = 0.938, Fig. 7). We found no change of the pooled estimate effect and heterogeneity after sensitivity

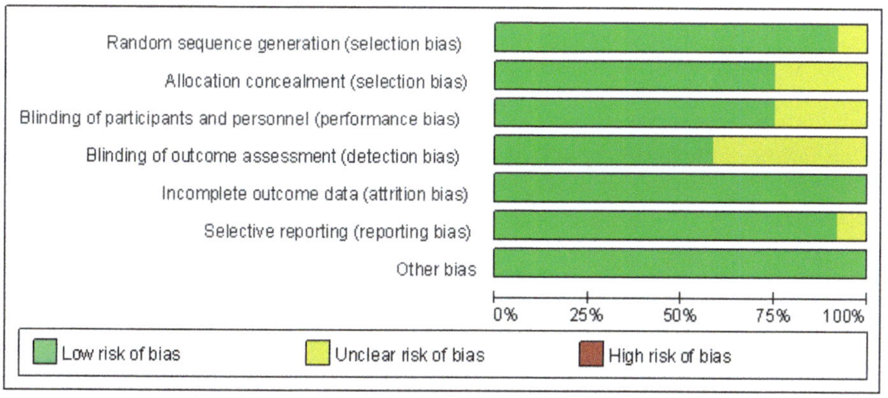

Fig. 2 Assessment of the risk of bias: bias of risk graph

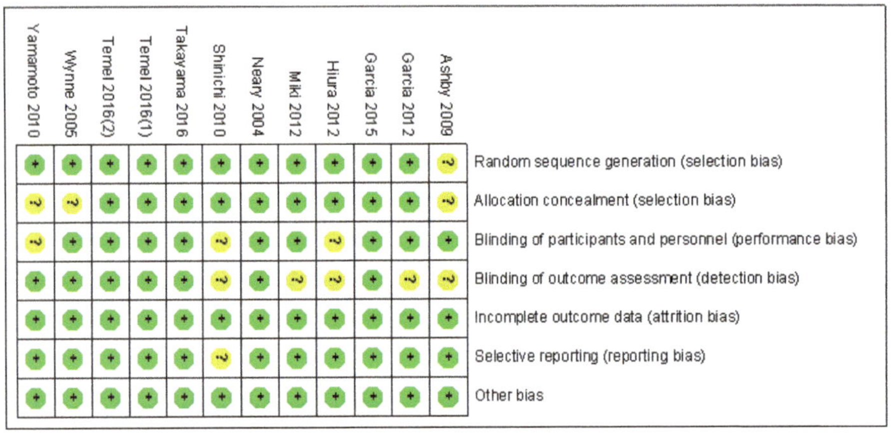

Fig. 3 Assessment of the risk of bias: bias of risk summary

analyses. Egger's test revealed no statistical significance ($P = 0.633$), showing that there is no publication bias.

Grip strength

A total of five studies comprising 1085 participants reported GS data: two of the studies measured handgrip strength on each side by using a hand-held dynamometer, while the other three only measured the handgrip strength of the non-dominant hand. The meta-analysis showed that administration of ghrelin receptor agonists could increase the GS in malnourished patients (WMD 0.31 kg, 95%CI 0.21 to 0.41, $P < 0.001$, Fig. 8). Sensitivity analyses showed no alterations of the main outcome after eliminating each study. However, we found no significant heterogeneity when we excluded the study by Garcia ($I^2 = 0\%$, $P = 0.43$), with a pooled WMD of 0.3 kg (95%CI 0.19 to 0.4, $P < 0.001$). Egger's test revealed no statistical significance ($P = 0.501$), indicating that there is no publication bias.

Discussion

In the present study, we demonstrated that administration of ghrelin receptor agonists could ameliorate the nutritional condition of patients with malnutrition by increasing their food intake, changing their body composition, and enhancing their muscle strength. These conclusions were strengthened by the fact that sensitivity analyses and the trim and fill method did not alter these outcomes, although there might be lack of power to detect differences with the limited sample size and other potential publications. There was significant heterogeneity in the pooled analyses of EI and LBM. Therefore, we used a subgroup analysis and sensitivity analysis to identify the causes of heterogeneity. When we excluded the

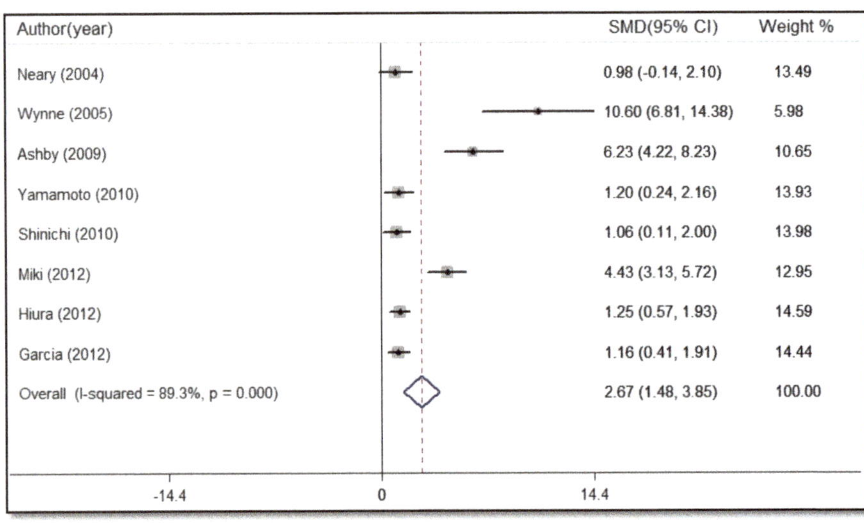

Fig. 4 Forest plot of energy intake

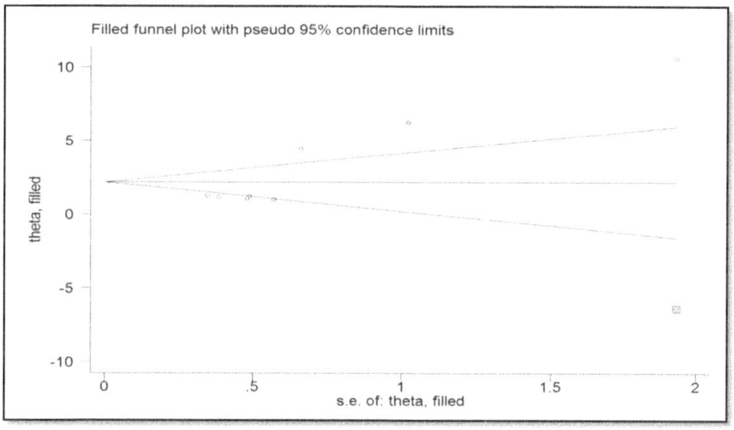

Fig. 5 Funnel plot with the trim and fill method for energy intake

studies that had no cancer patients enrolled, the high degree of heterogeneity vanished. Thus, the differences in patients' diseases might be the cause of the significant heterogeneity.

Loss of appetite appears in many patients with severe malnutrition, which is not only frequent, but is also associated with a poor prognosis and reduced quality of life [40]. In this study, we found that administration of ghrelin receptor agonists could increase energy intake, which confirms their well-established role in stimulating appetite and increasing food intake [41, 42]. Administration of exogenous ghrelin administration was first noted to promote food intake and weight gain in rats [43, 44]. These effects were independent of the effects of ghrelin on GH stimulation and the GH secretagogue receptor(GHS-R) and might be related to neuropeptide Y(NPY), as indicated by the increase of plasma NPY levels after IV bolus of ghrelin [45]. Another possible explanation is that ghrelin could inhibit the production of the anorectic proinflammatory cytokines such as interleukin-1β, interleukin-6, and tumour necrosis factors, as well as induce secretion of the anti-inflammatory cytokine interleukin-10 [46]. In contrast, in a randomized, double-cross-over clinical study, Strasser et al. used different doses of ghrelin in cancer patients and found that the nutritional intake did not increase following ghrelin administration [19]. Moreover, a single ghrelin infusion could not increase the food intake in patients with postvagotomy diarrhoea [22] and anorexia nervosa [23], although repeated infusions could stimulate hunger and food intake in these subjects [6, 32]. Thus, we postulated that the dose and frequency of ghrelin administration to the enrolled subjects would influence the actual clinical effect. Interestingly, the increase in energy

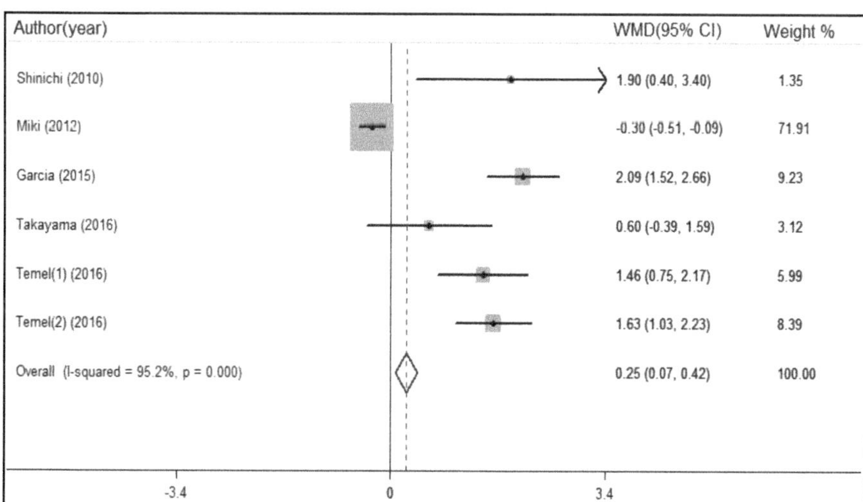

Fig. 6 Forest plot of lean body mass

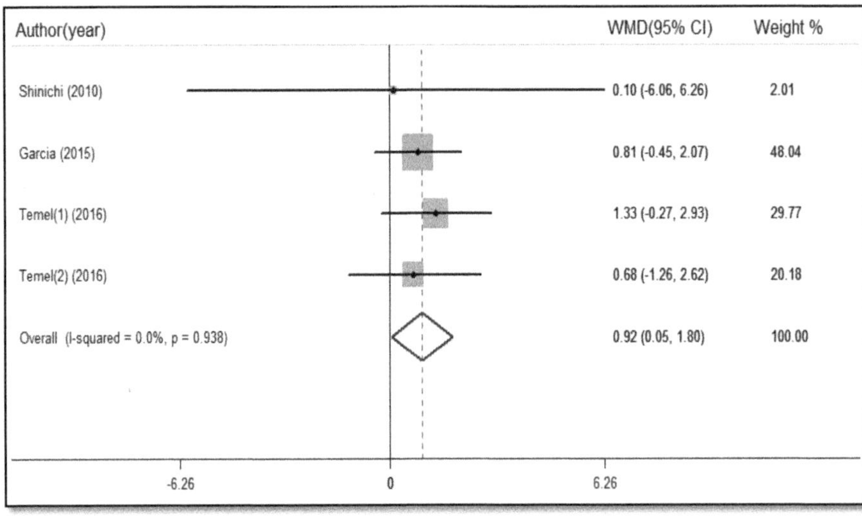

Fig. 7 Forest plot of fat mass

intake following ghrelin administration occurred without compensatory undereating [47] or evidence of tachyphylaxis [33]. However, the included studies evaluated EI by different methods, so we used SMD as the effect magnitude, which was less persuasive than WMD.

Changes in body composition that develop with chronic diseases are usually considered unwanted and are associated with the loss of muscle, fat mass, or both [48]. The loss of lean and fat tissue may be associated with weight loss; such involuntary weight loss has been termed cachexia [49]. Activation of the GHS-R exerted anabolic functions and could lead to weight gain [41]. Ghrelin receptor agonists could increase bodyweight by not only stimulating appetite but also by decreasing energy expenditure, the latter of which was relevant to cancer cachexia [50]. Our results validated the capacity of ghrelin receptor agonists in improving the body composition of patients with under-nutrition as indicated by the significant increase in LBM and FM. Low LBM was associated with a poor prognosis and could predict the toxic effects of treatment [51]. Increased FM reflected improved energy balance, although GH secretion induced by ghrelin receptor agonists may contribute to low adiposity [52]. Thus, the present study illuminated the beneficial effect of ghrelin receptor agonists on the positive changes in body composition and weight gain,

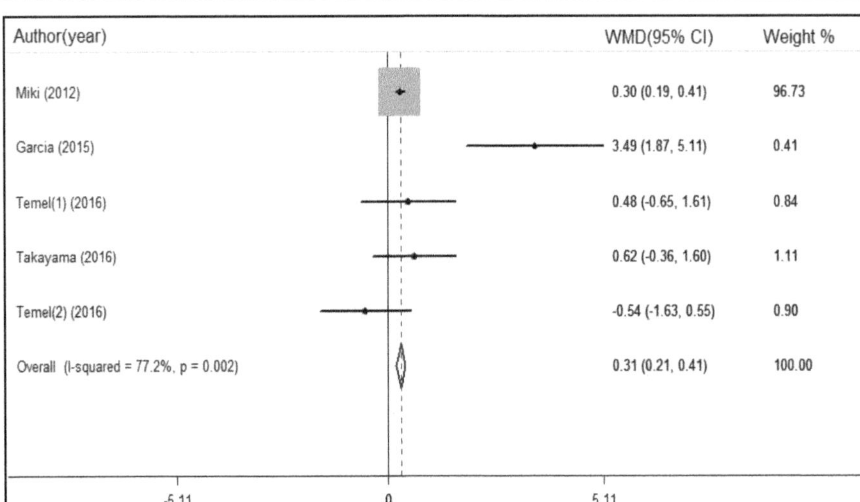

Fig. 8 Forest plot of grip strength

which would be promising for the treatment of malnutrition, as losses in body weight and sarcopenia are characteristic features of under-nutrition [53].

Theoretically, a valid treatment for cachexia-associated muscle wasting should increase muscle mass and, as a consequence, enhance muscle strength. However, muscle wasting in cachectic patients results from a variety of factors such as age-related muscle atrophy, therapies targeting the primary disease, comorbidity, and persistent systematic inflammation [24]. Contrary with corticosteroids [54] and progestational drugs [55], which were commonly prescribed as orexigenic agents and could only increase appetite and body weight, our findings verified that ghrelin receptor agonists could significantly enhance muscle strength. Activation using ghrelin receptor agonists induced GH secretion, thereby increasing the insulin-like growth factor-1 (IGF-1) concentration; GH and IGF-1 could promote muscle growth through a direct effect on the muscle and indirectly activating the production of both muscle-restricted IGF-1 and anti-cachectic cytokines [56]. However, our included studies investigated muscle function by measuring handgrip strength with either the dominant or non dominant hand, which measured upper-extremity strength and might not indicate a comprehensively physiological performance. Further studies using internationally validated methods to assess muscle strength are warranted.

An important concern with regard to the application of ghrelin receptor agonists in cancer cachexia is that they may increase the levels of growth factors such as GH and IGF-1 to promote tumour growth. In addition, ghrelin itself may have mitogenic potential. Northrup et al. evaluated ghrelin and anamorelin on tumour growth in mouse models of lung cancer, and found that neither compound could effect tumour growth until the end of the intervention despite the significantly increased GH and IGF-1 levels [57]. Additionally, clinical studies with anamorelin [58] and ghrelin [59] have also shown no significant effect on overall survival compared with placebo. Long-term, large-scale clinical trials are required to determine whether treatment with ghrelin receptor agonists could stimulate tumour growth [60].

There are some limitations in this meta-analysis. First, the basic characteristics of the included patients differed in some confounders. However, sensitivity analysis and the trim and fill method did not alter the results of our primary outcome, which lessened the adverse effect due to this limitation. Second, the sample size of included studies was small, the follow-up was short, and only two ghrelin receptor agonists were analysed among the variety of agonists in existence. Third, there were more male patients than females in each group, so the conclusions were less conclusive for female subjects. Further studies with more subjects, a longer follow-up period and implementation of different ghrelin receptor agonists are required to identify whether the administration of ghrelin receptor agonists would lead to long-term benefits such as reduced total medical cost, decreased hospital stay, and elevated quality of life and overall survival.

Conclusion

In conclusion, based on the results of our meta-analyses, we confirmed that administration of ghrelin receptor agonists could have beneficial effects on patients with malnutrition. This novel approach, which directly targets appetite stimulation, could have an important role in the future management and prevention of under-nutrition for malnourished patients.

Abbreviations

BMI: Body mass index; CI: Confidence interval; COPD: Chronic obstructive pulmonary disease; CRF: Chronic renal failure; DEXA: Dual energy x-ray absorptiometry; EI: Energy intake; FM: Fat mass; GH: Growth hormone; GHS-R: GH secretagogue receptor; GS: Grip strength; IGF-1: Insulin-like growth factor-1; LBM: Lean body mass; NPY: Neuropeptide Y; NR: Not reported.; RCT: Randomised controlled trial; SD: Standard deviation; SMD: Standard mean difference; WMD: Weighted mean difference

Acknowledgements

The authors appreciate the work of the editors and anonymous reviewers.

Funding

This work was supported by the project of critical care medicine of the key clinical specialty of Jiangsu Province.

Availability of data and material

Not applicable.

Authors' contributions

JS, SZ and WH conceived and designed the study. JS, JG, JB, YT, ML, HY, and YH performed the study. JS and JG analysed the data. JS wrote the paper. JS and YH critically revised the manuscript. All authors read and approved the final manuscript.

Competing interest

The authors declare that they have no competing interests.

Consent for publication

Not applicable.

Ethics approval and consent to participate

We performed all analyses based on the previously published studies; thus, no ethical approval and informed consent were required.

Author details

[1]Department of Geriatric Intensive Care Unit, The First Affiliated Hospital, Nanjing Medical University, Guangzhou road 300, Nanjing 210029, China. [2]Department of Geriatric Medicine, Wuxi NO.2 People's Hospital, Nanjing Medical University, Zhongshan road 68, Wuxi 214002, China. [3]Department of Cardiology, Huai'an First People's Hospital, Nanjing Medical University, Beijingxi road 6, Huai'an 223300, China.

References

1. Stratton RGC, Elia M. Scientific criteria for defining malnutrition. Disease related malnutrition: an evidence-based approach to treatment. UK: CABI Publishing; 2003.

2. Akashi YJ, Springer J, Anker SD. Cachexia in chronic heart failure: prognostic implications and novel therapeutic approaches. Curr Heart Fail Rep. 2005;2:198–203.
3. Nagaya N, Kojima M, Kangawa K. Ghrelin, a novel growth hormone-releasing peptide, in the treatment of cardiopulmonary-associated cachexia. Intern Med. 2006;45:127–34.
4. Bossola M, Tazza L, Giungi S, Luciani G. Anorexia in hemodialysis patients: an update. Kidney Int. 2006;70:417–22.
5. Crawford J. Clinical results in cachexia therapeutics. Curr Opin Clin Nutr Metab Care. 2016;19:199–204.
6. Hotta M, Ohwada R, Akamizu T, Shibasaki T, Takano K, Kangawa K. Ghrelin increases hunger and food intake in patients with restricting-type anorexia nervosa: a pilot study. Endocr J. 2009;56:1119–28.
7. Akamizu T, Iwakura H, Ariyasu H, Hosoda H, Murayama T, Yokode M, Teramukai S, Seno H, Chiba T, Noma S, et al. Repeated administration of ghrelin to patients with functional dyspepsia: its effects on food intake and appetite. Eur J Endocrinol. 2008;158:491–8.
8. Akamizu T, Iwakura H, Ariyasu H, Murayama T, Sumi E, Teramukai S, Goto K, Ohnishi E, Akiyama H, Kawanabe K, et al. Effects of ghrelin treatment on patients undergoing total hip replacement for osteoarthritis: different outcomes from studies in patients with cardiac and pulmonary cachexia. J Am Geriatr Soc. 2008;56:2363–5.
9. Agarwal E, Miller M, Yaxley A, Isenring E. Malnutrition in the elderly: a narrative review. Maturitas. 2013;76:296–302.
10. Kojima M, Hosoda H, Date Y, Nakazato M, Matsuo H, Kangawa K. Ghrelin is a growth-hormone-releasing acylated peptide from stomach. Nature. 1999;402:656–60.
11. Ashitani J, Matsumoto N, Nakazato M. Effect of octanoic acid-rich formula on plasma ghrelin levels in cachectic patients with chronic respiratory disease. Nutr J. 2009;8:25.
12. Akamizu T, Takaya K, Irako T, Hosoda H, Teramukai S, Matsuyama A, Tada H, Miura K, Shimizu A, Fukushima M, et al. Pharmacokinetics, safety, and endocrine and appetite effects of ghrelin administration in young healthy subjects. Eur J Endocrinol. 2004;150:447–55.
13. Garcia JM, Friend J, Allen S. Therapeutic potential of anamorelin, a novel, oral ghrelin mimetic, in patients with cancer-related cachexia: a multicenter, randomized, double-blind, crossover, pilot study. Support Care Cancer. 2013;21:129–37.
14. Murphy MG, Plunkett LM, Gertz BJ, He W, Wittreich J, Polvino WM, Clemmons DR. MK-677, an orally active growth hormone secretagogue, reverses diet-induced catabolism. J Clin Endocrinol Metab. 1998;83:320–5.
15. Tack J, Janssen P. Emerging drugs for functional dyspepsia. Expert Opin Emerg Drugs. 2011;16:283–92.
16. Shin A, Wo JM. Therapeutic applications of ghrelin agonists in the treatment of gastroparesis. Curr Gastroenterol Rep. 2015;17:430.
17. Lembo A, Camilleri M, McCallum R, Sastre R, Breton C, Spence S, White J, Currie M, Gottesdiener K, Stoner E. Relamorelin Reduces Vomiting Frequency and Severity and Accelerates Gastric Emptying in Adults With Diabetic Gastroparesis. Gastroenterology. 2016.
18. Piccoli F, Degen L, MacLean C, Peter S, Baselgia L, Larsen F, Beglinger C, Drewe J. Pharmacokinetics and pharmacodynamic effects of an oral ghrelin agonist in healthy subjects. J Clin Endocrinol Metab. 2007;92:1814–20.
19. Strasser F, Lutz TA, Maeder MT, Thuerlimann B, Bueche D, Tschop M, Kaufmann K, Holst B, Brandle M, von Moos R, et al. Safety, tolerability and pharmacokinetics of intravenous ghrelin for cancer-related anorexia/cachexia: a randomised, placebo-controlled, double-blind, double-crossover study. Br J Cancer. 2008;98:300–8.
20. Miki K, Maekura R, Nagaya N, Nakazato M, Kimura H, Murakami S, Ohnishi S, Hiraga T, Miki M, Kitada S, et al. Ghrelin treatment of cachectic patients with chronic obstructive pulmonary disease: a multicenter, randomized, double-blind, placebo-controlled trial. PLoS One. 2012;7:e35708.
21. le Roux CW, Neary NM, Halsey TJ, Small CJ, Martinez-Isla AM, Ghatei MA, Theodorou NA, Bloom SR. Ghrelin does not stimulate food intake in patients with surgical procedures involving vagotomy. J Clin Endocrinol Metab. 2005;90:4521–4.
22. Huda MS, Dovey T, Wong SP, English PJ, Halford J, McCulloch P, Cleator J, Martin B, Cashen J, Hayden K, et al. Ghrelin restores 'lean-type' hunger and energy expenditure profiles in morbidly obese subjects but has no effect on postgastrectomy subjects. Int J Obes (Lond). 2009;33:317–25.
23. Miljic D, Pekic S, Djurovic M, Doknic M, Milic N, Casanueva FF, Ghatei M, Popovic V. Ghrelin has partial or no effect on appetite, growth hormone, prolactin, and cortisol release in patients with anorexia nervosa. J Clin Endocrinol Metab. 2006;91:1491–5.
24. Temel JS, Abernethy AP, Currow DC, Friend J, Duus EM, Yan Y, Fearon KC. Anamorelin in patients with non-small-cell lung cancer and cachexia (ROMANA 1 and ROMANA 2): results from two randomised, double-blind, phase 3 trials. Lancet Oncol. 2016;17:519–31.
25. Liberati A, Altman DG, Tetzlaff J, Mulrow C, Gotzsche PC, Ioannidis JP, Clarke M, Devereaux PJ, Kleijnen J, Moher D. The PRISMA statement for reporting systematic reviews and meta-analyses of studies that evaluate health care interventions: explanation and elaboration. Ann Intern Med. 2009;151:W65–94.
26. Higgins JPGS. Handbook for Systematic Reviews of Interventions. Wiley Online Library. 2008;5: .
27. Higgins JP, Thompson SG. Quantifying heterogeneity in a meta-analysis. Stat Med. 2002;21:1539–58.
28. Mantel N, Haenszel W. Statistical aspects of the analysis of data from retrospective studies of disease. J Natl Cancer Inst. 1959;22:719–48.
29. DerSimonian R, Laird N. Meta-analysis in clinical trials. Control Clin Trials. 1986;7:177–88.
30. Duval S, Tweedie R. Trim and fill: A simple funnel-plot-based method of testing and adjusting for publication bias in meta-analysis. Biometrics. 2000;56:455–63.
31. Egger M, Davey Smith G, Schneider M, Minder C. Bias in meta-analysis detected by a simple, graphical test. BMJ. 1997;315:629–34.
32. Adachi S, Takiguchi S, Okada K, Yamamoto K, Yamasaki M, Miyata H, Nakajima K, Fujiwara Y, Hosoda H, Kangawa K, et al. Effects of ghrelin administration after total gastrectomy: a prospective, randomized, placebo-controlled phase II study. Gastroenterology. 2010;138:1312–20.
33. Ashby DR, Ford HE, Wynne KJ, Wren AM, Murphy KG, Busbridge M, Brown EA, Taube DH, Ghatei MA, Tam FW, et al. Sustained appetite improvement in malnourished dialysis patients by daily ghrelin treatment. Kidney Int. 2009;76:199–206.
34. Garcia JM, Boccia RV, Graham CD, Yan Y, Duus EM, Allen S, Friend J. Anamorelin for patients with cancer cachexia: an integrated analysis of two phase 2, randomised, placebo-controlled, double-blind trials. Lancet Oncol. 2015;16:108–16.
35. Hiura Y, Takiguchi S, Yamamoto K, Takahashi T, Kurokawa Y, Yamasaki M, Nakajima K, Miyata H, Fujiwara Y, Mori M, et al. Effects of ghrelin administration during chemotherapy with advanced esophageal cancer patients: a prospective, randomized, placebo-controlled phase 2 study. Cancer. 2012;118:4785–94.
36. Neary NM, Small CJ, Wren AM, Lee JL, Druce MR, Palmieri C, Frost GS, Ghatei MA, Coombes RC, Bloom SR. Ghrelin increases energy intake in cancer patients with impaired appetite: acute, randomized, placebo-controlled trial. J Clin Endocrinol Metab. 2004;89:2832–6.
37. Takayama K, Katakami N, Yokoyama T, Atagi S, Yoshimori K, Kagamu H, Saito H, Takiguchi Y, Aoe K, Koyama A, et al. Anamorelin (ONO-7643) in Japanese patients with non-small cell lung cancer and cachexia: results of a randomized phase 2 trial. Support Care Cancer. 2016.
38. Wynne K, Giannitsopoulou K, Small CJ, Patterson M, Frost G, Ghatei MA, Brown EA, Bloom SR, Choi P. Subcutaneous ghrelin enhances acute food intake in malnourished patients who receive maintenance peritoneal dialysis: a randomized, placebo-controlled trial. J Am Soc Nephrol. 2005;16:2111–8.
39. Yamamoto K, Takiguchi S, Miyata H, Adachi S, Hiura Y, Yamasaki M, Nakajima K, Fujiwara Y, Mori M, Kangawa K, Doki Y. Randomized phase II study of clinical effects of ghrelin after esophagectomy with gastric tube reconstruction. Surgery. 2010;148:31–8.
40. von Haehling S, Anker SD. Treatment of cachexia: An overview of recent developments. Int J Cardiol. 2015;184:736–42.
41. Garcia JM, Polvino WJ. Effect on body weight and safety of RC-1291, a novel, orally available ghrelin mimetic and growth hormone secretagogue: results of a phase I, randomized, placebo-controlled, multiple-dose study in healthy volunteers. Oncologist. 2007;12:594–600.
42. Wren AM, Bloom SR. Gut hormones and appetite control. Gastroenterology. 2007;132:2116–30.
43. Nakazato M, Murakami N, Date Y, Kojima M, Matsuo H, Kangawa K, Matsukura S. A role for ghrelin in the central regulation of feeding. Nature. 2001;409:194–8.
44. Tschop M, Smiley DL, Heiman ML. Ghrelin induces adiposity in rodents. Nature. 2000;407:908–13.

45. Coiro V, Saccani-Jotti G, Rubino P, Manfredi G, Vacca P, Volta E, Chiodera P. Oxytocin inhibits the stimulatory effect of ghrelin on circulating neuropeptide Y levels in humans. J Neural Transm (Vienna). 2008;115:1265–7.
46. Dixit VD, Schaffer EM, Pyle RS, Collins GD, Sakthivel SK, Palaniappan R, Lillard Jr JW, Taub DD. Ghrelin inhibits leptin- and activation-induced proinflammatory cytokine expression by human monocytes and T cells. J Clin Invest. 2004;114:57–66.
47. Wren AM, Seal LJ, Cohen MA, Brynes AE, Frost GS, Murphy KG, Dhillo WS, Ghatei MA, Bloom SR. Ghrelin enhances appetite and increases food intake in humans. J Clin Endocrinol Metab. 2001;86:5992.
48. von Haehling S, Anker SD. Cachexia vs obesity: where is the real unmet clinical need? J Cachexia Sarcopenia Muscle. 2013;4:245–6.
49. Letilovic T, Perkov S, Mestric ZF, Vrhovac R. Differences in routine laboratory parameters related to cachexia between patients with hematological diseases and patients with solid tumors or heart failure - is there only one cachexia? Nutr J. 2013;12:6.
50. Jatoi A, Daly BD, Hughes VA, Dallal GE, Kehayias J, Roubenoff R. Do patients with nonmetastatic non-small cell lung cancer demonstrate altered resting energy expenditure? Ann Thorac Surg. 2001;72:348–51.
51. Tsai S. Importance of lean body mass in the oncologic patient. Nutr Clin Pract. 2012;27:593–8.
52. Kojima M, Kangawa K. Ghrelin: structure and function. Physiol Rev. 2005;85:495–522.
53. Evans WJ, Morley JE, Argiles J, Bales C, Baracos V, Guttridge D, Jatoi A, Kalantar-Zadeh K, Lochs H, Mantovani G, et al. Cachexia: a new definition. Clin Nutr. 2008;27:793–9.
54. Galvao DA, Taaffe DR, Spry N, Joseph D, Newton RU. Combined resistance and aerobic exercise program reverses muscle loss in men undergoing androgen suppression therapy for prostate cancer without bone metastases: a randomized controlled trial. J Clin Oncol. 2010;28:340–7.
55. Maccio A, Madeddu C, Mantovani G. Current pharmacotherapy options for cancer anorexia and cachexia. Expert Opin Pharmacother. 2012;13:2453–72.
56. Ali S, Chen JA, Garcia JM. Clinical development of ghrelin axis-derived molecules for cancer cachexia treatment. Curr Opin Support Palliat Care. 2013;7:368–75.
57. Northrup R, Kuroda K, Duus EM, Barnes SR, Cheatham L, Wiley T, Pietra C. Effect of ghrelin and anamorelin (ONO-7643), a selective ghrelin receptor agonist, on tumor growth in a lung cancer mouse xenograft model. Support Care Cancer. 2013;21:2409–15.
58. Temel J, Bondarde S, Jain M, Allen S, Mann W. Efficacy and safety of anamorelin HCl in NSCLC patients: Results from a randomized, double-blind, placebo-controlled, multicenter phase II study. Eur J Cancer. 2013;49:S269–70.
59. Lundholm K, Gunnebo L, Korner U, Iresjo BM, Engstrom C, Hyltander A, Smedh U, Bosaeus I. Effects by daily long term provision of ghrelin to unselected weight-losing cancer patients: a randomized double-blind study. Cancer. 2010;116:2044–52.
60. Sever S, White DL, Garcia JM. Is there an effect of ghrelin/ghrelin analogs on cancer? A systematic review. Endocr Relat Cancer. 2016;23:R393–409.

Fortified breakfast cereal consumed daily for 12 wk leads to a significant improvement in micronutrient intake and micronutrient status in adolescent girls

Hilary J. Powers[1*], Mark Stephens[1], Jean Russell[2] and Marilyn H. Hill[1]

Abstract

Background: Poor micronutrient status is reported among adolescents across Europe and USA. This may be related to the well-documented decline in the regular consumption of breakfast by this group. The regular consumption of a breakfast cereal offers a possible means to improve micronutrient status; fortified cereal is likely to have enhanced benefit. A study was conducted to determine the efficacy of the regular consumption of a fortified cereal with milk, compared with unfortified cereal, consumed either as a breakfast or a supper, in improving micronutrient intake and micronutrient status of adolescent girls.

Methods: A randomised, double-blind, placebo-controlled intervention trial was conducted in girls recruited at ages 16–19 years, from schools and colleges in Sheffield, UK. Girls were randomised to receive 50 g fortified or unfortified cereal, with 150 ml semi-skimmed milk, daily, for 12 weeks, as a breakfast or as a supper. Dietary intake was estimated using a 4-d food diary and blood collected for the assessment of nutritional status. Within-group changes were tested using a paired sample t test; two-way ANOVA was used to analyse effects of the intervention, with cereal type and time of consumption as factors, correcting for baseline values. The analysis was conducted on 71 girls who completed the study.

Results: Consumption of unfortified cereal elicited an increase in the intake of vitamins B_1, B_2 and B_6; consumption of fortified cereal elicited increases in vitamins B_1, B_2, B_6, B_{12}, folate and iron ($P < 0.001$) and of vitamin D ($P = 0.007$), all increases were significantly greater than for unfortified cereal. Consumption of the fortified cereal also led to a significant improvement in biomarkers of status for vitamins B_2, B_{12}, folate and of iron, compared with girls receiving the unfortified cereal, and maintained vitamin D status, in contrast with the girls receiving the unfortified cereal ($P < 0.001$).

Conclusions: The daily consumption of cereal with milk for 12 weeks by adolescent girls, increased intakes of micronutrients. The consumption of fortified cereal elicited greater increases than for unfortified cereal and improved biomarkers of micronutrient status. The findings justify strategies to encourage the consumption of fortified cereal with milk by adolescents, either as a breakfast or a supper.

Trial registration: Registered with Current Controlled Trials (Registration: ISRCTN55141306)

Keywords: Fortified cereal, Breakfast, Vitamin and mineral status, Micronutrients, Adolescents

* Correspondence: h.j.powers@sheffield.ac.uk
[1]Human Nutrition Unit, University of Sheffield, Sheffield, UK
Full list of author information is available at the end of the article

Background

Data from the National Diet and Nutrition Surveys (NDNS) of the UK indicate low intakes of some micronutrients and poor nutritional status among adolescent girls, with concern over vitamin B_2 (riboflavin), vitamin D, calcium and iron [1]. Dietary data from the National Health and Nutrition Examination Surveys (NHANES) in the USA also show that adolescents are at higher risk of nutritional deficiencies than other age groups in the population [2]. Some of these deficiencies may be of particular functional importance to adolescent females given that they are of childbearing age and that low micronutrient intakes in this group influence risk of anaemia, peak bone mass attainment and adverse effects in the offspring [3–7].

Breakfast consumption by children and adolescents has declined over recent decades in many developed countries [8–12]. Milk consumption by children and adolescents in developed countries is also falling, and this is thought to associate with the declining trend in breakfast cereal consumption [1, 13, 14] Studies of association have identified a number of correlates of breakfast consumption in adolescents. Cross sectional studies have reported associations between regular consumption of breakfast and parameters of a healthy lifestyle and some measures of nutritional status [15, 16]. Breakfast-skipping is associated with increased likelihood of being a smoker, of being a consumer of alcohol, of engaging in little exercise and having a higher BMI [17]. On the other hand, some studies report that breakfast consumers have higher energy consumption than non-consumers, and may be associated with an increase in the contribution of fat to total energy intake [18]. A cross–sectional study in Belgium showed that the type of breakfast consumed was associated with the overall dietary intake profile in adolescents [19]. There is some evidence that a breakfast of cereal may have particular value [20] although it is not clear whether associations reported between breakfast cereal consumption and various biomarkers of health are attributable to the consumption of breakfast cereals per se, as part of a daily diet, or the consumption of the cereal as part of a breakfast meal.

There is a definite gender bias in the decline of breakfast consumption, with girls significantly more likely to miss breakfast than boys [17, 20]. There is also an age-related decline in breakfast consumption, with older adolescents more likely to miss breakfast [21]. Reasons often cited are lack of time, loss of appetite in the morning, tiredness or personal choice [22]. Dieting and a desire to lose weight is another reason given for not eating breakfast [23, 24].

The lack of randomised controlled trials to examine hypotheses linking the regular consumption of breakfast cereals to particular health benefits is an obstacle to making specific dietary recommendations.

The study reports that the daily consumption of a fortified cereal with milk, either at breakfast time or supper time for twelve weeks, elicits an increase in micronutrient intake and improvement in biomarkers of micronutrient status in adolescent girls who regularly skip breakfast, that is significantly greater than that observed by the consumption of unfortified cereal with milk. In contrast with girls receiving the unfortified cereal, all girls consuming the fortified cereal achieved the Recommended Nutrient Intake (RNI) for vitamins B_2, B_6, B_{12} and folate, although they did not all achieve the RNI for iron, and no girl achieved the current RDA (USA) for vitamin D. The RNI reflects the intake considered to satisfy the requirements of 97.5 % of the age and gender-specific population group.

Study aim

This study aimed to investigate the efficacy of the regular consumption of fortified cereal with milk, compared with unfortified cereal, either as a breakfast or a supper, in improving micronutrient intake and micronutrient status of adolescent girls who self-report regularly skipping breakfast.

Hypotheses

We hypothesised that the regular consumption of a fortified breakfast cereal with milk by adolescent girls who often skip breakfast will elicit an increased intake of some micronutrients and improvement in biomarkers of micronutrient status, compared with unfortified cereal. We also hypothesised that the consumption of breakfast cereal at supper-time will elicit the same improvements in nutritional status as when consumed at breakfast time.

Methods

Study design

The study was a randomised, placebo-controlled, double-blind intervention trial conducted over a twelve-week period (Sheffield University Breakfast Study – SUBS).

Recruitment

Ethics approval and consent

Ethics approval was obtained from Sheffield University Research Ethics Committee (Ref. SMBRER 223). Informed written consent was taken at the screening visit for the whole study.

Recruitment

Adolescent girls aged 16–19 years were selected for this study because the National Diet and Nutrition Survey (NDNS) of the UK and data from other developed countries, show that poor nutritional status is prevalent in this group [1, 2]. Girls were recruited from schools, colleges and Universities within the Sheffield area. An Amazon voucher for £30 was offered on completion of the study.

Eligibility

Inclusion criteria

Participants had to be female, aged between 16 and 19 years at the time of recruitment, who self-reported missing breakfast at least 4 times a week. They had to have no diagnosed illness and have low measures of riboflavin status and haemoglobin, as these have previously been found to track well with self-reported breakfast skipping [3].

Exclusion criteria

Potential participants were not recruited if they used multivitamin or iron supplements, had donated blood in the previous 6 months, were pregnant or breast feeding or had an allergy to wheat, barley or milk.

Screening

Recruitment to the study used a website which invited girls who self-reported skipping breakfast at least four times a week. Girls who responded were then screened for low riboflavin status and poor iron status. A screening visit was held to confirm eligibility, to answer any queries and concerns, to take consent, to collect additional information (such as date of birth, address and medication usage) and to take a small finger prick sample (~100 μl) for the measurement of riboflavin and iron status. Consent was taken for both the screening and the main intervention study. Blood samples were analysed for riboflavin status using the erythrocyte glutathione reductase activation coefficient assay (EGRAC) and hemoglobin concentration measured on-site using a portable Hemocue device (Hemocue Hb 201+ DM System, Hemocure, AB, Sweden). EGRAC is the most commonly used biomarker for riboflavin status. Samples with a low riboflavin status have a higher EGRAC value. An EGRAC value of >1.30 is conventionally used to indicate poor riboflavin status [3]. In this study, girls with an EGRAC value >1.40 and a hemoglobin of <137 g/L were eligible for the main study.

Sample size

Sample size was based on improvement in riboflavin status following the consumption of a fortified cereal with milk. Findings from the RIBOFEM study [3] showed that a supplement of 2 mg riboflavin per day for 8 weeks in young women elicits a fall in EGRAC of 0.25. This cereal study would provide 1.7 mg riboflavin per day for 12 weeks to adolescent girls, in addition to habitual dietary intake. It was anticipated that the intervention would achieve a similar fall in EGRAC and that the baseline SD would be ~ 0.20 on the basis of the RIBOFEM study. Standardised effect size was estimated to be 1.56. It was estimated that we would need 17 girls for each of 4 groups (cereal type and time of intervention) allowing for a possible 25 % dropout in this age and gender group. We therefore aimed to recruit 70 girls to the study.

Cereal

The cereal, supplied by Kellogg Marketing and Sales Company, was a wheat, rice and barley-based flake similar to their Special K cereal supplied in the UK. Unfortified and fortified cereal was provided and the identity of each was blinded to the researchers and participants. Participants were provided with an equal amount of plain and fruit cereal to add variety and improve compliance. Table 1 shows the estimated macronutrient and micronutrient intakes achieved from the consumption of unfortified and fortified cereal with milk.

Intervention and randomisation

Girls who were eligible for the main intervention study were invited to attend three clinics over a period of 12 weeks at the Clinical Research Facility at the Hallamshire Hospital, Sheffield. Prior to attending the first intervention clinic visit, girls were sent a study guide with instructions for the study, a timetable for the scheduled visits and a 4-d food diary to complete. They were also provided with a colour portion guide

Table 1 Nutrient and energy supplied by the cereal and milk intervention

Nutrient	50 g fortified cereal +150 ml milk	50 g unfortified cereal +150 ml milk
Energy (kcal)	257	257
Fat (g)	3.1	3.1
Carbohydrate (g)	47.8	47.8
Sugars (g)	15.9	15.9
Vitamin D (μg)	4.15	0.2
Vitamin C (mg)	51.5	1.5
Vitamin B_1 (mg)	1.21	0.36
Vitamin B_2 (mg)	1.71	0.61
Niacin (mg)	17.8	1.4
Vitamin B_6 (mg)	1.74	0.64
Folic Acid (μg)	176	18
Vitamin B_{12} (μg)	1.45	0.60
Iron (mg)	6.5	0.75
Calcium (mg)	215	215

From Windiets and Kellogg's published data (http://www.kelloggs.co.uk/en GB/special-k-html)
Values are averages of the berry and original varieties

booklet to facilitate portion size estimation. Girls were instructed to record dietary information for four consecutive days, including one weekend day.

Volunteers were randomised in blocks of twelve to receive a daily intake of either fortified or unfortified cereal (50 g) with semi-skimmed milk (150 ml) for 12 weeks, to be consumed at breakfast time or at supper-time. Volunteers were provided with a graduated measuring jug that indicated the cereal and milk portion sizes. 'Breakfast' refers to the first meal of the day, after an overnight fast; 'supper' refers to the last food consumed in the day, generally after an earlier complete meal, usually considered as 'dinner'. Previous experience had indicated that daily consumption of this amount of cereal and milk would be acceptable to volunteers.

Visit 1 (week 0)

The purpose of this visit was to collect baseline data and blood samples, to review completed pre-intervention food diaries, and to give the volunteers the first six weeks cereal supply. The girls were weighed using a digital Salter scale and their height measured using a stadiometer for adults. A fasted venous blood sample (6–7 ml) was collected. Girls were given instructions as to how and when to consume the cereal and milk and given tick sheets to record if and when they ate the cereal, for compliance assessment. At this visit, girls were given their next food diary to complete one week prior to visit 2.

Visit 2 (week 6)

At this visit the second diet diary was reviewed and girls were given the remainder of the cereal for the study. Any cereal that was not eaten was collected and weighed and used as a second measure of compliance.

Visit 3 (week 12)

At this final visit girls provided another venous blood sample and their height and weight were recorded. Any remaining cereal was collected for estimating compliance.

Blood collection

Blood was collected by venepunture from fasted volunteers in the morning, for plasma biochemical analysis (4.5 ml, EDTA vacutainer) and for routine hematology measurements (2 ml, EDTA vacutainer). Blood cells and plasma were separated by centrifugation, and the plasma divided into aliquots and stored at –80 °C for biochemical analysis. A hemolysate was prepared from the red blood cell pellet and stored at –80 °C for EGRAC measurements [3], to determine vitamin B_2 status.

Hematological measurements

Hemoglobin, hematocrit, MCV and red cell number were measured in the hematology laboratory at the Royal Hallamshire Hospital, Sheffield. If the laboratory report indicated 'suggestive of iron deficiency' at baseline, on the basis of low hemoglobin, ferritin and MCV, subjects were informed and withdrawn from the study.

Biochemical techniques

The choice of biochemical measurements of micronutrient status was informed primarily by those nutrients for which there is evidence of poor intake and/or status in adolescent girls, and which might therefore be expected to be influenced by the regular consumption of a fortified cereal.

Plasma ferritin for estimating iron stores

Plasma ferritin was measured by ELISA using a commercially available kit (Spectro Ferritin Kit, ATi Atlas Ltd. Chichester, UK). An external quality control was used to monitor accuracy and precision (Randox). The intra-batch coefficient of variation (CV) for QC1 (14 ng/mL) was 3.4 % and for QC2 (80 ng/mL) was 13.1 %. The inter-batch CV for QC1 (14 ng/mL) was 1.6 % and for QC2 (80 ng/mL) was 8.5 %. If the CV for sample replicates was greater than 10 %, these measurements were repeated.

Plasma holotranscobalamin (holoTC) for vitamin B_{12} status

Vitamin B_{12} status was assessed as its active form, holotranscobalamin, in plasma, using an ELISA kit (Active-B12 supplied by AXIS-SHIELD). The intra-batch CV for QC1 (25 nmol/L) was 3.1 % and for QC2 (60 nmol/L) was 12.5 %. The inter-batch CV for QC1 (25 nmol/L) was 5.1 % and for QC2 (60 nmol/L) was 3.5 %. If the CV for sample replicates was greater than 15 %, these measurements were repeated.

Plasma 5-methyltetrahydrofolate(5-MeTHF) for folate status

Plasma 5-MeTHF was measured by reverse-phase HPLC with fluorescence detection using a method described by Loehrer [25]. 5-MeTHF was detected fluorometrically at excitation and emission wavelengths of 295 nm and 365 nm, respectively. The intra-batch CV for the QC was 2.2 % and the inter-batch CV was 4.6 %.

Plasma 25-hydroxyvitamin D (25(OH)D for vitamin D status

The Bone Metabolism Group in the Faculty of Medicine, Dentistry and Health at Sheffield University measured plasma total 25-hydroxyvitamin D using an electrochemiluminescence binding method on a COBAS e 411auto analyser (Roche Diagnostics, Germany). The inter assay CV for total vitamin D was 5.7 %.

Erythrocyte glutathione reductase activation coefficient (EGRAC) for vitamin B_2 status

The activity of erythrocyte glutathione reductase (EC 1.6.4.2) was measured in haemolysates using the method described by Glatzle et al. [26], and modified by Hill et al. [27] for use on the Cobas Autoanalyser, (Roche Diagnostica). Results were expressed as an activation coefficient, EGRAC. The intra batch CV was 2.9 % and the inter batch CV was 1.25 %.

Dietary assessment

In order to monitor any changes in diet during the intervention and to assess dietary habits in this population of girls, dietary information was collected prior to and during the study. Four-day estimated food intake diaries were used, modified from those developed by the Institute of Food Research (IFR), Norwich, UK. The volunteers were also given food portion booklets developed by IFR and (based on the Ministry of Agriculture, Fisheries and Food (MAFF) food atlas [28] to assist in the recording of portion sizes. Data from the food diaries were analyzed for micronutrient and macronutrient contents with Windiets Research software (version 2010; Robert Gordon University, Aberdeen, United Kingdom).

Compliance

Two measures were used to assess compliance with the intervention. The completed tick sheets were used to assess self-reported compliance, which is a measure of occasions on which the cereal was consumed. The weight of cereal returned at the end of the study was used to estimate cereal consumed as a percentage of that requested.

Statistical analysis

Data sets did not deviate significantly from the normal distribution (Kolmogorov-Smirnov test). Data are therefore presented as mean ± SD. Analysis of the effects of the intervention on nutrient and energy intake and biomarkers of nutritional and haematological status, was by two-factor ANOVA (*F* test), with cereal type and time of consumption as factors, correcting for baseline values. When ANOVA indicated a significant difference according to cereal type or time of consumption, a Kruskal-Wallis multiple-comparison z value test was carried out, to identify where the differences lay. Within-group differences between baseline and follow-up were analysed using a paired sample *t* test. Comparison of percentage of girls falling outside normal thresholds for nutritional status was determined using Chi square test. Statistical analysis was performed using SPSS v.20 (IBM, Hampshire, UK). Significance was taken as $P < 0.05$.

Results

Subject recruitment, retention and compliance

Recruitment

Figure 1 details the flow of participants through the study. 198 girls were screened for moderate riboflavin and iron status, of whom 101 were eligible for the intervention trial. Of these, 78 girls agreed to take part in the main study. Five girls failed to complete the main study (one was withdrawn because of iron deficiency anaemia diagnosed by the Royal Hallamshire Hospital Haematology Department). Data are shown and analyses were conducted on data from 71 girls for whom there was a complete dataset. Of these, 37 girls had been randomised to receive unfortified cereal, 34 to receive fortified cereal. The main study was run alongside the screening and took place over 11 months between July 2012 and May 2013.

Compliance

On the basis of self-reported occasions on which cereal was consumed, compliance (mean ± SD) to the intervention was 91 ± 7.1 % ($n = 63$ responders). On the basis of the weight of cereal returned, compliance to the cereal consumption was 102 ± 10.3 % ($n = 71$); indicating that some girls consumed more than the weight of cereal they were asked to. Using this metric, compliance was lower in the girls receiving the unfortified cereal (98 ± 10.2 %) than the girls receiving the fortified cereal (105 ± 9.2 %), $P = 0.004$. Girls who consumed their cereal as a 'breakfast' had a

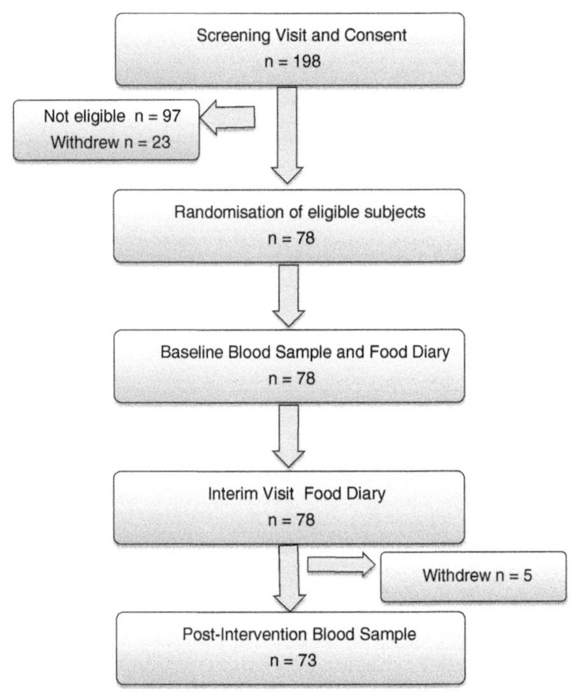

Fig. 1 Study protocol

median time of consumption of 0930 h, the median time of consumption as a 'supper' was 2130 h. Time of consumption (as breakfast or supper), did not influence compliance, by either metric.

Subject characteristics

Table 2 shows subject ages, weight, height and BMI, according to cereal type and time of consumption. The age distribution of girls completing the study was as follows: 5 at 16y, 7 at 17y, 22 at 18y, 36 at 19y and 1 who turned 20y between screening and starting the intervention. Analysis of variance revealed no significant differences in these variables between the randomisation groups.

Baseline biochemistry

Markers of micronutrient and hematological status

Table 2 also shows values for biochemical and hematological variables at baseline, according to cereal type and time of consumption. Analysis of variance revealed no differences in any of these variables between randomisation groups at baseline. Mean (±SD) EGRAC was higher (1.63 ± 0.21 vs 1.52 ± 0.20) and mean plasma ferritin (20 ± 13.4 vs 28 ± 22.9 μg/L) and hemoglobin concentrations were lower (128 ± 8.1 vs 131 ± 8.78 g/L) than the means (±SD) for girls of this age group in the UK, reported in NDNS [1]. Mean (±SD) plasma 25(OH)D concentration (40.8 ± 25.9) was comparable with the NDNS mean (±SD) of 42.5 ± 21.5 nmol/L.

Adequacy of micronutrient status

All girls fell above the conventional threshold of >1.30 for EGRAC, indicating low riboflavin status. 46 % the girls had evidence of low vitamin B_{12} status (plasma holoTC < 37 pmol/L and iron status (plasma ferritin < 15 ng/mL) whilst 32 % of the group had low vitamin D status (plasma 25(OH)D < 25 nmol/L).

Dietary intakes

Intakes of macronutrients and energy at baseline are shown in Table 3. There were no differences in any variable between cereal groups or according to time of consumption but there was an interaction between these factors for non-milk extrinsic sugars (NMES) sugars (g), sugars (% energy), total carbohydrate (g) and carbohydrate (% energy).

Intakes of micronutrients are shown in Table 4. There were no differences in intakes between cereal groups or according to time of consumption but there was an interaction between these factors for folate intake. At least half of the girls had intakes of vitamin B_2 and B_6, folate, iron and calcium lower than both the UK Recommended Nutrient Intakes (RNIs) and the Dietary Reference Intakes (DRIs) for USA. There are currently no DRV's for vitamin D for people between the ages of 4 and 65y in the UK [29], and therefore comparison was made with the recommendation from the Institute of Medicine (IOM) [30]. Intakes of vitamin D were lower

Table 2 Baseline characteristics of girls who completed the intervention

	Unfortified cereal				Fortified cereal				*P* value[e]		
	Morning (*n* = 21)		Evening (*n* = 16)		Morning (*n* = 18)		Evening (*n* = 16)		Cereal type	Timing	Interaction
	Mean	SD	Mean	SD	Mean	SD	Mean	SD			
Height (cm)	165	6.25	165	4.06	164	6.44	164	6.95	0.383	0.853	0.639
Weight (kg)	59.6	5.94	59.5	7.50	62.5	11.35	60.2	10.87	0.397	0.575	0.627
BMI (kg/m^2)	21.8	2.08	22.0	3.00	23.3	3.34	22.0	2.73	0.178	0.578	0.370
Age (y)	19.0	1.06	19.1	0.70	18.6	1.09	19.1	0.74	0.494	0.225	0.304
Biochemical and hematological status values											
EGRAC[a]	1.71	0.27	1.63	0.22	1.58	0.15	1.59	0.11	0.071	0.519	0.361
Plasma holoTC[b] (pmol/L)	40.6	16.90	40.08	15.95	34.6	12.68	34.1	14.12	0.143	0.806	0.839
Plasma 5MeTHF[c] (nmol/L)	14.1	7.74	17.1	8.45	17.0	9.50	17.2	6.18	0.364	0.328	0.557
Plasma 25(OH)D[d] (nmol/L)	37.1	20.72	42.6	25.63	33.8	21.87	50.3	33.34	0.632	0.062	0.316
Plasma ferritin (ng/ml)	23.9	13.57	18.8	15.41	19.7	11.03	17.9	13.69	0.519	0.360	0.511
Hemoglobin (g/L)	127	7.9	128	8.3	129	6.9	129	9.5	0.235	0.641	0.882
Hematocrit	0.38	0.03	0.38	0.03	0.38	0.02	0.39	0.03	0.967	0.153	0.377
Mean cell volume (fl)	85.8	3.67	84.1	5.01	83.9	3.41	84.4	4.49	0.348	0.451	0.348

[a]erythrocyte glutathione reductase activation coefficient
[b]holotranscobalamin
[c]5-methyltetrahydrofolate
[d]25-hydroxyvitamin D
[e]differences between groups according to cereal type, timing of consumption, and interactions

Table 3 Daily intakes of macronutrients and energy at baseline[a]

	Unfortified cereal				Fortified cereal				*P* value[d]		
	Morning (*n* = 21)		Evening (*n* = 16)		Morning (*n* = 18)		Evening (*n* = 16)		Cereal type	Timing	Interaction
	Mean	SD	Mean	SD	Mean	SD	Mean	SD			
Energy (kJ)	6756	2203	7318	2196	7712	2144	6426	2108	0.921	0.521	0.092
Fat (g)	61	26.2	65	25.6	71	25.0	61	24.6	0.644	0.696	0.253
Fat (% energy)	33.6	6.33	32.5	6.32	32.9	6.16	34.1	6.04	0.793	0.975	0.453
Protein (g)	59	19.8	57	10.0	63	19.2	58	18.9	0.567	0.471	0.809
Carbohydrate (g)	196	67.3	229	67.3	238	65.3	187	64.3	0.963	0.582	0.011
Carbohydrate (% energy)	46.3	6.24	50.8	6.00	49.9	71.28	46.8	6.85	0.870	0.693	0.010
Sugars (g)	72	37.3	96	36.7	101	36.3	70	36.0	0.814	0.749	0.003
Sugars (% energy)	16.7	6.02	20.1	5.96	21.9	5.79	17.0	5.69	0.394	0.662	0.006
Starch (g)	113	42.9	122	4.2	126	41.7	104	41.0	0.806	0.452	0.114
NMES[b] (g)	50	33.5	75	33.0	75	32.6	48	27.6	0.947	0.945	0.002
NSP[c] (g)	8.9	3.72	9.9	3.71	11.1	3.68	9.7	3.64	0.251	0.813	0.184
Alcohol (g)	11.9	12.22	8.6	12.0	6.33	11.9	6.0	11.69	0.190	0.574	0.557
Alcohol (% energy)	5.1	5.20	2.5	5.47	2.89	5.26	3.14	5.65	0.403	0.592	0.231

[a]energy and nutrient intakes determined using 4-day estimated diet diaries, aided by the use of portion size booklets
[b]non-milk extrinsic sugars
[c]non-starch polysaccharides
[d]differences according to cereal type, time of consumption and interaction

than the IOM Estimated Average Requirement (EAR) of 10 μg per day in all of the girls.

Effects of the intervention

Effects of the intervention on nutritional status and haematological biomarkers

The effects of the intervention on biochemical and hematological variables are shown in Table 5. Data are presented for values before and after intervention, according to cereal type. Two-way ANOVA revealed no effect of the time of consumption of the cereal on any variable and therefore the table shows results for morning and evening consumption combined, for the fortified and unfortified cereal.

Paired sample *t* test revealed a significant fall (improvement) in EGRAC, and a significant increase in plasma holo-transcobalamin, plasma 5-MeTHF and plasma ferritin after the intervention in the girls receiving the fortified cereal. Plasma 25(OH)D concentration fell in the girls receiving the unfortified cereal, but was maintained at the pre-intervention value in the group receiving the fortified cereal. Mean cell volume fell in both groups. When the

Table 4 Daily intakes of micronutrients at baseline[a]

	Unfortified cereal				Fortified cereal				*P* value[b]		
	Morning (*n* = 21)		Evening (*n* = 16)		Morning (*n* = 18)		Evening (*n* = 16)		Cereal type	Timing	Interaction
	Mean	SD	Mean	SD	Mean	SD	Mean	SD			
Vitamin B_1 (mg)	1.08	0.46	1.09	0.44	1.33	0.46	0.98	0.44	0.490	0.109	0.095
Vitamin B_2 (mg)	0.97	0.41	1.06	0.40	1.28	0.42	0.98	0.4	0.200	0.366	0.068
Niacin (mg)	24.2	9.71	25.0	9.68	28.3	9.58	26.2	9.40	0.228	0.830	0.576
Vitamin B_6 (mg)	1.17	0.51	1.27	0.48	1.50	0.46	1.21	0.48	0.321	0.334	0.065
Vitamin B_{12} (μg)	3.32	1.66	2.76	1.64	2.83	1.64	2.70	1.60	0.541	0.438	0.539
Folate (μg)	138	61	161	60	189	60	148	59	0.176	0.606	0.039
Vitamin D (μg)	1.55	1.33	1.51	1.32	1.93	1.30	1.53	1.28	0.501	0.525	0.620
Calcium (mg)	676	283	677	282	771	280	631	274	0.637	0.360	0.358
Sodium (mg)	2373	805	2480	804	2449	794	2167	776	0.609	0.725	0.365
Iron (mg)	8.06	2.57	8.51	2.60	9.54	2.56	7.45	2.52	0.699	0.207	0.050

[a]nutrient intakes determined using 4-day estimated diet diaries, aided by the use of portion size booklets
[b]differences according to cereal type, time of consumption, and interaction

Table 5 Nutritional status and hematological biomarkers following intervention

Analyte	Unfortified cereal ($n = 37$)		Fortified cereal ($n = 34$)		P value[a]
	Pre-intervention	Post-intervention	Pre-intervention	Post-intervention	
	Mean (SD)	Mean (SD)	Mean (SD)	Mean (SD)	
EGRAC[b]	1.68 (0.25)	1.65 (0.18)	1.58 (0.13)	1.38 (0.15)*	<0.001
Plasma holoTC[c] (pmol/L)	40.7 (16.27)	39.4 (7.44)	35.3 (12.94)	42.8 (13.66)**	<0.001
Plasma 5MeTHF[d] (nmol/L)	15.4 (8.09)	14.1 (6.90)	17.3 (7.96)	32.9 (16.16)**	<0.001
Plasma 25(OH)D[e] (nmol/L)	39.4 (22.77)	30.6 (18.74)*	42.5 (29.21)	43.7 (28.22)	<0.001
Plasma ferritin (ng/ml)	21.7 (14.42)	18.4 (11.63)	19.3 (12.38)	22.1 (16.73)**	<0.001
Hemoglobin (g/L)	128 (8.03)	128 (6.63)	130 (7.96)	130 (7.68)	0.876
Hematocrit	0.38 (0.03)	0.38 (0.02)	0.38 (0.02)	0.38 (0.02)	0.687
Mean cell volume (fl)	85.0 (4.31)	84.1 (4.33)*	84.0 (3.84)	83.2 (3.82)*	0.876

*significantly lower than value pre-intervention (paired t test; $P < 0.05$)
**significantly higher than value pre-intervention (paired t test; $P < 0.05$)
[a]significance of difference between cereal groups after intervention, corrected for baseline (ANOVA)
[b]erythrocyte glutathione reductase activation coefficient
[c]holotranscobalamin
[d]5-methyltetrahydrofolate
[e]25-hydroxyvitamin D

effect of the intervention was compared between cereal types, girls eating the fortified cereal showed a significant improvement in biomarkers of vitamin B_2, vitamin B_{12}, folate, and vitamin D status and of plasma ferritin, compared with girls receiving the unfortified cereal.

Effects of intervention on the percentage of girls with nutrient biomarkers below the lower limits for normality

Table 6 shows the percentage of girls who would be considered as 'deficient' in specific micronutrients, according to the stated threshold for each biomarker. Data are shown as percentages before and after the intervention, according to cereal type. Three thresholds are used for EGRAC; the conventional threshold is 1.30 but it has been suggested that a higher threshold should be used to reflect a functional deficiency [3], therefore 1.40 and 1.60 are used too. For girls receiving the fortified cereal, there was a significant decrease in the percentage with biomarker values below the lower limit of normality (or above the EGRAC thresholds) when compared with girls receiving unfortified cereal, for vitamin B_2, vitamin B_{12} and folate.

Effects of intervention on nutrient intakes

Macronutrients and energy

There were no significant differences in post-intervention values between consumers of unfortified and fortified cereal. Within-group analysis revealed a significant decrease from the pre-intervention value for fat and carbohydrate as a percentage of energy, and an increase in starch (Table 7).

Table 6 Effects of cereal intervention on percentage of girls falling below[a] biochemical thresholds for normality

Analyte	Threshold	Unfortified cereal		Fortified cereal	
		Pre-intervention	Post-intervention	Pre-intervention	Post-intervention
EGRAC[b]	>1.3	100	100	100	63*
EGRAC	>1.4	95	97	94	42*
EGRAC	>1.6	60	57	47	8*
Plasma HoloTC[c]	<37pmol/L	46	51	53	36*
Plasma 5MeTHF[d]	<14 nmol/L	11	8	14	0*
Plasma 25(OH)D[e]	<25 nmol/L	32	46	31	31
Plasma ferritin	<15 ng/ml	46	49	50	44
Hemoglobin	<120 g/L	24	14	11	15
Mean cell volume (fl)	<84 fl	27	49	46	53

*significantly different from girls in the unfortified group (Chi Squared test; $P < 0.05$)
[a]above threshold values for EGRAC
[b]erythrocyte glutathione reductase activation coefficient
[c]plasma holotranscobalamin
[d]plasma 5-methyl tetrahydrofolate
[e]plasma 25-hydroxyvitamin D

Table 7 Intakes of macronutrients and energy following intervention[a]

Nutrient	Unfortified cereal ($n = 37$)		Fortified cereal ($n = 34$)		P-value[d]
	Pre-intervention Mean (SD)	Post-intervention Mean (SD)	Pre-intervention Mean (SD)	Post-intervention Mean (SD)	
Energy (kcals)	1665 (526)	1732 (377)	1695 (534)	1743 (329)	0.952
Fat (g)	63 (23)	62 (18)	67 (29)	58 (19)	0.269
Fat (% energy)	33 (6)	31 (5)*	33 (7)	29 (6)*	0.078
Protein (g)	59 (19)	70 (16)**	61 (20)	67 (17)	0.357
Carbohydrate (g)	210 (66)	230 (53)	214 (74)	242 (45)**	0.351
Carbohydrate (% energy)	48 (6)	51 (6)**	48 (7)	53 (6)**	0.063
Sugars (g)	82 (41)	81 (32)	87 (37)	92 (32)	0.173
Sugars (% energy)	18 (6)	18 (5)	20 (7)	20 (6)	0.086
NMES[b] (g)	61 (37)	55 (27)	63 (34)	63 (32)	0.273
Starch (g)	116 (32)	142 (32)**	115 (53)	137 (30)**	0.441
NSP[c] (g)	9 (3)	10 (3)	10 (4)	10 (3)	0.734
Alcohol (g)	11 (15)	4 (7)*	6 (8)	5 (8)	0.304
Alcohol (% energy)	4 (6)	2 (3)*	3 (4)	2 (3)*	0.359

*significantly lower than value pre-intervention (paired t test; $P < 0.05$)
**significantly higher than value pre-intervention (paired t test; $P < 0.05$)
[a]energy and nutrient intakes determined using 4-day estimated diet diaries, aided by the use of portion size booklets
[b]non-milk extrinsic sugars
[c]Non-starch polysaccharides
[d]significance of differences between cereal groups, corrected for baseline

An increase in protein and carbohydrate was observed which reached statistical significance for the consumers of unfortified and fortified cereal, respectively. Alcohol intake as a percentage of energy showed a decrease from baseline in response to cereal intervention; there was no effect of cereal type.

Vitamins, minerals and trace elements

Within-group analysis showed that consuming the unfortified cereal improved intake of vitamins B_1, B_2 and B_6, and consuming the fortified cereal improved intakes of all fortificants - vitamins B_1, B_2, niacin, B_6, B_{12}, C, D, folate and iron (Table 8). The intake of these nutrients was significantly greater than for girls receiving unfortified cereal; there was no effect of time of consumption. There was no difference between groups in the effect of the interventions on calcium intakes, although within-group analysis showed an increase in the girls receiving the milk with unfortified cereal.

Table 8 Daily intake of micronutrients following intervention[a]

Nutrient	Unfortified cereal ($n = 37$)		Fortified cereal ($n = 34$)		P value[b]
	Pre-intervention Mean (SD)	Post-intervention Mean (SD)	Pre-intervention Mean (SD)	Post-intervention Mean (SD)	
Vitamin B_1 (mg)	1.1 (0.40)	1.3 (0.35)**	1.2 (0.50)	2.2 (0.36)**	<0.001
Vitamin B_2 (mg)	1.0 (0.41)	1.4 (0.35)**	1.2 (0.43)	2.7 (0.50)**	<0.001
Niacin (mg)	25 (8.1)	27 (9.0)	27 (11.1)	41 (10.3)**	<0.001
Vitamin B_6 (mg)	1.2 (0.45)	1.8 (0.40)**	1.3 (0.53)	3.0 (0.64)**	<0.001
Vitamin B_{12} (μg)	3.1 (1.81)	2.8 (1.09)	2.8 (1.44)	4.1 (1.78)**	<0.001
Folate (μg)	148 (55)	151 (61)	171 (69)	314 (54)**	<0.001
Vitamin D (μg)	1.5 (1.35)	1.6 (0.91)	1.8 (1.28)	5.5 (1.32)**	0.007
Calcium (mg)	677 (282)	822 (248)**	713 (282)	775 (177)	<0.001
Sodium (mg)	2419 (7367)	2528 (631)	2335 (863)	2576 (637)	0.628
Iron (mg)	8.3 (2.47)	7.7 (2.37)	8.9 (2.86)	13.1 (2.31)**	<0.001

**significantly higher than pre-intervention (paired t test; $P < 0.05$)
[a]nutrient intakes determined using 4-day estimated diet diaries, aided by the use of portion size booklets
[b]significance of difference between cereal groups corrected for baseline values (ANOVA)

Effect of intervention on percentage of girls with intakes below recommended intakes

Intakes of micronutrients following the intervention were compared with RNIs for the UK and DRIs for USA. After intervention with fortified cereal all girls had intakes of vitamins B_2 and B_6 that exceeded both sets of recommendations. Intakes of folate and vitamin B_{12} also achieved UK recommendations but fell short of DRIs; no girl achieved the recommended DRI for folate (Table 9). A high percentage of girls in this group still had iron intakes below both sets of recommendations, but none of the girls had an iron intake less than the Lower Reference Nutrient Intake (LRNI) for the UK, which represents an intake that satisfies the requirement of only 2.5 % of the population. In contrast, after intervention with unfortified cereal, micronutrient intakes less than both sets of recommendations persisted across all micronutrients with the exception of vitamin B_6. Although calcium was not a fortificant, the cereal and milk intervention increased calcium intakes but overall, intakes fell short of RNIs and DRIs in at least 50 % of girls, after the intervention. Although vitamin D intakes increased significantly in the fortified group, and were higher in the fortified group post-intervention, than the unfortified group, intakes still fell short of the EAR of 10 μg proposed by IOM [30].

Two-way ANOVA, correcting for baseline showed no effect of cereal type or time of consumption on weight or BMI. However, analysis of weight and BMI for all evening consumers, regardless of whether the cereal was fortified or not, showed a small but significant increase in weight (mean ± SD, 0.93 ± 1.96 kg) over the intervention period ($P = 0.012$), which was not seen in girls consuming the cereal in the morning (mean ± SD, 0.27 ± 1.64 kg).

Discussion

The consumption of fortified cereal with milk elicited very clear benefits in terms of increased intakes of some vitamins and iron, and significant improvements in biomarkers of nutritional status. The beneficial effects were seen whether the cereal with milk was consumed in the morning or the evening. The consumption of unfortified cereal with milk also showed some benefit but this was restricted to a few nutrients and was modest compared with the fortified cereal. This observation is important because previous statements about the health benefits of breakfast consumption in any age group have relied almost entirely on observational studies, which could only show associations. Girls taking part in the study had micronutrient intake and status profiles comparable with those reported in the NDNS, so the findings can be considered relevant to their gender and age group.

After 12 weeks of consuming a fortified cereal with milk each day all girls achieved intakes of at least RNI for all micronutrients except for iron and calcium. Intakes were still lower than the DRI for folate and vitamin D for all the girls. Several observational studies have shown that regular breakfast consumption among young people is associated with higher intakes of some micronutrients, including folate, vitamin D, calcium, iron and zinc [31, 32], although details of the type of breakfast consumed are often lacking. Concern has been expressed about a low intake of vitamin D in some sections of the UK population, and there is evidence for poor vitamin D status in some groups [1]; low intakes of this vitamin in adolescents are reported for several other European countries [33]. Vitamin D intake increased significantly in the girls receiving the fortified cereal and this was sufficient to maintain vitamin D status over the period of the intervention, in contrast with the girls receiving the unfortified cereal, in whom vitamin D status fell during the study. This is important because there are few good dietary sources of vitamin D [34] and people living in the Northern hemisphere generally show a decline in plasma concentrations of 25(OH)D during the winter months [35]. The study was conducted during winter and summer months, when potential for dermal

Table 9 Effect of intervention on percentage of girls with micronutrient intakes below recommendations

Diet	% below RNI Unfortified cereal		% below RNI Fortified cereal		% below DRI/RDA[a] Unfortified cereal		% below DRI/RDA[a] Fortified cereal	
	Pre	Post	Pre	Post	Pre	Post	Pre	Post
Vitamin B-2	62.2	18.9	50	0	62.2	18.9	50	0
Vitamin B-6	54.1	9.5	50	0	54.1	9.5	50	0
Vitamin B-12	18.9	13.5	25	0	35.1	35.1	44.1	14.7
Folate	78.4	86.5	72.2	0	100	100	100	100
Iron	97.3	100	97.2	82.9	97.3	100	97.2	82.9
Calcium	70.3	48.6	66.7	60	97.3	94.6	97.1	97.1
Vitamin D[a]	N/A	N/A	N/A	N/A	100	100	100	100

pre, post refer to values before and after intervention, *RNI* recommended nutrient intake (UK), *DRI* Dietary Reference Intake (USA) [a]RDA (Recommended Dietary Allowance) from the Institute of Medicine Report (31)

synthesis of vitamin D would have been different but the block randomisation method would have minimised differences in any seasonal effect on vitamin D synthesis between the groups. The regular consumption of a cereal fortified with vitamin D could make a useful contribution to dietary vitamin D and evidently has the potential to mitigate the seasonal deterioration in vitamin D status.

This simple intervention had a clear beneficial effect in terms of nutrient intake in this vulnerable group. This was true whether the cereal was consumed in the morning or the evening, offering potentially important flexibility in terms of a public health message.

There is very limited evidence that the consumption of a fortified breakfast cereal leads to an improvement in micronutrient status, due to the lack of randomised controlled trials. Tucker and colleagues [36] conducted a study in adults aged 50-85y, focussed on effects of fortified cereal on plasma homocysteine concentration. They reported improvements in vitamin B_6, B_{12} and folate status as well as a decrease in homocysteine concentration. Whilst this is of interest, adolescents are more likely to skip breakfast [16, 21, 22], making it particularly important to demonstrate beneficial effects of breakfast cereal consumption in this group. In our trial, compared with the girls receiving unfortified cereal, consumption of the fortified cereal led to significant improvements in biomarkers of vitamin B_2, B_{12}, vitamin D and folate status as well as plasma ferritin, a biomarker of hepatic iron stores. Despite the increase in iron stores elicited by the fortified cereal intervention compared with the unfortified cereal, no increase in hemoglobin was observed and there was no difference in hemoglobin concentration between the two groups following the intervention. An increase in iron stores following the intervention would suggest that iron delivery to the site of hemoglobin synthesis was adequate, and that hemoglobin synthesis was not compromised at the outset. Additional available iron in the diet would then be stored as hepatic iron. There were no differences in mean hemoglobin at baseline between the cereal groups but fewer girls receiving fortified cereal had low hemoglobin (<12 g/L), which may have influenced ferritin responses in this group. An intervention study carried out in New Zealand among women with low iron stores, demonstrated a beneficial effect on iron status of consuming an iron-fortified breakfast cereal together with kiwi fruit, which has a high vitamin C content, compared with cereal consumed with banana [37]. Although a direct comparison of this study with the present study is difficult to make, given differences in age of the women, and iron status at the outset, the results suggest that the vitamin C content of fortified cereal may be inadequate to maximise absorption of cereal iron.

There is very little information available regarding the nutritional status of adolescent breakfast consumers compared with non-consumers. The majority of studies have paid more attention to obesity and measures of metabolic health than biomarkers of nutritional status. A recent study of younger children in Cyprus reported no difference in plasma ferritin concentration between consumers and non-consumers [38].

Despite the unequivocal improvement in micronutrient status in the girls receiving fortified cereal, and the decrease in the percentage of girls falling below the biomarker thresholds for normality, the improvement was insufficient to bring all girls into the normal range for conventional biomarkers of status except for folate. The normalisation of folate status is of particular relevance to this study population, given the importance of good folate status to healthy pregnancy [39].

Girls consuming cereal in the evening showed a small but significant increase in weight, which was not seen in the girls consuming cereal in the morning. The two-way ANOVA, correcting for baseline values, did not reveal any difference between groups, suggesting that undue emphasis should not be placed on the within-group finding. It is possible that cereal consumed in the evening is less likely to displace other foods, but this was not reflected in a significant increase in energy intake in the evening consumers. Others have explored effects of breakfast habits on energy intake and there have been several reports that breakfast skipping causes a compensatory increase in energy intake later in the day [40]. There may be differences in physical activity following cereal consumed as a breakfast or as a supper. Betts et al. [41] recently reported that daily breakfast consumption was associated with an increase in energy expenditure during the morning of the breakfast. The mean weight gain reported in our study was small and it will be important to know whether this was maintained or lost if evening cereal consumption was sustained over a longer period.

The cereal and milk intervention led to a modest but significant decrease in the proportion of dietary fat as a percentage of total energy intake and an increase in the proportion of energy derived from carbohydrate. This, together with the lack of increase in energy intake suggests that the cereal may have displaced fat-rich foods from the diet of these girls. This is compatible with the findings of Deshmuk-Taskar et al. [42], who reported a lower intake of fat and a higher intake of carbohydrate in children and adolescents who consumed ready to eat breakfast cereal (RTEC) compared with non-consumers. There is also a small literature suggesting that breakfast consumption may influence snacking behaviour such as to reduce energy intake from snacks and reduce snacking frequency [43]. Utter et al. [44] reported that skipping breakfast is associated with a greater frequency of snacking in New Zealand teenagers. It is possible that the cereal and milk intervention had the effect of reducing the consumption of fat-rich snacks; this is the subject of further investigation. Before the intervention, analysis indicated a significant interaction between various measures of carbohydrate intake; this seemed to be a result of between-group differences in mean values (not-significant) for these variables at baseline. The interaction was not evident post-intervention and we do not ascribe particular significance to the observation.

In conclusion, the daily consumption of a micronutrient-fortified breakfast cereal for 12 weeks, in the morning or the evening, by adolescent girls in the UK, improved status indices for vitamins B_2, B_{12}, folate, and iron. For each of these micronutrients this effect was significantly greater than benefits of consuming a non-fortified cereal. Vitamin D status was maintained in girls consuming fortified cereal in contrast with a decline seen in girls consuming unfortified cereal. Consuming cereal in the evening, whether fortified or non-fortified, elicited a modest weight gain but this was not associated with an increase in energy intake. To our knowledge this is the only randomised controlled trial of cereal intervention in adolescents reporting on dietary intake and micronutrient status. These findings are relevant across age and gender groups but have particular importance during the transition from childhood to adolescence, which is generally associated with less healthy dietary choices. The findings contribute to our understanding of the value of developing strategies to encourage the regular consumption of breakfast cereal in adolescents.

Limitations of the study

Dietary intake was estimated using 4-day diet diaries, supported by food portion booklets; the use of weighed records would have produced more reliable data but the additional burden would probably have reduced ease of recruitment to the study and jeopardised compliance. In retrospect it would have been useful to have determined energy expenditure before and during the intervention, given the reported influence of breakfast consumption on morning energy expenditure. However, this would have entailed a significant demand on participants and may have reduced compliance. It may also have been useful to have explored the prevalence of mis-reporting of dietary data, although this is a complex subject to examine and the randomisation design should have minimised the impact on the main findings.

Strengths of the study

To our knowledge this is the only randomised placebo controlled intervention trial that has attempted to determine the effects of consuming breakfast cereal and milk on micronutrient intake and status in adolescents. The separation of the intervention into a morning and an evening consumption added value in that this allowed us to demonstrate the potential benefits of consuming cereal with milk in an evening as an alternative to morning consumption.

Acknowledgements

The Kelloggs Company of Great Britain provided the cereal for the study and financial support for the research. They had no role whatsoever in the design and execution of the study, in the writing of the manuscript, the data analysis or the interpretation of the results. The salary of HJP and JR was provided by the University of Sheffield, that of MHH by Kelloggs Company of Great Britain. MS was a Master's student with no income.

Authors' contributions

The study was conceived and designed by HJP, MHH and JR; MHH and MS carried out the day to day work; JR carried out the statistical analysis; HJP drafted the manuscript, all authors contributed to the final version. All authors read and approved the final manuscript.

Competing interests

The authors declare that they have no competing interests.

Author details

[1]Human Nutrition Unit, University of Sheffield, Sheffield, UK. [2]Corporate Information and Computing Services, University of Sheffield, Sheffield, UK.

References

1. Public Health England and Food Standards Agency. National Diet and Nutrition Survey:Results from Years 1 to 4 (combined) of the Rolling programme for 2008/2009 to 2011/2012. https://www.gov.uk/government/uploads/system/uploads/attachment_data/file/310995/NDNS_Y1_to_4_UK_report.pdf Published May 2014 PHE publications gateway number:2014051. Accessed 24 Oct 2016.
2. Second National Report on Biochemical Indicators of Diet and Nutrition In the US PopulationCDC2012 (www.cdc.gov/nutritionreport/pdf/ExecSummary_Web_032612.pdf). 24 Oct 2016.
3. Powers HJ, Hill MH, Mushtaq S, Dainty JR, Majsak-Newman G, Williams EA. Correcting a marginal riboflavin deficiency improves hematological status in young women in the United Kingdom (RIBOFEM). Am J Clin Nutr. 2011;93(6):1274–84.
4. Aranda N, Ribot B, Garcia E, Viteri FE, Arija V. Pre-pregnancy iron reserves, iron supplementation during pregnancy and birth weight. Early Hum Dev. 2011;87(12):791–7.
5. Chesnut 3rd CH. Is osteoporosis a pediatric disease? Peak bone mass attainment in the adolescent female. Public Health Rep. 1989;104 Suppl:50–4.
6. Faulkner RA, Bailey DA. Osteoporosis: a pediatric concern? Med Sport Sci. 2007;51:1–12.
7. Young BE, McNanley TJ, Cooper EM, McIntyre AW, Witter F, Harris ZL, et al. Maternal vitamin D and calcium interact to affect fetal growth in utero in pregnant adolescents. Am J Clin Nutr. 2012;95(5):1103–12.
8. Dror DK, Allen LH. Dairy product intake in children and adolescents in developed countries: trends, nutritional contribution, and a review of association with health outcomes. Nutr Rev. 2013;72(2):68–81.
9. Pearson N, Biddle SJ, Gorely T. Family correlates of breakfast consumption among children and adolescents. A systematic review. Appetite. 2009;52(1):1–7.
10. Pearson N, MacFarlane A, Crawford D, Biddle SJH. Family circumstances and adolescent behaviours. Appetite. 2009;52(3):668–74.
11. Rampersaud GC, Pereira MA, Girard BL, Adams J, Metzl JD. Breakfast habits, nutritional status, body weight, and academic performance in children and adolescents. J Am Diet Assoc. 2005;105(5):743–60.
12. Siega-Riz AM, Popkin BM, Carson T. Trends in breakfast consumption in the United States from 1965–1991. Am J Clin Nutr. 1998;67:S748–56.
13. Bowman SA. Beverage choices of young females: changes and impact on nutrient intakes. J Am Diet Assoc. 2002;102:1234–9.
14. Lioret S, Dubuisson C, Dufour A, Touvier M, Calamassi-Tran G, Maire B, et al. Trends in food intake in French children from 1999 to 2007: results from the

INCA (etude Individuelle Nationale des Consommation Alimentaires) dietary surveys. Brit J Nutr. 2010;103(4):585–601.
15. Sandercock GR, Voss C, Dye L. Associations between habitual school-day breakfast consumption, body mass index, physical activity and cardiorespiratory fitness in English schoolchildren. Eur J Clin Nutr. 2010; 64(10):1086–92.
16. Sjoberg A, Hallberg L, Hoglund D, Hulthen L. Meal pattern, food choice, nutrient intake and lifestyle factors in The Goteborg Adolescence Study. Eur J Clin Nutr. 2003;57(12):1569–78.
17. Keski-Rahkonen A, Kaprio J, Rissanen A, Virkunnen M, Rose RJ. Breakfast skipping and health-compromising behaviours in adolescents and adults. Eur J Clin Nutr. 2003;57:842–53.
18. Belderson P, Harvey I, Kimbell R, O'Neill J, Russell J, Barker ME. Does breakfast-club attendance affect children's nutrient intake? A study of dietary intake at three schools. Br J Nutr. 2003;90:1003–6.
19. Matthys C, De Henauw S, Bellemans M, De Maeyer M, De Backer G. Breakfast habits affect overall nutrient profiles in adolescents. Public Health Nutr. 2007;10(4):413–21.
20. Barr SI, DiFranceso L, Fulgoni III VL. Consumption of breakfast and the type of breakfast consumed are positively associated with nutrient intakes and adequacy of Canadian adults. J Nutr. 2013;143:86–92.
21. Gibson S, Gunn P. What's for breakfast? Nutritional implications of breakfast habits: insights from the NDNS dietary records. Nutr Bull. 2011;36:78–86.
22. Raaijmakers LG, Bessems KM, Kremers SP, van Assema P. Breakfast consumption among children and adolescents in the Netherlands. Eur J Public Health. 2010;20:318–24.
23. Reddan J, Wahlstrom K, Reicks M. Children's perceived benefits and barriers in relation to eating breakfast in schools with or without Universal School Breakfast. J Nutr Educ Behav. 2002;34(1):47–52.
24. Shaw ME. Adolescent breakfast-skipping: an Australian study. Adolescence. 1998;33(132):851–61.
25. Loehrer FM, Angst CP, Haefeli WE, Jordan PP, Ritz R, Fowler B. Low whole-blood S-adenosylmethionine and correlation between 5-methyltetrahydrofolate and homocysteine in coronary artery disease. Arterioscler Thromb Vasc Biol. 1996;16(6):727–33.
26. Glatzle D, Korner WF, Christeller S, Wiss O. Method for the detection of a biochemical riboflavin deficiency. Stimulation of NADPH2-dependent glutathione reductase from human erythrocytes by FAD in vitro. Investigations on the vitamin B-2 status in healthly people and geriatric patients. Int Z Vitaminforsch. 1970;40(2):166–83.
27. Hill MH, Bradley A, Mushtaq S, Williams EA, Powers HJ. Effect of methodological variation on assessment of riboflavin status using the erythrocyte glutathione reductase coefficient assay. Br J Nutr. 2009;102(2):273–8.
28. Nelson M, Atkinson M, Meyer J. Food portion sizes: a photographic atlas: food standards agency. 2002.
29. Department of Health. Dietary reference values for food energy and nutrients for the United Kingdom. Report on health and social subjects; 41. London: Her Majesty's Stationary Office; 1991.
30. IOM (Institute of Medicine). Dietary reference intakes for calcium and vitamin D. Washington DC: The National Academies Press, 2011. .
31. Barton BA, Eldridge AL, Thompson D, Affenito SG, Striegel-Moore RH, Franko DL, et al. The relationship of breakfast and cereal consumption to nutrient intake and body mass index: the National Heart, Lung, and Blood Institute Growth and Health Study. J Am Diet Assoc. 2005;105(9):1383–9.
32. Michels N, de Henauw S, Briedenassel C, Censi L, Cuenca-Garci M, Gonzales-Gross M, et al. European adolescent ready-to-eat-cereal (RTEC) consumers have a healthier dietary intake and body composition compared with non-RTEC consumers. Eur J Nutr. 2015;54:653–64.
33. Mensink GBM, Fletcher R, Gurinovic M, Huybrechts I, Lafay L, Serra-Majem L, et al. Mapping low intakes of micronutrients across Europe. Br J Nutr. 2013;110(4):755–73.
34. Black LJ, Walton J, Flynn A, Kiely M. Adequacy of vitamin D intakes in children and teenagers from the base diet, fortified foods and supplements. Public Health Nutr. 2014;17:721–31.
35. Logan VF, Gray AR, Peddie MC, Harper MJ, Houghton LA. Long-term vitamin D3 supplementation is more effective than vitamin D2 at maintaining 25-hydroxy vitamin D status over the winter months. Br J Nutr. 2013;109(6):1082–8.
36. Tucker KL, Olson B, Bakun P, Dallal GE, Selhub J, Rosenberg IH. Breakfast cereal fortified with folic acid, vitamin B-6 and vitamin B-12 increases vitamin concentrations and reduces homocysteine concentrations: a randomised trial. Am J Clin Nutr. 2004;79(5):805–11.
37. Beck K, Conlon CA, Kruger R, Coad J, Stonehouse W. Consumption of an iron-fortified breakfast cereal together with kiwifruit improved iron status in women with low iron stores compared with consuming with a banana. Br J Nutr. 2011;105(1):101–9.
38. Lazarou C, Matalas A-L. Breakfast intake is associated with nutritional status, Mediterranean diet adherence, serum iron and fasting glucose: the CYFamilies study. Public Health Nutr. 2015;18(7):1308–16.
39. Obeid R, Koletzko B, Pietrzik K. Critical evaluation of lowering the recommended intake of folate. Clin Nutr. 2014;33(2):252–9.
40. Astbury NM, Taylor MA, MacDonald IA. Breakfast consumption affects appetite, energy intake and the metabolic and endocrine responses to foods consumed later in the day in male habitual breakfast eaters. J Nutr. 2011;141(7):1381–9.
41. Betts JA, Richardson JD, Chowdhury EA, Holman GD, Tsintzas K, Thompson D. The causal role of breakfast in energy balance and health: a randomised controlled trial in lean adults. Am J Clin Nutr. 2014;100:539–47.
42. Deshmukh-Taskar PR, Nicklas TA, O'Neil CE, Keast DR, Radcliffe JD, Cho S. The relationship of breakfast skipping and type of breakfast consumption with nutrient intake and weight status in children and adolescents: the National Health and Nutrition Examination Survey 1999–2006. J Am Diet Assoc. 2010;110960:869–78.
43. Schlundt DG, Hill JO, Sbrocco T, Pope-Cordle J, Sharp T. The role of breakfast in the treatment of obesity: a randomised clinical trial. Am J Clin Nutr. 1992;55(3):645–51.
44. Utter J, Scragg R, Mhurchu CN, Schaaf D. At-home breakfast consumption among New Zealand children: associations with body mass index and related nutrition behaviours. J Am Diet Assoc. 2007;107(4):570–6.

Comparison of multi-modal early oral nutrition for the tolerance of oral nutrition with conventional care after major abdominal surgery: a prospective, randomized, single-blind trial

Da-Li Sun[1,2,3†], Wei-Ming Li[2†], Shu-Min Li[2,3†], Yun-Yun Cen[2,3], Qing-Wen Xu[2,3], Yi-Jun Li[2,3], Yan-Bo Sun[2,3], Yu-xing Qi[2,3], Yue-ying Lin[2,3], Ting Yang[2,3], Qi-Ping Lu[1*] and Peng-Yuan Xu[2,3*]

Abstract

Background & aims: Early oral nutrition (EON) has been shown to improve recovery of gastrointestinal function, length of stay and mortality after abdominal surgery; however, early oral nutrition often fails during the first week after surgery. Here, a multi-modal early oral nutrition program is introduced to promote recovery of gastrointestinal function and tolerance of oral nutrition.

Methods: Consecutive patients scheduled for abdominal surgery were randomized to the multimodal EON group or a group receiving conventional care. The primary endpoint was the time of first defecation. The secondary endpoints were outcomes and the cost-effectiveness ratio in treating infectious complications. The rate of infectious-free patients was regarded as the index of effectiveness.

Results: One hundred seven patients were randomly assigned to groups. Baseline characteristics were similar for both groups. In intention-to-treat analysis, the success rate of oral nutrition during the first week after surgery in the multimodal EON group was 44 (83.0%) versus 31 (57.4%) in the conventional care group ($P = 0.004$). Time to first defecation, time to flatus, recovery time of bowel sounds, and prolonged postoperative ileus were all less in the multimodal EON group ($P < 0.05$). The median postoperative length of stay in the multimodal EON group was 8 days (6, 12) versus 10 days (7, 18) in the conventional care group ($P < 0.001$). The total cost of treatment and nutritional support were also less in the multi-modal early oral nutrition group ($P < 0.001$). The effectiveness was 84.9 and 79.9% in the multimodal EON and conventional care group, respectively ($P = 0.475$). However, the cost-effectiveness ratio was USD 537.6 (506.1, 589.3) and USD 637.8 (593.9, 710.3), respectively ($P < 0.001$).

Conclusion: The multi-modal early oral nutrition program was an effective way to improve tolerance of oral nutrition during the first week after surgery, decrease the length of stay and improve cost-effectiveness after abdominal surgery.

Trial registration: Registration number: ChiCTR-TRC-14004395. Registered 15 March 2014.

Keywords: Multi-modal early oral nutrition (multimodal EON), Postoperative ileus (POI), Cost-effectiveness analysis

* Correspondence: ptwklqp111@163.com; destiny1978@163.com
The co-first authors (Wei-Ming Li and Shu-Min Li) who contributed equally to this paper
†Equal contributors
[1]Department of General Surgery, Wuhan Clinical School of Southern Medical University/Wuhan General Hospital of Guangzhou Military Command, Wuhan 430070, China
[2]Department of Gastrointestinal Surgery, Second Affiliated Hospital of Kunming Medical University, Kunming 650101, China
Full list of author information is available at the end of the article

Introduction

An early start of oral nutrition is promoted in most patients undergoing abdominal surgery and is an core component that enhances recovery after surgery [1, 2]. An early start of oral nutrition within the first 24 h postoperatively is beneficial and has even been associated with a reduced mortality rate in comparison to no caloric intake [3]. However, the early start of oral nutrition is not successful *per se* in all patients after major abdominal surgery [2, 3] and is commonly delayed due to gastrointestinal dysfunction, including postoperative nausea, vomiting and bloating [3]. Most of these patients have to accept total parenteral nutrition to meet nutritional requirements because of intolerance of early oral nutrition during the first week after surgery [4]. Intolerance of early oral nutrition is also associated with prolonged hospital stays and increased costs [4, 5].

A multi-modal approach is introduced here to pave the way for early start of oral nutrition and improving gastrointestinal function. Through this concept, it is possible to improve the tolerance and dose of early oral nutrition without using feeding tubes. Therefore, we designed a prospective, randomized, single blind, controlled study to assess the impact of our multi-modal EON on gastrointestinal dysfunction, tolerance of early oral nutrition, clinical outcomes and cost-effectiveness ratios.

Materials and methods

Between April 25, 2014 and April 1, 2016, 107 patients who were to undergo major abdominal surgery were enrolled in the clinical trial with a randomized, single-blind, controlled design. The protocol was approved by the ethics committee of the Second Affiliated Hospital of Kunming Medical University. The included patients were undergoing elective, radical oncologic surgery for gastric or colorectal cancer. The exclusion criteria were as follows: diabetes mellitus, severe pulmonary and cardiovascular disease and liver dysfunction, and Miles surgeries. Written informed consent was obtained before enrollment from each patient.

All patients had no pre-surgery medication or bowel preparation, and all patients fasted at least 8 h before surgery. Radical elective surgery was carried out by 3 senior surgeons. All of the patients received a standard anesthetic protocol and surgical management, prophylactic antibiotics, thoracic epidural for postoperative analgesia with patient controlled analgesia (fentanyl 50 µg/ml, 25 µg/ml per single dose in 6 min intervals) and restriction of intravenous fluid infusion. The nasogastric tube was inserted on the morning of surgery in all patients and was removed after the operation. No prokinetic pharmacotherapy was used in the 2 groups in the first 7 days postoperatively.

Randomization

After enrollment, we assigned the patients into 4 groups with stratified random sampling: (1) a radical gastrectomy group, (2) a radical colectomy and radical resection for rectal cancer group, (3) a right hepatic resection group, and (4) a pancreaticoduodenectomy group. The patients in each subgroup were then randomly assigned to our multi-modal early oral nutrition group or to a conventional care group after the operation (Table 1). A randomization sequence list was provided by the Statistics Department of Kunming Medical University using SPSS 17.0 software (SPSS, Chicago, IL, USA). A researcher who was not involved with clinical care determined the treatment allocation by sequentially opening consecutively numbered, opaque, sealed envelopes.

Interventions

The intervention was initiated on the first day after surgery and ended on the morning of the eighth day. The multimodal EON group received the following treatments (Table 1): (1) chewing sugar-free gum (30 min per session, 3 times per day) from the time the patients were

Table 1 Differences between groups in baseline characteristics

	Multimodal EON group ($n = 53$)	Conventional care group ($n = 54$)	*P*
Sex, M:F	27:26	32:22	0.440
Age, years (mean ± SD)	56 ± 10	55 ± 10	0.624
BMI (mean ± SD)	22.2 ± 2.2	21.4 ± 2.3	0.069
Blood loss, ml (IQR)	300 (200, 450)	350 (250, 450)	0.231
Duration of operation, h (IQR)	3.5 (3, 4)	3.5 (3, 4)	0.211
Duration of ICU stay, h (IQR)	0 (0, 16)	0 (0, 17)	0.654
Duration of mechanical ventilation, h (IQR)	0 (0, 3)	0 (0, 5.3)	0.398
Duration of postoperative analgesia, h (IQR)	48 (41, 56)	48 (44, 55)	0.722
Types of operation performed			0.903
Radical gastrectomy, n	14	15	
Radical colectomy, n	11	12	
Radical resection for rectal cancer, n	8	11	
Right hepatic resection, n	13	11	
Pancreatoduodenectomy, n	7	5	
Tumor stage			0.442
T0-1, n	1	1	
T2, n	15	8	
T3, n	23	28	
T4, n	14	16	

returned to the ward and were awakened to the time of first defecation; (2) appetite stimulation (including playing a favourite food-related media program [30 min per session, 3 times per day], seeing the colours of and tasting favourite foods [5 min per session, at least 3–4 times per day], and watching other people dine [15 min per session, 3 times per day], among other stimuli) from the time of waking to the time of first defecation; (3) drinking water immediately on waking and drinking 100 ml juice (orange juice, apple juice or grape juice, containing 30 g of glucose) 6 h after surgery, oral administration of 300 ml enteral nutrition suspension (Peptisorb liquid, Nutricia) divided into 4–5 administrations initiated 12 h after surgery; the volume of the enteral nutrition suspension was increased to 500 ml at 24 h after surgery, and oral intake was gradually increased until normal requirements were reached. In the conventional care group, patients received the following treatments: they were sent to the ward postoperatively, intake of water and 300 ml enteral nutrition suspension (Peptisorb liquid, Nutricia) that was divided into 4–5 administrations was commenced after the first defecation, and oral intake was gradually increased until normal requirements were reached. Intake of water was performed after the operation according to the patients' wishes.

Both regimens were isonitrogenous [0.2 g/kg (±0.01 Kcal) (±5%)] and isocaloric [24 Kcal/kg (±1.2 Kcal) (±5%)]. On the day of surgery, 6 h after the operation, parenteral nutrition was started in both groups. From day 2 postoperatively to day 7 postoperatively, if oral nutrition was not sufficient before 18 o'clock, then supplementation with parenteral nutrition was initiated after 18 o'clock. Vitamins and electrolytes were added as required. We recorded deviations to the protocol caused by a patient's wishes, medical reasons or adverse events.

Blinded assessment of discharge criteria was performed in all of patients after postoperative day 2. The physicians assessing the outcomes (including 1 senior surgeon and 2 resident doctors) were blinded to the group assignments throughout the study. All patients were followed for 1 month after discharge by calling patients and their relatives or searching the medical records database of our hospital.

The success rate of oral nutrition and recovery of gastrointestinal function

The primary endpoint was the success rate of oral nutrition, which was defined as the proportion of patients who tolerated oral nutrition supplying 80% full nutritional requirements and had no digestive symptoms (including vomiting, diarrhoea and abdominal distension) on day 7 postoperatively. First defecation, flatus, bowel sounds, bloating, vomiting, abdominal discomfort, postoperative ileus, time to tolerate ON supplying full nutritional requirements and reinsertion of the nasogastric tube also were recorded for the first 7 days postoperatively. The nasogastric tube was reinserted after two episodes of vomiting more than 100 ml over 24 h in the absence of bowel movements [6]. A postoperative ileus (POI) was defined as a transient cessation of coordinated bowel motility after surgical intervention that prevented effective transit of intestinal contents or tolerance of oral intake [7, 8]. POI was diagnosed when both criteria (passage of flatus or stool and tolerance of an oral diet) were not met before day 4 postoperatively [7]. A prolonged postoperative ileus was defined as a POI lasting more than 5 days for open surgery or more than 3 days for laparoscopic surgery [7, 8]. A recurrent postoperative ileus was defined as the occurrence of an ileus after an apparent resolution of the immediate postoperative POI [7, 8]. Intolerance of oral nutrition was defined as: (1) the presence of vomiting, diarrhoea, abdominal distension and/or an ileus after oral intake that led to halting oral intake [9]; and (2) oral nutrition supplying less than 80% of full nutritional requirements in 24 h [10].

Complications

The most common complications after abdominal surgery were described, such as pneumonia, SIRS, septicaemia, intra-abdominal abscess, wound infection, urinary tract infection, central catheter infection, anastomotic blood, anastomotic leakage, wound dehiscence, intestinal obstruction, and deep venous thrombosis. An infectious complication was defined as the presence of recognized pathogens in typically sterile body tissues as confirmed by culture results and supported by clinical, radiologic, or hematologic evidence of infection [11].

Length of stay (LOS)

Postoperative length of stay (PLOS) was defined as the duration between the date of operation and the date when discharge criteria were met. Discharge criteria included the ability to manage personal care and toilet activities, no fever, and no intravenous access [12]. When the patient's condition met the above objective criteria, hospital stay was no longer considered to be sensitive to nutritional support, and the patient was considered to be discharged from a nutritional sense [12]. The actual length of stay (ALOS) was recorded.

Cost

The cost of nutritional support was calculated as the total cost of all of the items related to nutritional support on the account statement, including nutritional products, disposal materials, consultation fee, infusion pumps, and catheters. The cost of infection-related complications (diagnosis and treatment by staff doctors who were unfamiliar with the protocol) was calculated as the total cost of all of the items related to the diagnosis and treatment of the infection on the account statement. The cost of the multimodal program was calculated as the total cost of all of the items (excluding nutritional support) related to the program, including fruit juice, fruits, the fee for preparation of individual multimedia materials (for playing food media programs), sugar-free gum, and other items. Indirect and intangible costs (pain and suffering) were not considered in this study. The total cost of treatment (C) = the cost of nutritional support and/or the cost of the multimodal program + the cost of infectious complications. Costs are expressed in USD (United States dollars). The cost-effectiveness analysis was performed from the payers' perspective as described elsewhere [13].

Sample size determination

Before the study was initiated, retrospective data ($n = 20$, unpublished results in patients with abdominal major surgeries in our hospital) indicated that the success rate of oral nutrition in the multi-modal EON care ($n = 12$) and conventional care ($n = 8$) were 9 (75.0%) and 4 (50.0%). We estimated that 100 patients would meet the inclusion criteria over the study period. If half of the patients were treated with the multi-modal EON, then according to a 2-sided alpha of 0.05, a sample size of 100 patients would provide more than 80% power to detect a relative reduction in the success rate of oral nutrition of 33.3% in the multi-modal early oral nutrition group compared to the conventional care group.

Statistical analysis

The statistical analysis was performed using SPSS 17.0 (SPSS Inc., Chicago, USA) by a statistician who was also blinded to the group allocation in the Statistics Department of Kunming Medical University. After the data had been entered and verified, the statistician conducting the analyses was notified as to which group had received the multimodal program. Normally distributed data were expressed as mean ± SD and non-normally distributed variables were expressed as medians and interquartile ranges (IQRs). For continuous variables, the distribution of the data was analyzed for normality. A Student's unpaired *t*-test was utilized for normally distributed numerical variables, and the Wilcoxon test was used for non-normally distributed numerical variables. Categorical data were analyzed using the chi-squared test or Fisher's exact test. All of the statistical tests were two sided, and $P < 0.05$ was considered statistically significant.

Results

Patients and baseline characteristics

During the study period, there were 178 eligible patients. Seventy-one patients were excluded for various reasons, resulting in 107 patients being entered into the randomized program. Protocol deviations are shown in Figs. 1 and 2. Intervention was discontinued in 12 patients. Among the 12 patients, 2 patients in the multimodal EON group suffered obvious bloating and vomiting and anastomotic blood within 2 postoperative days; 5 patients in the multimodal EON group suffered prolonged postoperative ileus and anastomotic leakage after 3 postoperative days; 1 patient with anastomotic blood and 4 patients with anastomotic leakage in the conventional care group were changed to receive PN to supply nutritional requirements after 4 postoperative days. Eight patients (3 cases in the multimodal EON group and 5 in the conventional care group) were not contacted by telephone successfully. We searched the databases of our hospital and obtained their hospitalization data. Among 8 patients, 4 patients were treated with chemotherapy in the oncology department, one patient suffered ureteral calculi and received percutaneous nephrolithotomy in the department of urology, 1 patient suffered from femoral fractures after a traffic accident and was treated in the trauma department, and two patients were hospitalized in the cardiac department of internal medicine due to coronary heart disease. According to the medical records database of our hospital, no records of complications and readmission were associated with the abdominal surgeries and multimodal programs. Finally, no patient dropped out of the study or was lost to follow-up (Fig. 1). All analyses were performed according to the intention-to-treat principle.

The differences in baseline characteristics between the multimodal EON group and conventional care groups are shown in Table 1. No differences were found in demographic characteristics, operative procedures, or stage of the cancer between groups ($P \geq 0.05$). The numbers of patients who underwent laparoscopic surgery in the multimodal EON group and the conventional care groups were 8 and 9, respectively ($P = 0.824$).

The success rate of oral nutrition and recovery of gastrointestinal function

The success rate of oral nutrition in the multimodal EON group was 44 (83.0%) versus 31 (57.4%) in the conventional care group ($P = 0.004$; Table 2). According to the types of operation, 4 subgroups were analyzed, as shown in Table 2. The Bonferroni method was used to account for multiple comparisons among subgroups, but there was no significant difference between subgroups ($P \geq 0.05$). In the conventional care group, we also did not find a significant difference between subgroups ($P \geq 0.05$). Two subgroups (including laparoscopic surgery and open surgery) were analyzed, as shown in Table 2. In the multimodal EON group, the success rate of oral nutrition was 87.5% ($n = 7$) in the subgroup of laparoscopic surgery versus 82.2% ($n = 37$) in the open surgery subgroup ($P = 1.000$). In the conventional care group,

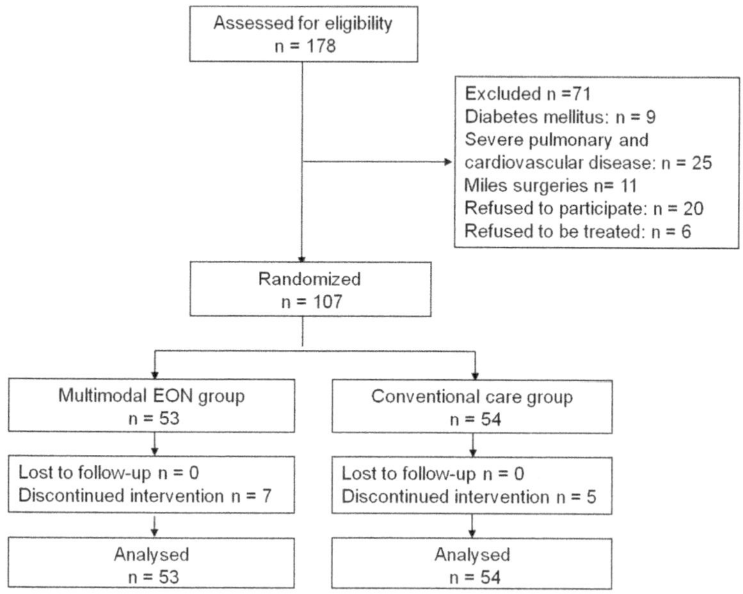

Fig. 1 Allocation of experimental and control groups

the success rate of oral nutrition was 66.7% ($n = 6$) in subgroup of laparoscopic surgery versus 55.6% ($n = 25$) in the open surgery group ($P = 0.717$).

The rates of patients that halted oral intake due to digestive symptoms in postoperative days 3, 4, 5, 6 and 7 in the two groups were not significantly different ($P = 0.202$, $P = 1.000$, $P = 0.119$, $P = 0.437$ and $P = 0.437$, respectively). However, there were significant differences in the rates of patients with ON supplying less than 80% of full nutritional requirements in postoperative days 3, 4, 5, 6 and 7 in the two groups ($P = 0.006$, $P = 0.005$, $P < 0.001$, $P = 0.001$ and $P = 0.028$, respectively).

The difference in recovery of gastrointestinal function between the two groups is shown in Table 3. Time to first defecation and time to flatus occurred earlier in the multimodal EON group ($P < 0.001$) and bowel sounds returned sooner ($P < 0.001$). The number of patients with a prolonged postoperative ileus in the multimodal EON group was 5 (9.4%) versus 13 (24.1%) in the conventional care group ($P = 0.043$). There were no differences in the recurrent postoperative ileus and nasogastric tube reinsertion rates ($P \geq 0.05$).

Complications and length of stay

There was no decrease in the incidence of infectious complications in the multimodal EON group (8 of 53, 15%) compared with the conventional care group (11 of 54, 20%; $P = 0.475$). No significant differences were found between the two groups in the incidence of intraoperative complications and non-infectious complications ($P \geq 0.05$; Table 4). There were a few minor intraoperative complications (including 2 cases of ecchymoma in the left arms in the multimodal EON group and 1 case of subcutaneous emphysema in the conventional care group) during the procedures. Only one death occurred (in the conventional care group) due to pneumonia and myocardial infarction. No patients who suffered any complications related to the last hospitalization in either group were readmitted within 30 days after discharge. The PLOS in the multimodal EON group was 8 (6, 12) days versus 10 (7, 18) days in the conventional care group ($P < 0.001$). There was no significant difference in ALOS between the multimodal EON group (26 [21.5–31.5] days) and the conventional care group (26 [26.0–29.3] days; $P \geq 0.05$).

Cost and cost/effectiveness

The differences between groups in cost and cost/effectiveness (C/E) in the treatment of infectious complications are shown in Table 5. Both the total cost of treatment/patient and the cost of nutritional support in the multimodal EON group were significantly less than in the conventional care group (10.4 and 9.4% less on average). For the multimodal EON group and the conventional care group, the rate of infectious complication-free patients was 84.9 and 79.9% ($P = 0.475$). The cost-effectiveness ratio was also less for the multimodal EON group than for the conventional care group ($P < 0.001$); therefore, the multimodal EON group was more cost effective than the conventional care.

To evaluate the reliability of the above findings, we conducted a sensitivity analysis by increasing the price

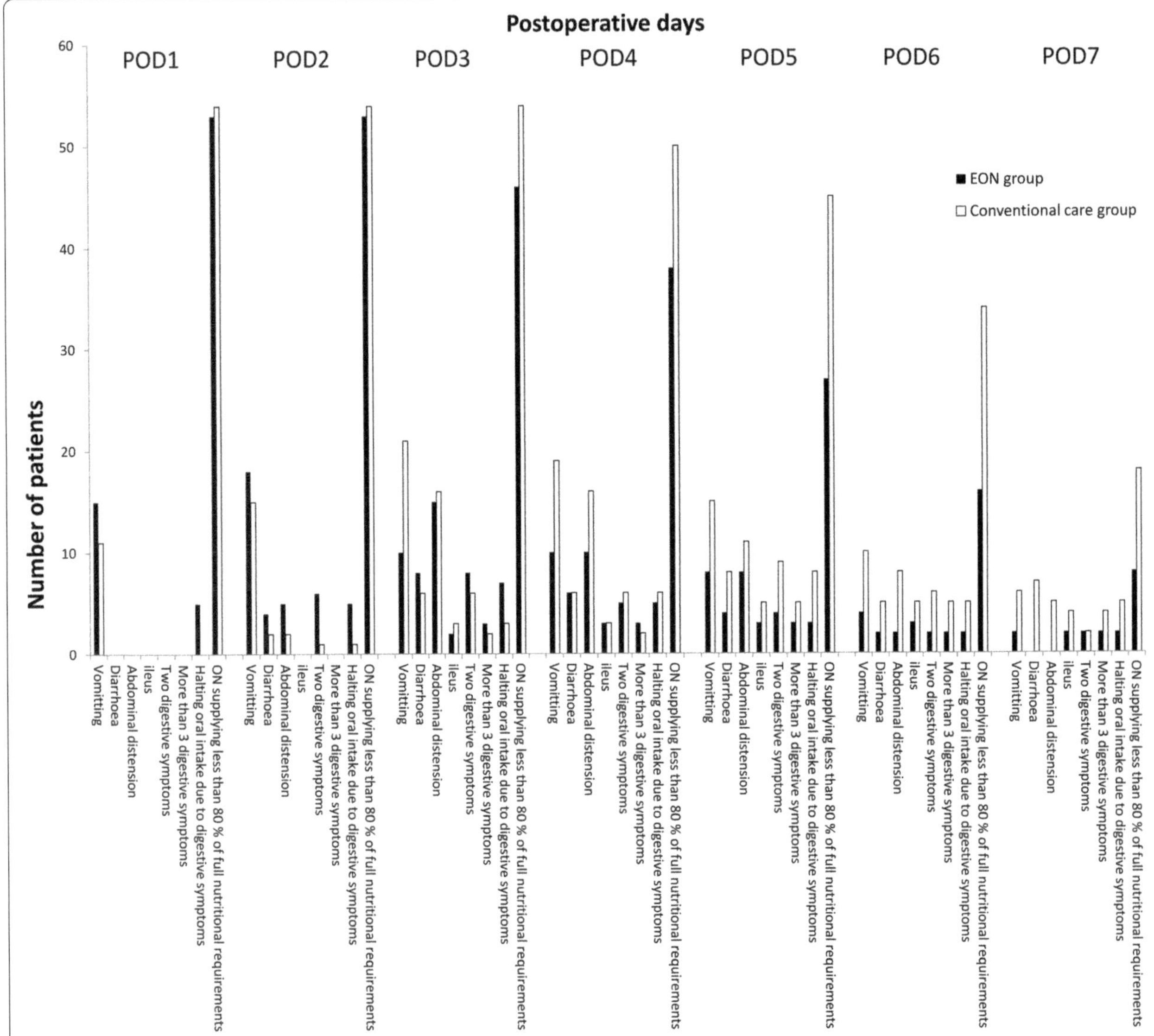

Fig. 2 Intolerance of oral nutrition in the 2 groups

of the preparations by 5% and observed that the results were consistent with the results provided in Table 5.

Discussion

Multi-modal early oral nutrition increased the success rate of oral nutrition during the first week after surgery, and significantly decreased LOS and the cost of treatment. Thus, it was more cost-effective.

The success rate of oral nutrition was used to reflect tolerance of oral nutrition in our study, which included 2 aspects: (1) the gastrointestinal tract had the capacity to receive enough nutrition (at least 80% full nutritional requirements); and (2) the digestive ability of the gastrointestinal tract was also good, which did not cause digestive symptoms (including vomiting, diarrhoea and abdominal distension). The beneficial effects of multimodal early oral nutrition on the success rate of oral nutrition and recovery of gastrointestinal function in this study were remarkable. Background mechanisms are thought to include the fact that several components of the multimodal protocol appeared to improve recovery of gastrointestinal function. Watching food-related media programs, perceiving the color and taste of favorite foods, watching other people dining, drinking small amounts of fruit juice, chewing gum, and the early provision of oral nutrition can stimulate the early brain phase and mouth and stomach phase, induce centrally mediated vagal effects [14], and promote the recovery from splanchnic nerve inhibition of motor activity due to surgery. In addition, early provision of oral nutrition may decrease inflammation and consequently decrease the duration of POI [15, 16]. In our study, SIRS in the

Table 2 Differences between groups in the success rates of oral nutrition

	Multimodal EON group (*n* = 53)	Conventional care group (*n* = 54)	*P* value
Types of operations			
Radical gastrectomy, n	10/14 (71.4%)	7/15 (46.7%)	0.176
Radical resection for colorectal cancer, n	18/19 (94.7%)	15/23 (65.2%)	0.027
Right hepatic resection, n	12/13 (92.3%)	7/11 (63.6%)	0.142
Pancreatoduodenectomy, n	4/7 (57.1%)	2/5 (40.0%)	1.000
Laparoscopic or open surgery			
Laparoscopic surgery	7/8 (87.5%)	6/9 (66.7%)	0.576
Open surgery	37/45 (82.2%)	25/45 (55.6%)	0.006
The total success rate of oral nutrition, n (%)	44/53 (83.0%)	31/44 (57.4%)	0.004

EON early oral nutrition

first postoperative week was decreased significantly by multi-modal EON (Table 4). Chewing gum containing hexitol can produce an osmotic laxative effect [17, 18]. This hypothesis on background mechanisms was not investigated in this study.

In the subgroup analysis on the success rate of oral nutrition (Table 2), we analyzed the differences in the success rates of oral nutrition between different types of operations (including radical gastrectomy, radical resection for colorectal cancer, right hepatic resection and pancreatoduodenectomy). In the multimodal EON group, the success rates of oral nutrition in the subgroup of radical resection for colorectal cancer and the subgroup of right hepatic resection were more than 90%; but the success rates of oral nutrition were 71.4 and 57.1% in the radical gastrectomy subgroup and

Table 3 Differences between groups in recovery of gastrointestinal function

Variables	Multimodal EON group (*n* = 53)	Conventional care group (*n* = 54)	*P* value
Time to first defecation, h (mean ± SD)	49 ± 7	62 ± 5	<0.001
Time to flatus, h (mean ± SD)	32.8 ± 5.3	42.9 ± 4.8	<0.001
Recovery time of bowel sounds, h (IQR)	24 (21, 27)	35 (31, 37)	<0.001
Prolonged postoperative ileus, n (%)	5 (9.4%)	13 (24.1%)	0.043
Recurrent postoperative ileus, n (%)	3 (5.7%)	6 (11.1%)	0.489
The nasogastric tube reinsertion rate, n (%)	4 (9.4%)	8 (14.8%)	0.359

EON early oral nutrition, IQR interquartile ranges

Table 4 Differences between groups in complications

	Multimodal EON group (*n* = 53)	Conventional care group (*n* = 54)	*P* value
No. of patients with infectious complications, n (%)	8 (15.1%)	11 (20.4%)	0.475
Pneumonia, n (%)	7 (13.2%)	9 (16.7%)	0.616
SIRS, n (%)	2 (3.8%)	9 (16.7%)	0.028
Septicaemia, n (%)	4 (7.5%)	3 (5.6%)	0.716
Intra-abdominal abscess, n (%)	2 (4.0%)	1 (1.9%)	1.000
Wound infection, n (%)	5 (9.4%)	4 (7.4%)	0.742
No. of patients with non-infectious complications, n (%)	10 (18.9%)	9 (16.7%)	0.766
Anastomotic blood, n (%)	2 (4.0%)	1 (1.9%)	1.000
Anastomotic leakage, n (%)	7 (13.2%)	6 (11.1%)	0.740
Wound dehiscence, n (%)	1 (1.9%)	1 (1.9%)	0.495
Intestinal obstruction, n (%)	0 (0.0%)	1 (1.9%)	1.000
Deep venous thrombosis, n (%)	2 (3.8%)	0 (0.0%)	0.243
No. of intraoperative complications, n (%)	2 (4.0%)	1 (1.9%)	1.000

EON early oral nutrition, SIRS indicates systemic inflammatory response syndrome

pancreatoduodenectomy subgroup. Even if we did not find a statistically significant difference, the differences in the success rates of oral nutrition in different types of operations were significant. Compared with resection for colorectal cancer and hepatic resection, reconstruction of the upper gastrointestinal tract after gastrectomy and pancreatoduodenectomy is more complicated, which also causes more disorder in the secretion of the digestive tract and more severe damage in nerves of the gastrointestinal tract. In theory, the tolerance of early oral nutrition in patients with upper digestive tract surgery was lower than that of the lower digestive tract.

Subgroup analysis on the success rate of oral nutrition in laparoscopic surgery and open surgery was also performed. In the multimodal EON group, the success rate of oral nutrition was 87.5% in the subgroup of laparoscopic surgery, which was slightly higher than that in the subgroup of open surgery (82.2%). This difference was not statistically significant. In previous studies, researchers found that laparoscopic surgery had an earlier return of bowel function when compared with open surgery [19–22]. The reduced use of opioid drugs during the operation, decreased intestinal manipulation and operation-related inflammation in laparoscopic surgery contributed to the result [21, 23, 24]. Whether it is able to increase the tolerance of early oral nutrition remains controversial. In a prospectively case-controlled study on effect of laparoscopic and open gastric bypass surgery on bowel function, the results showed the return of bowel movement and the time to first passage of gas in the

Table 5 Differences between groups of cost and cost/effectiveness(C/E) in the treatment of infectious complications

	Multimodal EON group ($n = 53$)	Conventional care group ($n = 54$)	*P* value
Median cost of nutritional support/patient (IQR)	450.0 (426.7, 462.8)	496.8 (466.9, 526.4)	<0.001
Median cost of nutritional support/patient/day (IQR)	69.7 (61.8, 79.9)	67.2 (53.1, 78.6)	0.497
Median total cost of treatment/patient (C) (IQR)	456.4 (429.7, 500.3)	509.6 (474.5, 567.5)	<0.001
Effectiveness (E)	84.9%	79.9%	0.475
Cost/effectiveness (C/E) (IQR)	537.6 (506.1, 589.3)	637.8 (593.9, 710.3)	<0.001
Incremental cost-effectiveness ratio	1064		

EON early oral nutrition, IQR interquartile ranges, C cost, E effectiveness

laparoscopic group were shorter than that in the open surgery group ($P < 0.05$), but there was no significant difference in the time to oral food intake between the laparoscopic and open gastric bypass surgery groups ($P = 0.06$) [21]. In a meta-analysis on the clinical efficacy of laparoscopic and open surgery for rectal cancer [25], consuming liquid food data from 4 RCTs were pooled. The results indicated the time of consuming liquid food was 1.04 days earlier in the laparoscopic group than that in the open surgery group ($P < 0.05$). The inconsistent results from these studies, including our study, were related to the types of operations (the upper gastrointestinal tract or the lower digestive tract), the contents of early oral nutrition (normal food, fluid food, or enteral nutrition emulsion) and the different assessment methods for tolerance of oral nutrition.

However, it is prudent to qualify these results in subgroups because of inadequate sample sizes. In future research, expanding the sample sizes for different subgroups will further validate this result.

In our study, we found that multi-modal EON tended to reduce the risk of post infectious and non-infectious complications, but individual clinical complications failed to reach statistical significance, except for SIRS. These results are similar to the results of two recent meta-analyses of early enteral nutrition versus later commencement of feeding [26, 27]. In a meta-analysis [26], 14 RCTs represented 1,224 patients who underwent gastrointestinal surgery. The direction of the effect indicated that earlier feeding may reduce the risk of post-surgical complications without reaching statistical significance. Mortality was the only outcome showing a significant benefit, but was not necessarily associated with early commencement of feeding, as the reported cause of death was anastomotic leakage, reoperation, and acute myocardial infarction. In our study, one patient died due to pneumonia and myocardial infarction in the conventional care group, which was also not related to EON. In a meta-analysis including 7 RCTs with a total of 587 patients undergoing elective colorectal surgery [27], the researchers found that the risk of anastomotic dehiscence, pneumonia, wound infection, the rate of nasogastric tube reinsertion, vomiting, or mortality were not different between early enteral nutrition and later commencement of feeding. The total complications tended to be reduced EON ($P = 0.04$). Therefore, early enteral nutrition is safe in patients undergoing major abdominal surgeries, even if our protocol was moderately different from previous studies since it increased the multi-modal program to help the administration of EON.

In our study, PLOS under the multimodal protocol was on average 2 days less than that of patients managed with conventional care, which was consistent with the results of two meta-analyses [26, 27]. In previous studies, the PLOS was used as one of the evaluation indexes of early oral feeding [28–30], and PLOS was determined according to the discharge criteria [12, 28, 29]. Many factors might affect the length of stay. Some of these factors are altered by nutritional support, including mobilization and infectious complications, and some are not affected by nutritional support, including a planned admission for medical insurance policy reasons, delay until initiation of homecare or patient wishes [12] These factors may explain why there was no difference between the two groups regarding the ALOS.

Even if the incidence of infectious complications was not decreased by the multi-EON, it significantly improved the cost-effectiveness ratio in the treatment of infectious complications. Because the cost of oral nutrition was less than that of PN, the cost of nutritional support in the multimodal EON group was significantly decreased relative to that of the conventional care group (Table 5). The recovery of gastrointestinal function might also improve the treatment of infectious complications, thereby significantly decreasing the total cost of treatment per patient. Therefore, the multi-modal EON had a better therapeutic effect (Table 5). Compared with previous studies, the total cost of treatment was significantly low. The main reason was the total cost of treatment only included the cost of nutritional support (and/or the cost of the multimodal program) and the cost of infectious complications postoperatively in this study. This choice was made because infectious complications could be modified by nutritional support and non-infectious complications; e.g., deep venous thrombosis and anastomotic blood, were not sensitive to nutritional support. [12] Other hospitalization fees (related to operations, anesthesia, preoperative examinations and treatment, and the cost of non-infectious complications, etc.) were not calculated in the total cost of treatment. The secondary reason was that the incidence of infectious complications was 17.8% in all patients, which means that part of the cost of infectious complications in 82.2% of the patients was zero.

The present study had several methodologic differences from previous studies. *First,* in our multimodal protocol, we added new measures to stimulate appetite, such as watching favorite food-related media or other people dining and seeing, tasting favorite foods. *Second, we* also used a single-blind design, but we blinded those who assessed outcomes and the statisticians. However, due to the characteristics of intervention programs, we could not blind the researchers and subjects. This strategy increased the power of the intervention. *Third,* we estimated the sample size before developing the study design and showed that it could effectively evaluate the effects of the multimodal protocol on the success rate of oral nutrition and recovery of gastrointestinal function. *Fourth,* we described the total range of costs in detail and used cost-effectiveness ratios to evaluate the pros and cons of the multimodal protocol for the success rate of oral nutrition and recovery of gastrointestinal function from a health economics perspective.

There were limitations in our study. First, even if some markers of recovery of gastrointestinal function (including time to first defecation, time to flatus and recovery time of bowel sounds) and the diagnosis of POI were commonly used in previous studies, these markers were somewhat subjective, which might cause inaccurate assessment of recovery regarding gastrointestinal function and incidence of POI. In a recent systematic review about the diagnosis of POI, the authors found that postoperative defecation together with tolerance of diet seemed to be the best clinical endpoint of POI and computed tomography had the best differential diagnostic value between POI and other complications [31]. Certainly, gastrointestinal motility monitoring and abdominal X-rays are also important affiliated means to diagnose POI. In future studies, relatively objective indicators, especially computed tomography, should be designed to accurately assess recovery of gastrointestinal function and POI. Second, we did not include a separate early oral nutrition group and a chewing gum group; therefore, we could not evaluate whether the multimodal protocol was more effective than early oral nutrition or chewing gum alone. In the multimodal protocol, we believe that each component may independently promote the recovery of gastrointestinal function via a different mechanism. Therefore, we suggest that any single component is unlikely to exceed the effect of the multimodal protocol on recovery of gastrointestinal function as an integrated process. Third, the cost was calculated based on a hospital computerized list for which the patients paid directly for the multimodal program and nutritional support, and the cost for treating infectious complications was also included. The other costs, such as the side effects of PN and/or EN, would probably affect the results, and the assessment of intangible costs (such as pain and suffering due to illness) would probably expand our findings. In addition, the economic parameters in our study may differ from country to country depending on the type of health care system and insurance reimbursement systems.

In this study, multi-modal EON was superior to conventional care in improving gastrointestinal function and tolerance of oral nutrition during the first week after surgery, decreasing the length of stay and improving cost-effectiveness. Therefore, we propose the use of multi-modal EON. We suggest a preoperative plan for multi-modal EON in patients with major abdominal surgery.

Abbreviations

ALOS: Actual length of stay; C: Cost; C/E: Cost/Effectiveness; E: Effectiveness; EON: Early oral Nutrition; IQR: Interquartile range; ON: Oral nutrition; PLOS: Postoperative length of stay; PN: Parental Nutrition; PN: Parental nutrition; POI: Postoperative ileus; USD: United States Dollars

Acknowledgements

The authors thank Xiongzhi Chen, Liya An and Dongyong Li, who were blinded to the protocol and who judged and recorded all of the endpoints; the finance section of Second Affiliated Hospital of Kunming Medical University, which provided the cost information; and the Medical Records Division of Second Affiliated Hospital of Kunming Medical University, which helped review case information.

Funding

This study was supported by the Foundation of Research Center for Surgical Clinical Nutrition in Yun-Nan Province (No. 2014NS089), the Professor Yang Hua Research Station in Yun-Nan Province and The National Natural Science Fund (No. 81160114). We used the funding to collect the data and revise the manuscript.

Availability of data and materials

All authors wish to share our data, but the data belong to the shared multicentre database of Research Center for Surgical Clinical Nutrition in Yun-Nan Province. The Multi-Centre Cooperative Clinical Study Group does not allow these data to be released until the multi-centre papers have been published.

Authors' contribution

D-LS, W-ML, S-ML, Q-PL and P-YX designed the study; Y-YC, Q-WX, Y-JL, Y-BS, Y-XQ, Y-YL and TY performed the experiments and collected the data; D-LS and W-ML analysed the data; D-LS, S-ML, Q-PL and P-YX wrote the paper. All authors read and approved the final manuscript.

Competing interests

The authors declare that they have no competing interests.

Consent for publication

Not applicable.

Ethics approval and consent to participate

This prospective randomized controlled study was approved by the Ethics Committee at the Second Affiliated Hospital of Kunming Medical University (approval no. 2014–06). The study was performed in accordance with the Declaration of Helsinki. All patients enrolled in the study provided informed consent.

Author details

[1]Department of General Surgery, Wuhan Clinical School of Southern Medical University/Wuhan General Hospital of Guangzhou Military Command, Wuhan 430070, China. [2]Department of Gastrointestinal Surgery, Second Affiliated Hospital of Kunming Medical University, Kunming 650101, China. [3]Research Center for Surgical Clinical Nutrition in Yun-Nan Province, Kunming 650101, China.

References

1. Kehlet H, Wilmore DW. Evidence-based surgical care and the evolution of fast-track surgery. Ann Surg. 2008;248(2):189–98.
2. Fearon KC, Ljungqvist O, Von Meyenfeldt M, Revhaug A, Dejong CH, Lassen K, et al. Enhanced recovery after surgery: a consensus review of clinical care for patients undergoing colonic resection. Clin Nutr. 2005;24(3):466–77.
3. Lewis SJ, Andersen HK, Thomas S. Early enteral nutrition within 24 h of intestinal surgery versus later commencement of feeding: a systematic review and meta-analysis. J Gastrointest Surg. 2009;13(6):1163–5.
4. Klaver YL, Nienhuijs SW, Nieuwenhuijzen GA, Rutten HJ, de Hingh IH. Omentoplasty in rectal cancer surgery prolongs post-operative ileus. Int J Colorectal Dis. 2008;23(2):165–9.
5. Blaser AR, Starkopf J, Kirsimägi Ü, Deane AM. Definition, prevalence, and outcome of feeding intolerance in intensive care: a systematic review and meta-analysis. Acta Anaesthesiol Scand. 2014;58(8):914–22.
6. Balayla J, Bujold E, Lapensée L, Mayrand MH, Sansregret A. Early versus delayed postoperative feeding after major gynaecological surgery and its effects on clinical outcomes, patient satisfaction, and length of stay: a randomized controlled trial. J Obstet Gynaecol Can. 2015;37(12):1079–85.
7. Vather R, Trivedi S, Bissett I. Defining postoperative ileus: results of a systematic review and global survey. J Gastrointest Surg. 2013;17(5):962–72.
8. Bragg D, El-Sharkawy AM, Psaltis E, Maxwell-Armstrong CA, Lobo DN. Postoperative ileus: recent developments in pathophysiology and management. Clin Nutr. 2015;34(3):367–76.
9. Reignier J, Mercier E, Le Gouge A, Boulain T, Desachy A, Bellec F, Clavel M, Frat JP, Plantefeve G, Quenot JP, Lascarrou JB, Clinical Research in Intensive Care and Sepsis (CRICS) Group. Effect of not monitoring residual gastric volume on risk of ventilator-associated pneumonia in adults receiving mechanical ventilation and early enteral feeding: a randomized controlled trial. JAMA. 2013;309:249–56.
10. Woodcock NP, Zeigler D, Palmer MD, Buckley P, Mitchell CJ, MacFie J. Enteral versus parenteral nutrition: a pragmatic study. Nutrition. 2001;17(1):1–12.
11. American College of Chest Physicians/Society of Critical Care Medicine. Consensus conference. Definitions for sepsis and organ failure and guidelines for the use of innovative therapies in sepsis. Crit Care Med. 1992; 20(6):864–74.
12. Johansen N, Kondrup J, Plum LM, Bak L, Nørregaard P, Bunch E, et al. Effect of nutritional support on clinical outcome in patients at nutritional risk. Clin Nutr. 2004;23(4):539–50.
13. Braga M, Gianotti L. Preoperative immunonutrition: cost-benefit analysis. J Parenter Enteral Nutr. 2005;29(1 Suppl):S57–61.
14. Zaghiyan K, Felder S, Ovsepyan G, Murrell Z, Sokol T, Moore B, et al. A prospective randomized controlled trial of sugared chewing gum on gastrointestinal recovery after major colorectal surgery in patients managed with early enteral feeding. Dis Colon Rectum. 2013;56(3):328–35.
15. Boelens PG, Heesakkers FF, Luyer MD, van Barneveld KW, de Hingh IH, Nieuwenhuijzen GA, et al. Reduction of postoperative ileus by early enteral nutrition in patients undergoing major rectal surgery: prospective, randomized, controlled trial. Ann Surg. 2014;259(4):649–55.
16. Lubbers T, de Haan JJ, Luyer MD, Verbaeys I, Hadfoune M, Dejong CH, et al. Cholecystokinin/cholecystokinin-1 receptor-mediated peripheral activation of the afferent vagus by enteral nutrients attenuates inflammation in rats. Ann Surg. 2010;252(2):376–82.
17. Tandeter H. Hypothesis: hexitols in chewing gum may play a role in reducing postoperative ileus. Med Hypotheses. 2009;72(1):39–40.
18. Bauditz J, Norman K, Biering H, Lochs H, Pirlich M. Severe weight loss caused by chewing gum. BMJ. 2008;336(7635):96–7.
19. Schippers E, Ottinger AP, Anurov M, Polivoda M, Schumpelick V. Laparoscopic cholecystectomy: a minor abdominal trauma? World J Surg. 1993;17(4):539–43.
20. Chen HH, Wexner SD, Iroatulam AJ, Pikarsky AJ, Alabaz O, Nogueras JJ, Nessim A, Weiss EG. Laparoscopic colectomy compares favorably with colectomy by laparotomy for reduction of postoperative ileus. Dis Colon Rectum. 2000;43(1):61–5.
21. El Shobary H, Christou N, Backman SB, Gvocdic B, Schricker T. Effect of laparoscopic versus open gastric bypass surgery on postoperative pain and bowel function. Obes Surg. 2006;16(4):437–42.
22. Morneau M, Boulanger J, Charlebois P, Latulippe JF, Lougnarath R, Thibault C, Gervais N. Comité de l'Évolution des Pratiques en Oncologie. Laparoscopic versus open surgery for the treatment of colorectal cancer: a literature review and recommendations from the Comité de l'évolution des pratiques en oncologie. Can J Surg. 2013;56(5):297–310.
23. Schwarz NT, Beer-Stolz D, Simmons RL, Bauer AJ. Pathogenesis of paralytic ileus: intestinal manipulation opens a transient pathway between the intestinal lumen and the leukocytic infiltrate of the jejunal muscularis. Ann Surg. 2002;235(1):31–40.
24. Liu SS, Carpenter RL, Mackey DC, Thirlby RC, Rupp SM, Shine TS, Feinglass NG, Metzger PP, Fulmer JT, Smith SL. Effects of perioperative analgesic technique on rate of recovery after colon surgery. Anesthesiology. 1995; 83(4):757–65.
25. Zhao JK, Chen NZ, Zheng JB, He S, Sun XJ. Laparoscopic versus open surgery for rectal cancer: results of a systematic review and meta-analysis on clinical efficacy. Mol Clin Oncol. 2014;2(6):1097–102.
26. Andersen HK, Lewis SJ, Thomas S. Early enteral nutrition within 24 h of colorectal surgery versus later commencement of feeding for postoperative complications. Cochrane Database Syst Rev. 2006;4:CD004080.
27. Zhuang CL, Ye XZ, Zhang CJ, Dong QT, Chen BC, Yu Z. Early versus traditional postoperative oral feeding in patients undergoing elective colorectal surgery: a meta-analysis of randomized clinical trials. Dig Surg. 2013;30(3):225–32.
28. El Nakeeb A, Fikry A, El Metwally T, Fouda E, Youssef M, Ghazy H, Badr S, Khafagy W, Farid M. Early oral feeding in patients undergoing elective colonic anastomosis. Int J Surg. 2009;7:206–9.
29. da Fonseca LM, Profeta da Luz MM, Lacerda-Filho A, Correia MI, Gomes da Silva R. A simplified rehabilitation program for patients undergoing elective colonic surgery – randomized controlled clinical trial. Int J Colorectal Dis. 2011;26:609–16.
30. Dag A, Colak T, Turkmenoglu O, Gundogdu R, Aydin S. A randomized controlled trial evaluating early versus traditional oral feeding after colorectal surgery. Clinics (Sao Paulo). 2011;66:2001–5.
31. Wu Z, Boersema GS, Dereci A, Menon AG, Jeekel J, Lange JF. Clinical endpoint, early detection, and differential diagnosis of postoperative ileus: a systematic review of the literature. Eur Surg Res. 2015;54(3–4):127–38.

Impact of nutritional support that does and does not meet guideline standards on clinical outcome in surgical patients at nutritional risk

Da-Li Sun[1,2,3], Wei-Ming Li[2,3], Shu-Min Li[2,3], Yun-Yun Cen[2,3], Yue-ying Lin[2,3], Qing-Wen Xu[2,3], Yi-Jun Li[2,3], Yan-Bo Sun[2,3], Yu-xing Qi[2,3], Ting Yang[2,3], Qi-Ping Lu[1*] and Peng-Yuan Xu[2,3*]

Abstract

Objective: To investigate the impact of nutritional support on clinical outcomes in patients at nutritional risk who receive nutritional support that meets guideline standards and those who do not.

Methods: This prospective cohort study enrolled hospitalized patients from the Second Affiliated Hospital of Kunming Medical University from February 2010 to June 2012. The research protocols were approved by the university's ethics committee, and the patients signed informed consent forms. The clinical data were collected based on nutritional risk screening, administration of enteral and parenteral nutrition, surgical information, complications, and length of hospital stay.

Results: During the study period, 525 patients at nutritional risk were enrolled in the cohorts. Among patients who received nutritional support that met the guideline standards (Cohort 1), the incidence of infectious complications was lower than that in patients who did not meet guideline standards (Cohort 2) (17.1 % vs. 26.9 %, $P = 0.01$). Subgroup analysis showed that individuals who received a combination of parenteral nutrition (PN) and enteral nutrition (EN) for 7 or more days had a significantly lower incidence of infectious complications ($P = 0.001$) than those who received only PN for 7 or more days or those who received nutritional support for less than 7 days or at less than 10 kcal/kg/d. Binary logistic regression analysis showed that, after adjusting for confounding factors, nutritional support that met guideline standards for patients with nutritional risk was a protective factor for complications (OR: 0.870, $P < 0.002$).

Conclusions: In patients at nutritional risk after abdominal surgery, nutritional support that meets recommended nutrient guidelines (especially regimens involving PN + EN ≥ 7 days) might decrease the incidence of infectious complications and is worth recommending; however, well-designed trials are needed to confirm our findings. Nutritional support that does not meet the guideline standards is considered clinically undesirable.

Keywords: Nutritional risk, Outcome, Guidelines, Abdominal surgery patients, Logistic regression analysis

* Correspondence: ptwklqp111@163.com; destiny1978@163.com; pyxu778@sina.com

[1]Department of General Surgery, Wuhan Clinical School of Southern Medical University/Wuhan General Hospital of Guangzhou Military Command, Wuhan 430070, China

[2]Department of Gastrointestinal Surgery, Second Affiliated Hospital of Kunming Medical University, Kunming 650101, China

Full list of author information is available at the end of the article

Background

Nutritional support has been in clinical use for approximately 40 years, and several countries have developed specific nutritional guidelines [1, 2]. However, in practice, many patients still receive nutrients that do not meet guideline standards, including the use of amino acids or fat emulsion only or nutritional support of insufficient amount or duration [3–5].

The reference standards for the amount of energy, nitrogen, and trace elements recommended by nutritional support guidelines are based on the theoretical amounts suitable to ameliorate a human disease state [1, 2]. Nutritional support that meets guideline standards leads to significantly better improvements in clinical outcome than no support in patients who are at nutritional risk or are malnourished [6–8]. However, permissive low-nutrient intake has been shown to result in better clinical outcomes than standard nutritional support in patients after stomach surgery and is considerably less costly [9]. The question of whether nutrition support with nutrient intake between no nutritional support and permissive low-nutrient intake (defined as nutritional support that does not meet guideline standards) can result in clinical outcomes comparable to those of patients who receive full nutritional support has not been addressed.

Current nutritional support guidelines do not explicitly state how long perioperative nutritional support should be administered to patients at nutritional risk. Although certain guidelines and related studies have suggested that patients with severe preoperative malnutrition should receive total parental nutrition (TPN) for at least seven days to improve clinical outcomes [1, 8], this is clinically unrealistic for most patients at nutritional risk. This approach can delay surgery, prolong hospital stays, and increase hospital costs, placing it at odds with the concept of ethics and health care reform. Consequently, postoperative nutritional support is currently used in clinical practice, and nutritional support lasting at least 7 days is thought to be effective. Nutritional support for less than 7 days is considered inadequate to meet guideline standards.

There is a need for research comparing the impact of nutritional support on clinical outcomes in at-risk patients who receive guideline-recommended nutritional support and those who do not. Although a randomized controlled study can provide high-level evidence with which to evaluate clinical interventions, there are serious ethical issues in designing and implementing a randomized controlled study that compares clinical outcomes between patients who receive recommended levels of nutritional support guideline standardsand those who do not. A rigorous cohort study was therefore considered the most feasible approach for the current study. The reality is that some Chinese clinicians in certain parts of China have yet to fully implement nutritional support in accordance with standardized nutrition guidelines, and some departments cannot adequately prepare the standard nutrient solutions due to poor hospital conditions. This situation creates two de facto treatment groups of patients at nutritional risk who are receiving nutrients: those receiving full nutritional support as stipulated in guidelines and those receiving partial support. Partial support may involve fewer calories, less nitrogen, or a shorter duration of nutritional support (<7 days) than recommended. These two groups make it possible to conduct a cohort study at this stage among patients receiving nutritional support that does not meet guideline-recommend standards.

This prospective cohort study was designed to compare the impact of nutritional support on clinical outcome in patients at nutritional risk who had undergone major abdominal surgery and received guideline-recommended nutritional support (involving two nutritional support programs, parenteral nutrition [PN] and a combination of PN and enteral nutrition [EN]) and those who did not (in two categories, those who received <10 kcal/kg/d and those whose nutritional support lasted <7 days).

Methods

This prospective cohort study was registered at www.chictr.org, identifier ChiCTR-OOC-16008782, and approved by the ethics committee at the Second Affiliated Hospital of Kunming Medical University (approval no. 2010-08). The study was performed in accordance with the Declaration of Helsinki [10]. All patients enrolled in the study provided informed consent.

The study enrolled patients from 5 general surgery departments with a total of 200 beds at the Second Affiliated Hospital of Kunming Medical University. Continuous sampling was performed to collect research data from February 2010 to June 2012.

The study subject inclusion criteria were as follows: (1) undergoing major abdominal surgery confirmed by clinicians, including partial gastrectomy, full stomach resection, colorectal resection, pancreaticojejunostomy, biliary-enteric anastomosis, hepatectomy, biliary exploratory surgery, duodenal resection, and small-bowel resection and being (2) ≥18 years of age, <90 years of age; (3) willing to participate in this study; (4) capable of communicating with researchers; (5) screened for nutritional risk according to Nutritional Risk Screening-2002 (NRS-2002) with a resulting nutritional risk ≥3 points; and (6) hospitalized for more than 7 days.

Study exclusion criteria were as follows: (1) being pregnant or lactating; (2) having impaired cognitive function; (3) not undergoing a face-to-face examination within 48 h of admission; (4) having severe illness or being transferred from the intensive care unit or other medical institutions; (5) undergoing emergency surgery; and (6) receiving more calories or nitrogen than recommended by guidelines or receiving nutritional support for only one day.

The patients were evaluated in person for the first time within 48 h of admission to obtain their informed consent, assess nutritional risk, and collect baseline information.

The inpatient nutritional risk screening method recommended by the European Society of Parenteral and Enteral Nutrition (ESPEN) and the Chinese Society for Parenteral and Enteral Nutrition (CSPEN), NRS-2002, was used within 48 h of admission to screen the nutritional risk of patients who met the inclusion criteria, and patients whose total score was ≥3 were considered at nutritional risk and included in the follow-up programme.

All patients who completed the first assessment and met the selection criteria received follow-up 4 times a week until discharge to ensure the prospective nature of the study. Each patient's medical records, nursing records, and face-to-face interviews were used to gather information about their complications and nutritional support and to record the discharge date and discharge outcomes. In all cases, the assessment and collection of information were completed by specialized researchers with the help of doctors and nurses in the inpatient department.

Justification and definition of nutritional support

In this study, the nutritional support programme was selected by the patients' attending physicians rather than being randomly determined or affected by the researchers. The physicians' selection of nutritional support programme was determined primarily by the following factors: (1) the physician's clinical nutrition knowledge; (2) attitudes toward and awareness of nutritional support of the patients and their families; (3) Medicare coverage; and (4) nutritional support routinely practiced by the department. Because the attending physicians were blind to the nutritional risk screening results, the results did not affect their selction of nutritional support programme.

During the study period, the physicians at the Second Affiliated Hospital of Kunming Medical University had not yet started following the clinical practice guidelines for nutritional support recommended by the CSPEN. Although the hospital had nutritional support and consultation groups and nutrition-preparation rooms to provide standard nutritional technology and support, some clinicians and departments did not use the prepared nutrient solution and followed departmental or personally preferred methods of nutritional support, such as administering insufficient quantity of amino acids, fat emulsion alone or support for a limited duration. For the subjects included in this study, different levels of nutrients (at a minimum, glucose and amino acids) were administered instead of a glucose saline solution (i.e., no nutritional support).

The ESPEN and CSPEN standards were used to define the concept of nutritional support.

PN: The ESPEN and Chinese Medical Association Clinical Practice Guidelines served as the reference. PN was defined as administration of sugar/fat and amino acids at a dose of 15–30 kcal/kg/d (non-protein) and ≥0.8 g/kg/d of amino acids, with continuous application for ≥7 days at intervals of no more than 48 h [1, 2, 9]. The PN formulation used in this study was in a three-chamber bag (Cavan Kabiven, Huarui Pharmaceuticals, Wuxi, China) and prepared in a sterile room in the hospital (TPN preparation room). In this study, PN was administered through the surrounding central vein/central vein (internal jugular vein/subclavian vein). Continuous infusion of PN lasted at least 16 h a day.

EN was also administered in accordance with the ESPEN and the Chinese Medical Association Clinical Practice Guidelines. The treatment, which was administered via a parenteral route (oral or tube feeding), consisted of industrialized enteral nutrition, such as whole protein and peptides, including nutritional products from SSPC and Nutricia. The calories were maintained at 15–30 kcal/kg/d (≥1 g/kg/d of protcin), with continuous adminstration for ≥7 days at intervals of no more than 48 h of receiving EN [2, 9, 11]. The continuous tube feeding time was at least 16 h per day, with 100 ml per hour of oral EN.

The combination of PN and EN consisted of the above-mentioned PN and EN methods, and the total number of calories could reach 15–30 kcal/kg/d (≥0.8 g/kg/d of amino acids), with continuous administration for ≥7 days, at intervals of no more than 48 h. If the patients also continued normal dietary intake, the parenteral or enteral nutrition support would provide more than 80 % of the patient's total energy to meet the requirements described above and to be included in the nutritional support cohort.

Nutrient supplementation programmes did not meet the recommended guidelines if (1) the calories or proteins in the PN, EN, or PN + EN met the standards but the treatment lasted ≤6 days or (2) the calories or nitrogen were lower than the PN or EN mentioned above but lasted ≥2 days.

Complications

The most common complications after abdominal surgery in the patients were pneumonia, septicaemia, intra-abdominal abscess, wound infection, urinary tract infection, central catheter infection, anastomotic blood, anastomotic leakage, wound dehiscence, intestinal obstruction, organ dysfunction, pulmonary embolism, bleeding due to duodenal ulcer, abdominal bleeding, severe electrolyte imbalance, deep venous thrombosis and pleural effusion/pneumothorax. The primary endpoint was the incidence of infectious complications. Infectious complications were defined as the appearance of pathogens in the sterile tissue within the body confirmed by pathogen culture results or by evidence of infection corresponding to clinical signs and symptoms, radiological results, or haematology [12]. Infection of the incisional wound was defined as purulent exudate in the wound with a positive bacterial culture. Clinical signs of pneumonia and radiographic evidence and/or a positive bacterial culture of tracheal aspirate, blood or brush were considered to indicate pneumonia. An intra-abdominal abscess was defined as an abscess diagnosed by radiographic examination that required operative or percutaneous drainage. Anastomotic leakage was defined as clinical suspicion of leakage of anastomosis, confirmed by radiographic examination, or a visually dehiscent anastomosis during reoperation. A catheter-related infection was defined as a positive culture of a catheter combined with a positive bacterial culture.

Postoperative hospital stay

Because nutritional support was administered after surgery in all the included patients, the analysis of postoperative hospital stay could accurately indicate the impact of nutritional support on the length of stay. Postoperative hospital stay was defined as the duration between the date of operation and the date when discharge criteria were met. Discharge criteria included the ability to manage personal care and toilet activities, absence of fever, and no intravenous access [13].

Sample-size determination

Before the study was initiated, retrospective data from 100 at-risk patients who had undergone major abdominal surgery showed that the infection complication rate among patients who received calories or nutritional support that did not meet guideline standards was approximately 30 %. Nutritional support that did meet guideline standards was considered an efficient method of reducing the incidence of infectious complications. During the study period, an estimated 500 patients at nutritional risk were expected to meet the inclusion criteria. If 2/3 of the patients were given nutritional support that met guideline standards, then, using a 2-sided alpha of 0.05, 500 patients would provide 80 % power to detect a 40 % reduction in infectious complications in the cohort given nutritional support that met guideline standards (15.5 %) relative to the cohort given nutritional support that did not (26 %).

Statistical analysis

In this study, EpiData software 3.0 was used to establish the database. Excel 2010 was used to organize the data. The χ^2 test and Fisher's exact test were used to compare the categorical variables. Normally distributed data were expressed as the mean ± SD, and non-normally distributed variables were expressed as medians and interquartile ranges (IQRs). For continuous variables, the distribution of the data was analysed for normality. Student's unpaired *t*-test was used for normally distributed numerical variables, and Wilcoxon test was used for non-normally distributed numerical variables. Binary logistic regression analysis was used to analyse the risk factors (gender, age, BMI, weight loss, reduced food intake, nutrition support, energy and nitrogen) for infectious complications. SPSS18.0 (SPSS Inc, Chicago, IL, US) software was used for the statistical analysis. $P < 0.05$ indicated statistical significance, and $P < 0.01$ indicated statistical significance.

Results

General information regarding the study subjects

During the study period, there were a total of 22,453 patients in the five wards, and the inclusion process was as described in the flowchart (Fig. 1). Of the 1824 patients who were treated with NRS 2002, 1285 with NRS-2002 scores <3 were excluded; 539 patients were found to be at nutritional risk, and 14 of these patients were excluded because they were hospitalized for <5 days. Ultimately, 525 patients at nutritional risk were analysed in the study. Although nutritional support should have been administered to patients at nutritional risk (NRS-2002 score ≥3), only 39.05 % (205/525) of such patients received nutritional support that met the recommended guidelines. The other 60.95 % received caloric and nutritional support that did not meet recommended guidelines (320/525).

The demographic characteristics and baseline information for the subjects are shown in Table 1. Significant differences were found between cohorts in gender, age, body weight loss >5 %, average calories, average amount of N and diagnosis ($P < 0.05$). There were no differences in nutritional risk, BMI, food intake < 75 %, or postoperative hospital stay between cohorts ($P \geq 0.05$).

Complications

Differences in complications in the 2 cohorts are shown in Table 2. Of the 525 patients at nutritional risk, 126 experienced complications: 121 of these were infectious complications and 17 were non-infectious (including 12 cases of co-infection complications). Caloric or

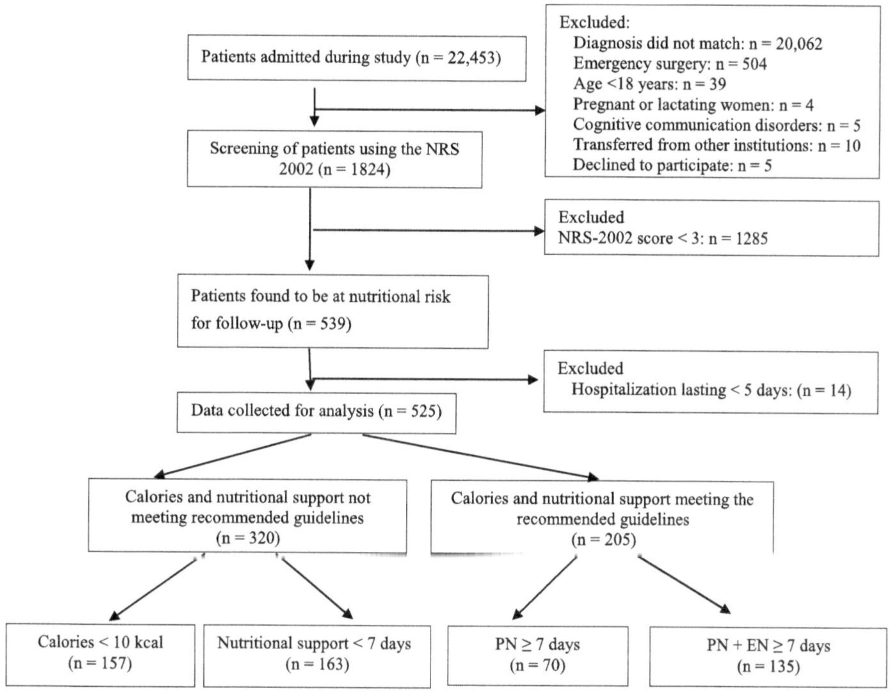

Fig. 1 Flowchart of subject inclusion process

Table 1 Baseline characteristics of patients in cohorts receiving and not receiving nutritional support meeting guideline standard

	Calories or nutritional support not meeting guideline standards (n = 320)	Calories and nutritional support meeting guideline standards (n = 205)	P value
Male (percentage)	188 (58.7 %)	100 (48.8 %)	0.025
Age (mean ± SD)	66.43 ± 11.73	62.86 ± 13.99	0.006
Nutritional risk (mean ± SD)	4.09 ± 0.90	4.08 ± 0.93	0.134
BMI (mean ± SD)	21.09 ± 2.51	20.80 ± 2.56	0.687
Body weight loss >5 %	126 (39.4 %)	117 (57.1 %)	<0.001
Food intake <75 %	240 (75.0 %)	142 (69.3 %)	0.150
Average calories (kcal/person/day)	15.35 ± 2.44	22.67 ± 1.48	< 0.001
Average N amount (g/person/day)	0.66 ± 0.51	1.15 ± 0.09	< 0.001
Duration of nutritional support (days)	——	10.5 ± 2.6	——
Postoperative hospital stay (days)	15 (13,19)	15 (12, 20)	0.609
Diagnosis[a] (n)			< 0.001
A1	11 (3.4 %)	6 (2.9 %)	
A2	123 (38.4 %)	117 (57.1 %)	
B1	129 (40.3 %)	60 (29.3 %)	
B2	57 (17.8 %)	22 (10.7 %)	

[a] A1 = benign gastrointestinal diseases: gastric ulcer, duodenal ulcer, gastric stromal tumours, jejunum stromal tumours, congenital megacolon, lengthy colon, rectal polyps, colonic diverticulitis; A2 = gastrointestinal cancer: gastric cancer, colon cancer, colorectal cancer, duodenal cancer, small intestine cancer, non-Hodgkin's lymphoma; B1 = benign disease of the liver, bile ducts and pancreas: bile duct stones, bile duct stricture, Mirizzi syndrome, bile duct cyst, liver haemangioma, pancreas cystadenoma, papillary tumour of the pancreas, pancreatic pseudocyst; B2 = malignant cancer of the liver, bile ducts and pancreas: cholangiocarcinoma, gallbladder cancer, liver cancer, pancreatic cancer

Table 2 Differences in complications between cohorts receiving and not receiving nutritional support meeting guideline standard

	Calories or nutritional support not meeting guideline standards (*n* = 320)	Calories or nutritional support meeting guideline standards (*n* = 205)	*P* value
(1) Infectious complications	86 (26.9 %)	35 (17.1 %)	0.009
Pneumonia	52 (16.3 %)	18 (8.8 %)	0.014
Urinary tract infection	4 (1.3 %)	0 (0.0 %)	0.160
Sepsis	25 (7.8 %)	10 (4.9 %)	0.187
Septic shock	0 (0.0 %)	2 (1.0 %)	0.152
Catheter-related infection	1 (0.3 %)	0 (0.0 %)	1.000
Intra-abdominal abscess	6 (1.9 %)	10 (4.9 %)	0.051
Infection of incisional wound	11 (3.4 %)	1 (0.5 %)	0.034
Two or more infections	12 (3.8 %)	7 (3.4 %)	1.0
(2) Non-infectious complications	8 (2.5 %)	9 (4.4 %)	0.312
Organ dysfunction	2 (0.4 %)	1 (0.5 %)	1.000
Multiple organ failure	5 (1.6 %)	1 (0.5 %)	0.412
Pulmonary embolism	1 (0.3 %)	0 (0.0 %)	1.000
Bleeding due to duodenal ulcer	3 (0.9%)	0 (0.0 %)	0.285
Postoperative abdominal bleeding	1 (0.3 %)	1 (0.5 %)	1.000
Severe electrolyte imbalance	1 (0.3 %)	1 (0.5 %)	1.000
Anastomotic bleeding	1 (0.3 %)	0 (0.0 %)	1.000
Anastomotic leak	0 (0.0 %)	2 (1.0 %)	0.152
Pleural effusion/pneumothorax	0 (0.0 %)	1 (0.5 %)	0.390
Wound dehiscence/healing delay	0 (0.0 %)	1 (0.5 %)	0.390
Gastrointestinal obstruction/perforation	0 (0.0 %)	1 (0.5 %)	0.390
Deep vein thrombosis	1 (0.3 %)	1 (0.5 %)	1.000
Two or more non-infectious complications	5 (1.6 %)	1 (0.5 %)	0.412
Co-infectious complications	4 (1.3 %)	8 (3.9 %)	0.069
(3) Total complications	90 (28.1 %)	36 (17.6 %)	0.006
(4) Deaths	6 (1.9 %)	2 (1.0 %)	0.492

Chi-square tests or Fisher's exact test were used

nutritional support that met recommended guidelines was associated with a significantly lower incidence of total complications than caloric and nutritional support that did not meet the recommended guidelines (17.6 % vs. 28.1 %, $P = 0.006$). The incidence of infectious complications was lower (17.1 %) in the cohort given recommended levels of caloric or nutritional support than in the cohort that did not (26.9 %) ($P = 0.009$). There were no differences in non-infectious complications or mortality between the cohorts ($P \geq 0.05$). Eight

Table 3 Incidence of complications among subgroups

	Calories or nutritional support not meeting guideline standards (*n* = 320)		Calories or nutritional support meeting guideline standards (*n* = 205)		*P* value
	Nutritional support < 7 days (*n* = 163)	Calories < 10 kcal (*n* = 157)	PN + EN ≥ 7 days (*n* = 135)	PN ≥7 days (*n* = 70)	
Infectious complications	43 (26.3 %) [a]	43 (27.4 %) [a]	17 (12.6 %) [b]	18 (25.7 %) [a]	0.010
Non-infectious complications	3 (1.8 %) [a]	5 (3.2 %) [a]	3 (2.2 %) [a]	6 (8.6 %) [b]	0.050
Total complications	46 (28.2 %) [a]	44 (28.0 %) [a]	17 (12.6 %) [b]	19 (27.1 %) [a]	0.005
Death	2 (1.2 %) [a]	4 (2.5 %) [a]	0 (0.0 %) [a]	2 (2.8 %) a	0.025

Chi-square tests or Fisher's exact test were used

[a]denotes a subset of cohort categories whose column proportions did not differ significantly from each other, $P \geq 0.05$

[b]denotes a subset of cohort categories whose column proportions differed significantly from each other, $P < 0.05$

patients died: 3 with multiple-organ dysfunction, 1 with anastomotic leakage, 3 with lung infections and uremic syndrome, and 1 with septic shock.

The differences in complications between the 4 subgroups are shown in Table 3. There were significant differences between subgroups with respect to infectious complications, non-infectious complications, total complications and mortality rate ($P < 0.05$). The Bonferroni method was used to account for multiple comparisons among subgroups. The incidence of infectious complications and total complications was lower (12.6 %) in the subgroup receiving PN and EN combined nutritional support for ≥7 days than in the other subgroups ($P < 0.05$). The incidence of non-infectious complications was higher (8.6 %) in the subgroup receiving PN for ≥7 days than in the other subgroups ($P < 0.05$).

Binary logistic regression analysis was performed to identify the risk factors for infectious complications (Table 4). Infectious complications served as the dependent variable in the analysis, and gender, age, BMI, weight loss, reduced food intake, type of nutritional support, disease, and type of surgery were the independent variables. Binary logistic regression analysis conducted to identify the factors that influenced infectious complications showed that age, weight loss, and reduced food intake were risk factors for infectious complications and that nutritional support that met recommended guidelines was a protective factor.

Discussion

China is currently undergoing health care reform and improvements to the health care system; standardizing medical management and behaviour in medical institutions and promoting guidelines are two important objectives. Standard nutritional support for hospitalized patients at nutritional risk has been recommended by the Clinical Practice Guidelines [2], but our study showed that the actual situation was not congruent with these recommendations. This prospective cohort study showed that approximately 60.95 % of the patients at nutritional risk who underwent major abdominal surgery did not receive nutritional support consistent with recommended guidelines. Of all the patients in this study, 29.90 % were given only amino acids, at <10 kcal/kg/d, and 31.05 % received nutritional support for less than 7 days. The main reasons for these inadequate procedures were lack of screening for medical nutrition risk and lack of knowledge concerning nutritional support [14, 15]. The need for nutritional support was usually determined by a physician, based on insufficient food intake, hypoproteinemia, or general critical condition [14].

More importantly, we found that nutritional support that did not meet the standards in the guidelines (i.e., nutritional support for < 7 days and calories <10 kcal) was associated with a higher incidence of infectious complications and total complications than guideline-compliant nutritional support. However, it is prudent to qualify this result because possible confounding factors, such as gender, age, body weight loss, average calories, average amount of N and diagnosis, may have introduced bias. To adjust for the confounding factors as much as possible and more precisely evaluate the impact of nutritional support on the incidence of infectious diseases in patients at nutritional risk, binary logistic regression analysis was performed to account for these variables. The analysis showed that nutritional support that met the guideline standards was a protective factor for patients at nutritional risk. However, the OR value was 0.870, and the strength of the correlation was moderate. After adjusting for the confounding factors, higher age, weight loss, and reduced food intake were also found to increase the incidence of infectious complications (Table 4). These results confirmed the effects of nutritional support on clinical outcome and also demonstrated that nutritional deterioration was related to age and poorer clinical outcomes. This is consistent with the findings reported by Kondrup et al. [16].

In previous prospective cohort studies of nutritional support in patients at risk, nutritional support consisted mainly of PN and little to no PN combined with EN; therefore, the investigators were unable to conduct a complete statistical analysis [6, 8, 15]. In the present study, 65.85 % of patients with nutritional support lasting ≥7 days received combined

Table 4 Risk factors for infectious complications

Variable	Parameter	SEM	Wald value	*P* value	OR 95 % CI
Gender	0.224	0.249	0.809	0.368	1.251 (0.768, 2.037)
Age	0.029	0.012	5.963	0.015	1.030 (1.006, 1.055)
BMI	−0.027	0.05	0.284	0.594	0.974 (0.883, 1.074)
Body weight loss >5 %	0.093	0.045	4.306	0.038	1.097 (1.005, 1.198)
Food intake <75 %	0.449	0.19	5.594	0.018	1.567 (1.080, 2.273)
Nutritional support that met recommended guidelines	−0.139	0.045	9.394	0.002	0.870 (0.796, 0.951)
Energy	0.106	0.054	3.807	0.051	1.111 (0.998, 1.236)
Nitrogen	−1.446	0.753	3.685	0.055	0.235 (0.054, 1.031)

Binary logistic regression analysis was used

PN and EN nutritional support, which was suitable for data analysis. Previous studies included EN-only groups, mostly for nutritional support administered to patients with internal illness or nutritional support before abdominal surgery. PN was frequently used for postoperative nutritional support after abdominal surgery [6, 8, 15]. In this study, no EN-only groups were identified for the following reasons: (1) physicians lacked adequate knowledge regarding nutrition support and awareness of EN application methods; (2) surgical safety concerns of the clinician, such as administration of intestinal nutritional support after gastrointestinal surgery, increasing anastomotic tension and thus being unfavourable for anastomotic healing; and (3) the need for catheters and careful monitoring of the implementation process, such as adjusting the concentration, speed, and temperature, which is more complicated than the implementation of PN.

In this study, the incidence ratio of infectious complications between the groups given nutritional support that met guideline standards and those that did not was 1:1.6 (17.1 % vs. 26.9 %, $P = 0.01$), which was higher than the incidence ratio in previous studies (approximately 1:2) [6, 14]. The sub-cohort analysis (Table 3) showed a similar rate of infectious disease in patients given PN nutritional support for ≥ 7 days and those whose treatments did not meet the standards recommended in guidelines (i.e., nutritional support <7 days or calories <10 kcal). This was consistent with the conclusion that TPN for ≥7 days does not significantly reduce the rate of infectious complications compared with no nutritional support at all [17]. In the combined EN and PN group, along with other sub-groups of the cohorts (PN ≥ 7 days, nutritional support for <7 days and calories <10 kcal), the incidence of infectious complications was significantly lower, which was considered a benefit conferred by EN. However, these results need to be confirmed and supported by additional trials with sufficient sample sizes.

There are several limitations of this study. First, there were no previous studies to draw on for the calculation of sample size. Because infectious complications were extracted retrospectively from patient records, the results may not have been fully accurate. Second, the categorization of some variables in the logistic regression analysis was too general. Some valuable information may have been missed. Third, logistic regression analysis is notoriously unstable; therefore, the associations we found need to be confirmed in future studies. Although our study had these limitations, our findings might provide a useful reference for Chinese clinicians and policy makers to improve nutritional support practices.

Conclusions

This study demonstrated that nutritional support that did not meet the standards in recommended guidelines was associated with a higher incidence of infectious complications in patients at risk after abdominal surgery and is thus clinically undesirable. Nutritional support meeting the recommended nutrient guidelines was a protective factor for infectious complications, but the strength of the correlation was moderate. A support regimen involving PN + EN for ≥7 days generated significantly better outcomes and is therefore highly recommended. These positive findings in our study need to be confirmed and supported by additional well-designed trials.

Abbreviations

CSPEN, Chinese society for parenteral and enteral nutrition; EN, enteral nutrition; ESPEN, European society for parenteral and enteral nutrition; IQR, interquartile range; NRS-2002, nutritional risk screening-2002; PN, parental autrition; TPN, total parental nutrition

Acknowledgements

Not applicable.

Funding

This study was supported by the Foundation of Research Center for Surgical Clinical Nutrition in Yun-Nan Province (no. 2014NS089), the Professor Yang Hua Research Station in Yun-Nan Province and The National Natural Science Fund (no. 81160114). We used the funding to collect the data and revise the manuscript.

Availability of data and materials

All authors wish to share our data, but the data belong to the shared multicentre database of the Nutritional Support for Those at Risk of Undernutrition Outcomes and Cost-effectiveness study. The Multi-Center Co-operative Clinical Study Group does not allow these data to be released until the multi-centre papers have been published.

Authors' contributions

DLS, WML, QPL and PYX designed the study; YYC, YL, QWX, YJL, YBS, YQ and TY performed the research and collected the data; DLS and WML analysed the data; DLS, QPL and PYX wrote the paper. All authors read and approved the final manuscript.

Competing interests

The authors declare that they have no competing interests.

Consent for publication

Not applicable.

Ethics approval and consent to participate

This prospective cohort study was approved by the ethics committee at the Second Affiliated Hospital of Kunming Medical University (approval no. 2010-08). The study was performed in accordance with the Declaration of Helsinki. All patients enrolled in the study provided informed consent.

Author details

[1]Department of General Surgery, Wuhan Clinical School of Southern Medical University/Wuhan General Hospital of Guangzhou Military Command, Wuhan 430070, China. [2]Department of Gastrointestinal Surgery, Second Affiliated Hospital of Kunming Medical University, Kunming 650101, China. [3]Research Center for Surgical Clinical Nutrition in Yun-Nan Province, Kunming 650101, China.

References

1. Braga M, Ljungqvist O, Soeters P, et al. ESPEN Guidelines on Parenteral Nutrition: surgery. Clin Nutr. 2009;28:378–86.
2. Chinese Medical Association. Clinical Practice Guidelines Parenteral Enteral Nutrition Section. Beijing: People's Medical Publishing House; 2009. p. 16–8.

3. Yan JJ, Mou SY, Zhang H, et al. Analysis on nutritional risk and nutritional support status of patients with digestive diseases. Chinese Nurs Res (Chinese). 2013;27:4114.
4. Zhang M, Wang Y, Song GH, et al. Nutritional risk, undernutrition, and nutrition support among inpatients with early and middle stage gastrointestinal cancers in a tertiary hospital in Weifang, Shandong Province. Chinese J Clin Nutr (Chinese). 2012;20:345–50.
5. Zhang H, Mou SY, Tan RF. Prevalence of nutritional risks and malnutrition and application of nutritional support in the elderly inpatients of Chongqing. Laser J (Chinese). 2012;33:87–8.
6. Jie B, Jiang ZM, Nolan MT, et al. Impact of nutritional support on clinical outcome in patients at nutritional risk: a multicenter, prospective cohort study in Baltimore and Beijing teaching hospitals. Nutrition. 2010;26:1088–93.
7. The Veterans Affairs Total Parenteral Nutrition Cooperation Study Group. Perioperative total parenteral nutrition in surgical patients. N Engl J Med. 1991;325:525–32.
8. Jie B, Jiang ZM, Nolan MT, et al. Impact of preoperative nutritional support on clinical outcome in abdominal surgical patients at nutritional risk. Nutrition. 2012;28:1022–7.
9. Zhan WH, Jiang ZM, Tang Y, et al. Impact of hypocaloric and hypo-nitrogen parenteral nutrition on clinical outcome in postoperative patients: a multi-center randomized controlled trial of 120 cases. Zhonghua Yi Xue Za Zhi (Chinese). 2007;87:1729–33.
10. World Medical Association Declaration of Helsinki. Ethical principles for medical research involving human subjects. 59th WMA General Assembly. Seoul. 2008. Accessed at: http://www.wma.net/en/30publications/10policies/b3/index.html in March 5, 2009.
11. Weimann A, Braga M, Harsanyi L, et al. ESPEN Guidelines on Enteral Nutrition: Surgery including organ transplantation. Clin Nutr. 2006,25:224–244.
12. American College of Chest Physicians/Society of Critical Care Medicine Consensus Conference Committee. American College of Chest Physicians/Society of Critical Care Medicine Consensus Conference: definitions for sepsis and organ failure and guidelines for the use of innovative therapies in sepsis. Crit Care Med. 1992;20:864–74.
13. Johansen N, Kondrup J, Plum LM, et al. Effect of nutritional support on clinical outcome in patients at nutritional risk. Clin Nutr. 2004;23:539–50.
14. Pang D, Zheng FF, Zhou YJ, et al. Survey on and analysis of pre-operative nutritional risks and nutritional supports among patients and related knowledge among surgeons in general surgical wards. Parenter Enteral Nutr (Chinese). 2010;17:65–8.
15. Hui Zhang,Yang Wang, Zhu-Ming Jiang, et al. Effect of Nutrition Support on Clinical Outcome and Cost Effectiveness in Patients at Nutritional Risk by NRS 2002 Tool: A Prospective Cohort Study. http://pen.sagepub.com/content/suppl/2012/12/27/37.1.138.DC1/DS_10.1177_0148607112470611_all_abstracts.pdf
16. Kondrup J, Allison SP, Elia M, et al. ESPEN guidelines for nutrition screening 2002. Clin Nutr. 2003;22:415–21.
17. Koretz RL, Lipman TO, Klein S, et al. AGA technical review on parenteral nutrition. Gastroenterology. 2001;121:970–1001.

Behaviors of consumers, physicians and pharmacists in response to adverse events associated with dietary supplement use

Tsuyoshi Chiba[1*], Yoko Sato[1], Etsuko Kobayashi[1], Kazuki Ide[2], Hiroshi Yamada[2] and Keizo Umegaki[1]

Abstract

Background: The prevalence of dietary supplements has increased in Japan, and, as a consequence, the adverse events associated with dietary supplement use have become more prominent. Severe adverse events must be reported to the Japanese government via public health centers. However, the number of cases reported to the Japanese government is limited. To clarify this discrepancy, we conducted an internet questionnaire, and surveyed how consumers, physicians and pharmacists acted when they or their patients developed adverse events due to dietary supplement use.

Methods: This study was completed by 2732 consumers, 515 physicians, and 515 pharmacist via internet surveillance on November 2015.

Results: Although 8.8% of consumers developed adverse events including diarrhea, constipation, stomachache, headache, and nausea and vomiting, most of them did not report their adverse events to public health centers. However, some consumers went to hospitals because of adverse events. We also surveyed how physicians and pharmacists acted when their patients developed adverse events due to dietary supplement use. Most physicians and pharmacists did not report these cases to public health centers because they were unable to definitively prove the cause-and-effect relationship of these adverse events. Furthermore, some physicians and pharmacists did not know how or where to report these adverse events.

Conclusions: We clarified the reasons for the limited number of reports of adverse events to the Japanese government in this survey. It is important to encourage not only consumers, but also physicians and pharmacists to report adverse events to public health centers. In addition, an analyzing tool of cause-and-effect relationships might be helpful for physicians and pharmacists.

Keywords: Dietary supplements, Adverse events, Consumers, Physicians, Pharmacists

Background

The prevalence of dietary supplements, which are helpful to supply nutrients for health, has increased in Japan [1–3]. Consumers use not only vitamins and minerals, but also various other ingredients as dietary supplements. However, most consumers do not understand the properties of dietary supplements and their ingredients, which may be beneficial, but are also associated with a risk of adverse reactions, such as gastrointestinal and neurological complications, hepatotoxicity, and interactions with drugs [4–8]. The reasons for misunderstanding of consumers are that manufacturers tend to emphasize the key characteristics of their products and promote sales using attractive claims [9]. Furthermore, some dietary supplements have claimed beneficial effects for the treatment of several diseases, even though these claims are illegal in Japan. Under these conditions, consumers use dietary supplements inappropriately, thereby increasing the risk of adverse events.

There are several causes of adverse events due to dietary supplement use, the first of which is the use of low quality dietary supplements. For example, an excess amount of

* Correspondence: tyschiba@nih.go.jp
[1]Information Center, National Institute of Health and Nutrition, National Institutes of Biomedical Innovation, Health and Nutrition, 1-23-1 Toyama, Shinjuku-ku, Tokyo 162-8636, Japan
Full list of author information is available at the end of the article

heavy metals or unlabeled ingredients associated with allergies may contaminate products. Drug ingredients, such as sibutramine, sildenafil, and dexamethasone, are added to dietary supplements [10, 11]. A large number of studies have reported a relationship between adverse events and the use of these products. Another cause of adverse events is consumer characteristics. Some individuals develop allergic reactions to the ingredients of dietary supplements. Infants/children, pregnant and lactating women, and the elderly are influenced more by dietary supplements [12, 13]. In addition, patients, particularly those receiving medication, need to be more cautious of dietary supplement use [14]. A third cause of adverse events is the inappropriate use of dietary supplements including an excessive intake or the concomitant use of various dietary supplements and/or medicines. In the past few decades, a large number of ingredients have been shown to interact with drugs [15–21]; however, it currently remains unclear whether most ingredients in dietary supplements interact with drugs.

We previously reported that some dietary supplement users in Japan experienced adverse events [22, 23]. There are several ways by which to report the adverse events associated with dietary supplement use in Japan. Consumers report their adverse events to manufacturers or retail stores. In the US, dietary supplements are regulated by the Dietary Supplement Health and Education Act (DSHEA) [24, 25]. Under the DSHEA, the manufacturers, packers, and distributors of dietary supplements are required to submit the main associated adverse events to the US Food and Drug Administration (FDA)'s Center for Food Safety and Applied Nutrition Adverse Event Reporting System (CAERS) within 15 business days of receiving information on adverse events. On the other hand, manufacturers do not have a duty to report adverse events to the Ministry of Health, Labour and Welfare (MHLW) in Japan, which regulates adverse events associated with dietary supplement use. Therefore, the majority of complaints are handled by each manufacturer. Consumers also have the option of reporting adverse events to the Practical Living Information Online Network System (PIO-NET), which is the operating system of the National Consumer Affairs Center of Japan. Several hundred cases per year are reported to the PIO-NET [26]. However, most reports cannot define cause-and-effect relationships because the information obtained from consumers is not considered to be sufficient to define these relationships. Furthermore, consumers themselves or their physicians or pharmacists report severe adverse events associated with dietary supplement use to public health centers, which then report adverse events to the MHLW. However, only 20 adverse events per year are reported to the MHLW. Therefore, the Japanese government cannot take action against adverse events associated with dietary supplement use. The cause of the limited number of adverse events reported to the MHLW currently remains unclear.

In the present study, we surveyed how consumers behaved when they experienced adverse events associated with dietary supplement use. We also surveyed how physicians and pharmacists advised their patients and whether they reported adverse events to public health centers.

Methods

Definition of "dietary supplement"

In Japan, "dietary supplement" has no definition in the law, and some dairy or soybean products are recognized as dietary supplements even if they are in the form of common foods. Therefore, the meaning of the term "dietary supplement" differs for each individual. In this survey, "dietary supplement" was defined as those that consumers considered to have beneficial effects on their health (e.g., vitamins, minerals, fish oil, glucosamine, cereal) except for daily foods (e.g., vegetables, fruits, milk, tofu).

Internet survey

An internet-based questionnaire was conducted by Macromill, Inc. (Tokyo, Japan) with their research registrants (2 million registrants in 2015) between 13 November and 19 November 2015 on consumers, and between 13 November and 18 November 2015 on physicians and pharmacists. This study was conducted with the approval of the Research Ethics Committee of the National Institutes of Biomedical Innovation, Health and Nutrition (No.198-1, approved on Aug. 28, 2015) and in accordance with Declaration of Helsinki.

Preliminary survey for subjects who experienced adverse effects due to dietary supplement use

To extract consumers who experienced adverse events due to dietary supplement use, a preliminary survey was conducted with randomly selected 70,000 consumers from research registrants of Macromill, Inc. (Additional file 1). Of these, 24,295 subjects (34.7%) were currently using dietary supplements, 18,194 (26.0%) had used dietary supplements in the past, and 27,511 (39.3%) have never used dietary supplements. We asked current- and ex-users of dietary supplements whether they had experienced adverse events (diarrhea, constipation, stomachache, headache, nausea and vomiting, fatigue, anthema and itching, palpitations, worsening health examination data, or other symptoms) due to dietary supplement use. A total of 6129 subjects (8.8%) experienced adverse events, and a part of these consumers answered the full survey. Veterinary surgeons and dentists were excluded from the survey because they had few opportunities to be asked by patients about the adverse events associated with dietary supplement use.

Full survey

The full survey was conducted on 3095 consumers who experienced adverse events (Additional file 2). The questionnaire included the purpose of supplementation (maintenance of health, improvements to health, for beauty or weight loss, prevention of diseases, and treatment of diseases), types of dietary supplements, their responses to adverse events which associated by dietary supplement use, and their reasons if they did not report it to public institutes. Among physicians and pharmacists, the survey was conducted on 1030 subjects (515 physicians and 515 pharmacists) (Additional file 3). The questionnaire included their experiences of being asked by patients about adverse events associated with dietary supplement use, what advice they gave their patients, whether they reported it to public institutes, and their reasons if they did not report it to public institutes. The demographic characteristics (sex and age) were obtained from the research registrants' data of Macromill, Inc.

Statistical analysis

Differences among groups were tested using the χ^2 test. Statistical analyses were performed using HALBAU 7.5.1 (HALBAU R&D Co., Ltd., Tokyo). *P*-values less than 0.05 were considered significant.

Results

Characteristics

Characteristics of consumers, physicians and pharmacists are shown in Table 1. Consumers ($n = 3095$) were as follows: sex (male; 1340, female; 1755), age (20s; 468, 30s; 736, 40s; 634, 50s; 611, older than 60; 646). The characteristics of physicians and pharmacists ($n = 1030$) were as follows: sex (female; 379, male; 651), age (20s; 64, 30s; 248, 40s; 317, 50s; 289, older than 60; 112). Physicians (515) specialized in internal medicine; 214, pediatrics; 34, obstetrics and gynecology; 18, and others; 249. Pharmacists (515) worked in dispensing pharmacies; 416, drugstores; 24, and others; 75.

Table 1 Characteristics of consumers, physicians and pharmacists

	Consumers		Physicians		Pharmacists	
	n	%	n	%	n	%
All	3095		515		515	
Sex						
Male	1340	43.3	440	85.4	211	41.0
Female	1755	56.7	75	14.6	304	59.0
Age						
20–29	468	15.1	10	1.9	54	10.5
30–39	736	23.8	71	13.8	177	34.4
40–49	634	20.5	171	33.2	146	28.3
50–59	611	19.7	192	37.3	97	18.8
≥ 60	646	20.9	71	13.8	41	8.0

Purpose of dietary supplement use

The purposes indicated by consumers for the use of dietary supplements are shown in Table 2. The main reason that consumers used dietary supplement was for the maintenance of health. Other reasons were for improvements to health, for beauty, the prevention of diseases, weight loss, and the treatment of disease. The prevalence of the prevention of disease, weight loss, and treatment of disease was significantly higher in subjects who experienced adverse events in the full survey than in all subjects in the preliminary survey. This result suggests that dietary supplements for these purposes cause more adverse events.

In addition, ratio of who used dietary supplement to treat their diseases was greater in subject who experienced adverse events (7.2%) compared to all subject (4.0%). This data suggests that adverse events were more frequently occurred, when they used dietary supplements to treat their diseases.

Symptoms of adverse events

The symptoms of adverse events due to dietary supplement use are shown in Table 3. Diarrhea was the most frequent adverse event, followed by nausea and vomiting, fatigue, and constipation. Diarrhea, nausea and vomiting, headache, and stomachache were significantly more prevalent in younger consumers than in the elderly. On the other hand, anthema and itching and worsening health examination data were significantly more prominent in the elderly than in younger consumers.

Table 2 Purpose of dietary supplement use

	AE[a]		All[b]	
	n	%	n	%
Maintenance of health	2336	75.5	33,347	78.5
Improvements to health	936	30.2	9500	22.4
For beauty	841	27.2	9977	23.5
Prevention of diseases	742	24.0	7906	18.6
Weight loss	738	23.8	7014	16.5
Treatment of diseases	222	7.2	1714	4.0
Others	63	2.0	821	1.9

[a]subjects who experienced adverse events ($n = 3095$)
[b]all subjects who were using or used to use dietary supplement in preliminary survey ($n = 42{,}489$)

Table 3 Adverse events due to dietary supplement use ($n = 3095$)

	All (%)	20s (%)	30s (%)	40s (%)	50s (%)	Older than 60 (%)	*P*-value
Diarrhea	27.9	35.0	32.7	29.3	27.3	16.4	<0.001
Nausea & vomiting	19.1	23.7	22.8	21.3	17.3	11.0	<0.001
Fatigue	17.4	19.7	17.4	18.6	15.4	16.3	0.327
Constipation	17.0	17.7	16.4	15.6	15.5	20.0	0.189
Headache	15.6	22.4	19.0	15.9	13.7	8.4	<0.001
Stomachache	15.4	23.1	17.7	15.1	13.3	9.4	<0.001
Anthema & itching	15.0	11.8	13.0	14.8	14.1	20.6	<0.001
Worsening data of health examination	10.2	4.3	4.1	8.2	11.9	22.0	<0.001
Palpitations	5.5	4.5	5.7	5.7	5.6	5.7	0.895
Others	11.6	9.6	9.4	11.0	13.1	14.9	0.009

Statistical analysis were conducted among ages in each event. *P*-values were calculated using the χ^2 test

Details of dietary supplements potentially associated with adverse events

Details of dietary supplements potentially associated with adverse events are shown in Table 4. Among vitamins/minerals, multi-vitamins were more frequently associated with adverse events than multi-minerals or multi-vitamins and minerals. Individual mineral, such as Fe, Zn, and Ca, and individual vitamin, including vitamin B, vitamin C, and vitamin E also caused adverse events. Furthermore, various non-vitamin, non-mineral supplements were associated with the development of adverse events. *Coleus forskohlii*, which is one of the popular ingredients used to promote weight loss in Japan, was the top ingredient that caused adverse events at a rate that was more than two-fold that of glucosamine/chondroitin, garlic, sesamin, collagen, and other ingredients. In addition, weight loss supplements (except for *Coleus forskohlii*) were strongly associated with the development of adverse events.

Table 4 Details of dietary supplements potentially causing adverse events

	n	Percent
Vitamin/Mineral		
Multi-vitamins	117	3.8
Multi-minerals	20	0.6
Multi-vitamins and minerals	15	0.5
Individual vitamin (vitamin B, vitamin C, and vitamin E)	162	5.2
Individual mineral (Fe, Zn, and Ca)	214	6.9
Non-Vitamin, Non-Mineral (Top 10)		
Coleus forskohlii	183	5.9
Glucosamine/Chondroitin	87	2.8
Garlic	70	2.3
Sesamin	69	2.2
Collagen	64	2.1
Blueberry/Lutein	53	1.7
EPA/DHA/Fish oil/n-3 PUFA	50	1.6
Placenta	44	1.4
Enzymes	42	1.4
Royal jelly/Propolis	41	1.3
Weight loss supplements (except for *Coleus forskohlii*)	155	5.0

Responses of consumers to adverse events

Responses of consumers to adverse events are shown in Table 5. Almost half of consumers stopped using dietary supplements immediately. Adverse events are typically ameliorated by the discontinuation of dietary supplements. On the other hand, one-third of consumers did nothing. Only 5.8% of consumers reported adverse events to public institutes (5.1% to public health centers, 0.5% to the National Consumer Affairs Center of Japan or other consumer affairs centers, and 0.2% to the MHLW or Consumer Affairs Agency, Government of Japan). The reason why most consumers did not report to public institutes was "adverse events were not sufficiently severe to make a complaint (70.8%)". Other reasons were "there were other possibilities for adverse

Table 5 Responses of consumers to adverse events

	n	Percent
Stopped using dietary supplements immediately	1669	53.9
Did nothing	1164	37.6
Went to a hospital	184	5.9
Complained to manufacturers	167	5.4
Reported to public health centers	159	5.1
Complained to the retail store	42	1.4
Reported to the National Consumer Affairs Center of Japan or other consumer affairs centers	16	0.5
Reported to the MHLW or Consumer Affairs Agency, Government of Japan	6	0.2

MHLW Ministry of Health, Labour and Welfare

events (28.1%)" or "making a complaint to public institutes was considered to be too troublesome (13.5%)".

A total of 5.9% of consumers who experienced adverse effects went to a hospital. Physicians and pharmacists have a responsibility to report adverse events associated with dietary supplement use to public health centers.

Consultations regarding adverse events

We conducted a survey on physicians and pharmacists regarding consultations related to dietary supplements. The 57.3% (295/515) of physicians and 59.0% (304/515) of pharmacists were asked about dietary supplement use by their patients. Of these, 25.4% (131/515) of physicians and 19.6% (101/515) of pharmacists had consultations on adverse events with their patients (Table 6). Physicians had significantly more opportunities for consultations on adverse events as compared to pharmacists. Most consultations only occurred 1–2 times, whereas some were more than 3 times. A total of 11.5% (15/131) of physicians and 6.9% (7/101) of pharmacists had more than 10 consultations.

Responses of physicians and pharmacists to adverse events among their patients

Among physicians and pharmacists who had consultations on adverse events, most physicians (84.0%) and pharmacists (75.2%) advised their patients to stop using dietary supplements immediately (Table 7). On the other hand, only 12.3% of physicians and 17.5% pharmacists reported these events to public institutes (8.4 and 11.9% to public health centers, 3.1 and 5.9% to the National Consumer Affairs Center of Japan or other consumer affairs centers, and 0.8 and 1.0% to the Consumer Affairs Agency, Government of Japan). There were no significant differences in behaviors between physicians and pharmacists, except for ask manufactures. Pharmacists (18.8%) significantly more frequently asked manufactures about their products compared to Physicians (3.8%).

Table 6 Opportunity of consultations related to adverse reactions with their patients

	Physicians		Pharmacists		
	n	%	n	%	*P*-value
Yes, I have.	131	25.4	101	19.6	0.030
No, I have never.	384	74.6	414	80.4	
Number of times					
1–2	75	14.6	69	13.4	0.081
3–5	38	7.4	19	3.7	
6–9	3	0.6	6	1.2	
More than 10	15	2.9	7	1.4	

Physicians ($n = 515$), Pharmacists ($n = 515$), *P*-values were calculated using the χ^2 test

Table 7 Responses of physicians and pharmacists to adverse events among their patients

	Physicians		Pharmacists		
	n	%	n	%	*P*-value
Advice to stop using dietary supplements immediately	110	84.0	76	75.2	0.137
Nothing apart from a follow-up	32	24.4	24	23.8	1.000
Ask patients to report to other institutes by themselves	14	10.7	19	18.8	0.117
Ask manufacturers about their products	5	3.8	19	18.8	<0.001
Report to public health centers	11	8.4	12	11.9	0.510
Report to the National Consumer Affairs Center of Japan or other consumer affairs centers	4	3.1	6	5.9	0.455
Report to the Consumer Affairs Agency, Government of Japan	1	0.8	1	1.0	-
Others	4	3.1	3	2.3	-

Physicians ($n = 131$), Pharmacists ($n = 101$), *P*-values were calculated using the χ^2 test

Reasons why physicians and pharmacists did not report adverse events to public health centers

The reasons why physicians and pharmacists did not report adverse events to public health centers were similar (Table 8). They were unable to define case-and-effect relationships for adverse events. Furthermore, they did not know what level of severity needed to be reported. These two reasons were significantly higher in pharmacists than physicians. On the other hand, one third of physicians and pharmacists did not know to where to report adverse events. This reason was significantly higher in physicians than pharmacists.

Discussion

We previously reported that some patients used dietary supplements to treat their diseases [22], and concomitantly used dietary supplements and medicines [23]. The inappropriate usage of dietary supplements causes adverse events. The percentages of consumers who experienced

Table 8 Reasons why physicians and pharmacists did not report adverse events to public health centers

	Physicians		Pharmacists		
	n	%	n	%	*P*-value
It is difficult to define a cause-and-effect relationship	284	55.1	343	66.6	<0.001
It is not clear which case (severity) needs to be reported	214	41.6	249	48.3	0.033
It is not clear where to report	224	43.5	172	33.4	0.001
Cumbersome procedure to report	61	11.8	51	9.9	0.368
Others	18	3.5	11	2.1	0.258

Physicians ($n = 515$), Pharmacists ($n = 515$), *P*-values were calculated using the χ^2 test

adverse events were 3.3 and 8.4% in each report. Several hundred complaints about adverse events due to dietary supplement use are reported to the National Consumer Affairs Center of Japan or other consumer affairs centers every year [26]. However, our results showed that most consumers, physicians, and pharmacists did not report adverse events to public health centers. This is the main reason why the number of adverse events reported to the MHLW is limited.

In the US, dietary supplements are regulated by the DSHEA; however, the DSHEA does not work well. The FDA almost daily warns or recalls tainted dietary supplements, such as the sexual enhancement products containing sildenafil, tadalafil, or their analogues, the weight-loss products containing sibutramine and the laxative phenolphthalein, and the sports supplements containing 1,3-dimethylamylamine or anabolic steroids. On the other hand, manufacturers have to report adverse events to the FDA's CAERS [24, 25]. However, inadequate and poor-quality reports on adverse events associated with dietary supplements are the main limitations of safety monitoring [4, 27]. This condition is similar to Japan. Although several hundred cases per year are reported to the PIO-NET from consumers [26], most reports are inadequate and of insufficient quality to define cause-and-effect relationships. On the other hand, the number of adverse event reports from physicians and pharmacists is limited, but are based on clinical examinations. Therefore, it is important to increase the number of adverse event reports from physicians and pharmacists. However, some physicians and pharmacists have inadequate knowledge about dietary supplements and do not know how or where to report adverse events [28, 29]. Furthermore, 28.0% of physicians and 35.1% of pharmacists were using dietary supplements themselves, while 20.6% of physicians and 35.1% of pharmacists had previously used dietary supplements in this present survey. This result indicates that half of physicians and pharmacists might have a positive attitude towards dietary supplements and may pay less attention to the adverse events associated with their use.

There are some reports that most of patients did not inform their physicians/pharmacists about dietary supplement use, and communication between patients and physicians/pharmacists was important to avoid adverse events [22, 30]. On the other hand, there is no report whether there are differences in attitude towards dietary supplement use in their patients between physicians and pharmacists, and whether physicians and pharmacists discuss dietary supplement use in their patients each other. In our survey, there were some differences between physicians and pharmacists in opportunities for consultation, management of adverse events, and their own personal supplement use. In this regard, communication between physicians and pharmacists might be an important strategy to prevent adverse events and to increase the number of adverse event reports to public health centers.

Our survey also clarified the features of adverse events among generations. This difference might be attributed to the different types of dietary supplements used by each generation. The prevalence of anthema and itching was significantly higher among the elderly, who prefer to use glucosamine/chondroitin for arthralgia [31]. Glucosamine/chondroitin have been shown to induce an allergic reaction [32]. On the other hand, the prevalence of diarrhea was significantly higher in the younger generation, which prefers to use dietary supplements for weight loss. In Japan, most young women want to lose weight in order to maintain their appearance, even though being excessively thin is an important issue among this demographic [33]. A large number of dietary supplements for weight loss contain *Coleus forskohlii*, *Red pepper*, *Senna*, or other ingredients that may cause diarrhea [34–36]. However, it is difficult to define cause-and-effect relationships among them. A generation difference has also been reported in adverse events in the US [13]. Adverse events were associated with dietary supplements for weight loss or energy products in younger generations, and with micronutrients in older generations. Therefore, appropriative information to avoid adverse events are needed for each generation.

There are several limitations to the passive collection of adverse reactions associated with dietary supplements. Consumers, physicians, and pharmacists do not report to public health centers if adverse events are not severe. Furthermore, the numbers of reported adverse reactions that define cause-and-effect relationships are very low. Therefore, the MHLW cannot establish whether these cases are common or singular. However, a one-year prospective surveillance study on dietary supplement-related poison control center calls enabled the rapid detection of potentially harmful products [37]. In this regard, the active collection of adverse events associated with dietary supplements, such as an internet questionnaire, may be a useful method for the rapid detection of harmful products because a large number of consumers obtain information on dietary supplements via the internet [38]. In addition, 23.5% of consumers concomitantly used dietary supplements and medicines in this survey. There is a possibility that interaction of dietary supplements and medicines might cause adverse events. However, we could not estimate how it contributed to our results, because we did not ask in detail about their medications.

In this survey, we clarified that most of consumers did not report adverse events by their self, and physicians and pharmacists also did not report, because they could not define cause-and-effect relationships. So, the number of reports on adverse events to the MHLW are limited. There are two possible ways by which to improve this limitation. A large number of physicians and pharmacists are unable to define case-and-effect relationships for adverse events. In order to resolve this issue, easy-to-use assessment methods (a modified Naranjo scale and modified FDA algorithm) may be useful [39]. These methods enable cause-and-effect relationships for adverse events to be determined. Furthermore, although some physicians and pharmacists reported adverse events to public health centers, public health centers may not report adverse events to the MHLW. Public health centers may receive a large number of reports that include several levels of adverse events. Public health centers review these reports and only report severe adverse events to the MHLW. Therefore, a survey on public health centers is needed in order to clarify the extent to which public health centers receive reports on adverse events and what they report to the MHLW.

Conclusions

Our investigation revealed that a large number of consumers experienced adverse events due to dietary supplement use; however, most of these events were not severe. Although some consumers went to a hospital because of adverse events, physicians and pharmacists were unable to define cause-and-effect relationships for adverse events. Therefore, the reconsideration of a reporting system is needed in order for the MHLW to collect reports on adverse events. It is important that not only patients, but also physicians and pharmacists actively report adverse events to public health centers to decrease and prevent adverse events due to dietary supplement use.

Additional files

Additional file 1: Preliminary Survey for Consumers. (DOCX 15 kb)
Additional file 2: Full Survey for Consumers. (DOCX 15 kb)
Additional file 3: Survey for Physicians and Pharmacists. (DOCX 15 kb)

Abbreviations

DHA: Docosahexaenoic acid; DSHEA: Dietary Supplement Health and Education Act; EPA: Eicosapentaenoic acid; FDA: Food and Drug Administration; MHLW: Ministry of Health, Labour and Welfare; PUFA: Polyunsaturated fatty acid

Acknowledgements

Not applicable.

Funding

This work was supported by a grant from the Japanese Ministry of Health, Labour and Welfare (No. 24220501).

Availability of data and materials

All data generated or analysed during this study are included in this published article [and its supplementary information files].

Authors' contributions

TC, HY, and KU conceived and designed the experiments; TC performed the experiments; TC and YS analyzed the data; TC, EK, KI, and YS checked the data; TC wrote the manuscript. All authors read and approved the final manuscript.

Competing interests

The authors declare that they have no competing interests.

Consent for publication

Not applicable.

Ethics approval and consent to participate

This study was conducted with the approval of the Research Ethics Committee of the National Institutes of Biomedical Innovation, Health and Nutrition (No.198-1, approved on Aug. 28, 2015) and in accordance with Declaration of Helsinki.

Publisher's Note

Springer Nature remains neutral with regard to jurisdictional claims in published maps and institutional affiliations.

Author details

[1]Information Center, National Institute of Health and Nutrition, National Institutes of Biomedical Innovation, Health and Nutrition, 1-23-1 Toyama, Shinjuku-ku, Tokyo 162-8636, Japan. [2]Department of Drug Evaluation & Informatics, Graduate School of Pharmaceutical Sciences, University of Shizuoka, 52-1 Yada, Suruga-ku, Shizuoka 422-8526, Japan.

References

1. Hirayama F, Lee AH, Binns CW, Watanabe F, Ogawa T. Dietary supplementation by older adults in Japan. Asia Pac J Clin Nutr. 2008;17:280–4.
2. Ikuyama S, Imamura-Takase E, Tokunaga S, Oribe M, Nishimura J. Sixty percent of patients with rheumatoid arthritis in Japan have used dietary supplements or health foods. Mod Rheumatol. 2009;19:253–9.
3. Sato Y, Yamagishi A, Hashimoto Y, Virgona N, Hoshiyama Y, Umegaki K. Use of dietary supplements among preschool children in Japan. J Nutr Sci Vitaminol (Tokyo). 2009;55:317–25.
4. Wallace RB, Gryzlak BM, Zimmerman MB, Nisly NL. Application of FDA adverse event report data to the surveillance of dietary botanical supplements. Ann Pharmacother. 2008;42:653–60.
5. Teschke R, Wolff A, Frenzel C, Schulze J, Eickhoff A. Herbal hepatotoxicity: a tabular compilation of reported cases. Liver Int. 2012;32:1543–56.
6. Bjelakovic G, Gluud LL, Nikolova D, Bjelakovic M, Nagorni A, Gluud C. Antioxidant supplements for liver diseases. Cochrane Database Syst Rev. 2011;16:CD007749.
7. Pilkington K, Boshnakova A. Complementary medicine and safety: a systematic investigation of design and reporting of systematic reviews. Complement Ther Med. 2012;20:73–82.
8. Sadovsky R, Collins N, Tighe AP, Brunton SA, Safeer R. Patient use of dietary supplements: a clinician's perspective. Curr Med Res Opin. 2008;24:1209–16.
9. Morris CA, Avorn J. Internet marketing of herbal products. JAMA. 2003;290:1505–9.
10. Cohen PA. American roulette–contaminated dietary supplements. N Engl J Med. 2009;361:1523–5.
11. Cohen PA, Venhuis BJ. Adulterated sexual enhancement supplements: more than mojo. JAMA Intern Med. 2013;173:1169–70.
12. Picciano MF, Dwyer JT, Radimer KL, Wilson DH, Fisher KD, Thomas PR, Yetley EA, Moshfegh AJ, Levy PS, Nielsen SJ, Marriott BM. Dietary supplement use among infants, children, and adolescents in the United States, 1999–2002. Arch Pediatr Adolesc Med. 2007;161:978–85.
13. Geller AI, Shehab N, Weidle NJ, Lovegrove MC, Wolpert BJ, Timbo BB, Mozersky RP, Budnitz DS. Emergency department visits for adverse events related to dietary supplements. N Engl J Med. 2015;373:1531–40.
14. Pitkala KH, Suominen MH, Bell JS, Strandberg TE. Herbal medications and other dietary supplements. A clinical review for physicians caring for older people. Ann Med. 2016;48:586–602.

15. Madabushi R, Frank B, Drewelow B, Derendorf H, Butterweck V. Hyperforin in St. John's wort drug interactions. Eur J Clin Pharmacol. 2006;62:225–33.
16. Izzo AA, Ernst E. Interactions between herbal medicines and prescribed drugs: an updated systematic review. Drugs. 2009;69:1777–98.
17. Shord SS, Shah K, Lukose A. Drug-botanical interactions: a review of the laboratory, animal, and human data for 8 common botanicals. Integr Cancer Ther. 2009;8:208–27.
18. Hermann R, von Richter O. Clinical evidence of herbal drugs as perpetrators of pharmacokinetic drug interactions. Planta Med. 2012;78:1458–77.
19. Yokotani K, Chiba T, Sato Y, Taki Y, Yamada S, Shinozuka K, Murata M, Umegaki K. Hepatic cytochrome P450 mediates interaction between warfarin and Coleus forskohlii extract in vivo and in vitro. J Pharm Pharmacol. 2012;64:1793–801.
20. Muto S, Fujita K, Yamazaki Y, Kamataki T. Inhibition by green tea catechins of metabolic activation of procarcinogens by human cytochrome P450. Mutat Res. 2001;479:197–206.
21. Bamba Y, Yun YS, Kunugi A, Inoue H. Compounds isolated from Curcuma aromatica Salisb. inhibit human P450 enzymes. J Nat Med. 2011;65:583–7.
22. Chiba T, Sato Y, Nakanishi T, Yokotani K, Suzuki S, Umegaki K. Inappropriate usage of dietary supplements in patients by miscommunication with physicians in Japan. Nutrients. 2014;6:5392–404.
23. Chiba T, Sato Y, Suzuki S, Umegaki K. Concomitant use of dietary supplements and medicines in patients due to miscommunication with physicians in Japan. Nutrients. 2015;7:2947–60.
24. Wallace TC. Twenty years of the dietary supplement health and education act–How should dietary supplements be regulated? J Nutr. 2015;145:1683–6.
25. Young AL, Bass IS. The dietary supplement health and education act. Food Drug Law J. 1995;50:285–92.
26. Umegaki K, Yamada H, Chiba T, Nakanishi T, Sato Y, Fukuyama S. Information sources for causality assessment of health problems related to health foods and their usefulness. Shokuhin Eiseigaku Zasshi. 2013;54:282–9.
27. Gardiner P, Sarma DN, Low Dog T, Barrett ML, Chavez ML, Ko R, Mahady GB, Marles RJ, Pellicore LS, Giancaspro GI. The state of dietary supplement adverse event reporting in the United States. Pharmacoepidemiol Drug Saf. 2008;17:962–70.
28. Ashar BH, Rice TN, Sisson SD. Physicians' understanding of the regulation of dietary supplements. Arch Intern Med. 2007;167:966–9.
29. Cellini M, Attipoe S, Seales P, Gray R, Ward A, Stephens M, Deuster PA. Dietary supplements: physician knowledge and adverse event reporting. Med Sci Sports Exerc. 2013;45:23–8.
30. Tarn DM, Paterniti DA, Good JS, Coulter ID, Galliher JM, Kravitz RL, Karlamangla AS, Wenger NS. Physician-patient communication about dietary supplements. Patient Educ Couns. 2013;91:287–94.
31. Wold RS, Lopez ST, Yau CL, Butler LM, Pareo-Tubbeh SL, Waters DL, Garry PJ, Baumgartner RN. Increasing trends in elderly persons' use of nonvitamin, nonmineral dietary supplements and concurrent use of medications. J Am Diet Assoc. 2005;105:54–63.
32. Tallia AF, Cardone DA. Asthma exacerbation associated with glucosamine-chondroitin supplement. J Am Board Fam Pract. 2002;15:481–4.
33. Hayashi F, Takimoto H, Yoshita K, Yoshiike N. Perceived body size and desire for thinness of young Japanese women: a population-based survey. Br J Nutr. 2006;96:1154–62.
34. Bortolotti M, Coccia G, Grossi G, Miglioli M. The treatment of functional dyspepsia with red pepper. Aliment Pharmacol Ther. 2002;16:1075–82.
35. Langmead L, Rampton DS. Review article: herbal treatment in gastrointestinal and liver disease–benefits and dangers. Aliment Pharmacol Ther. 2001;15:1239–52.
36. Sivarajah V, Abdul Q, Pardoe H, Lunniss P. Ulcerative colitis associated with the herbal weight loss supplement Hydroxycut. BMJ Case Rep. 2013;2013:1-3.
37. Haller C, Kearney T, Bent S, Ko R, Benowitz N, Olson K. Dietary supplement adverse events: report of a one-year poison center surveillance project. J Med Toxicol. 2008;4:84–92.
38. Saldanha LG, Dwyer JT, Andrews KW, Bailey RL, Gahche JJ, Hardy CJ, Holden JM, Picciano MF, Roseland JM, Thomas PR, Wolf WR: Online dietary supplement resources. J Am Diet Assoc. 2010;110:1426, 1428, 1430–1.
39. Ide K, Yamada H, Kitagawa M, Kawasaki Y, Buno Y, Matsushita K, Kaji M, Fujimoto K, Waki M, Nakashima M, Umegaki K. Methods for estimating causal relationships of adverse events with dietary supplements. BMJ Open. 2015;5:e009038.

18

Preoperative carbohydrate load and intraoperatively infused omega-3 polyunsaturated fatty acids positively impact nosocomial morbidity after coronary artery bypass grafting: a double-blind controlled randomized trial

Gibran Roder Feguri[1,2,3,8*], Paulo Ruiz Lúcio de Lima[4], Danilo de Cerqueira Borges[2], Laura Ramos Toledo[5], Larissa Nadaf Batista[2], Thaís Carvalho e Silva[2], Neuber José Segri[6] and José Eduardo de Aguilar-Nascimento[7]

Abstract

Background: A strategy of limited preoperative fasting, with carbohydrate (CHO) loading and intraoperative infusion of omega-3 polyunsaturated fatty acids (ω-3 PUFA), has seldom been tried in cardiovascular surgery. Brief fasting, followed by CHO intake 2 h before anesthesia, may improve recovery from CABG procedures and lower perioperative vasoactive drug requirements. Infusion of ω-3 PUFA may reduce occurrences of postoperative atrial fibrillation (POAF) and shorten hospital stays. The aim of this study was to assess morbidity (especially POAF) in ICU patients after coronary artery bypass grafting (CABG)/cardiopulmonary bypass (CPB) in combination, if preoperative fasts are curtailed in favor of CHO loading, and ω-3 PUFA are infused intraoperatively.

Methods: Fifty-seven patients undergoing CABG were randomly assigned to receive 12.5% maltodextrin (200 ml, 2 h before anesthesia), without infusing ω-3 PUFA (CHO, $n = 14$); water (200 ml, 2 h before anesthesia), without infusing ω-3 PUFA (controls, $n = 14$); 12.5% maltodextrin (200 ml, 2 h before anesthesia) plus intraoperative ω-3 PUFA (0.2 mcg/kg) (CHO + W3, $n = 15$); or water (200 ml, 2 h before anesthesia) plus intraoperative ω-3 PUFA (0.2 mcg/kg) (W3, $n = 14$). Perioperative clinical variables and mortality were analyzed, examining the incidence of POAF, as well as the need for inotropic vasoactive drugs during surgery and in ICU.

Results: Two deaths occurred (3.5%), but there were no instances of bronchoaspiration and mediastinitis. Neither ICU stays nor total postoperative stays differed by group ($P > 0.05$). Patients given preoperative CHO loads (CHO and CHO + W3 groups) experienced fewer instances of hospital infection (RR = 0.29, 95%CI 0.09–0.94; $P = 0.023$) and were less reliant on vasoactive amines during surgery (RR = 0.60, 95% CI 0.38–0.94; $P = 0.020$). Similarly, the number of patients requiring vasoactive drugs while recovering in ICU differed significantly by group ($P = 0.008$), showing benefits in patients given CHO loads. The overall incidence of POAF was 29.8% (17/57), differing significantly by group ($P = 0.009$). Groups given ω-3 PUFA (W3 and CHO + W3 groups) experienced significantly fewer instances of POAF (RR = 4.83, 95% CI 1.56–15.02; $P = 0.001$).

(Continued on next page)

* Correspondence: gibranrf@yahoo.com.br
[1]Federal University of Mato Grosso, Cuiabá, Brazil
[2]General University Hospital, Cuiabá, Brazil
Full list of author information is available at the end of the article

(Continued from previous page)

Conclusion: Preoperative curtailment of fasting was safe in this cohort. When implemented in conjunction with CHO loading and infusion of ω-3 PUFA during surgery, expedited recovery from CABG with CPB was observed.

Trial registration: NCT: 03017001

Keywords: Myocardial revascularization, CAGB, Perioperative care, POAF, Fasting, Metabolism

Background

Omega-3 polyunsaturated fatty acids (ω-3 PUFA) are likely involved in proper balance of host immunity postoperatively. Although most studies of nutrients implicated in immunity pertain to abdominal surgery, there is some evidence that ω-3 PUFA is beneficial for patients undergoing cardiac surgery as well [1]. A recent meta-analysis has shown that ω-3 PUFA may reduce the incidence of postoperative atrial fibrillation (POAF) and shorten hospital stays [2, 3].

POAF is among the most common complications after coronary artery bypass grafting (CABG), ranging from 10 to 40% in incidence. Such events are known to impact healthcare costs, morbidity and mortality, postoperative discomfort, and tachycardia, necessitating rhythm reversal and prolonging ICU stays or forcing readmission. Hence, perioperative strategies to minimize occurrences of POAF are of great importance and are constantly under study [4, 5].

On the other hand, an abbreviated period of preoperative fasting with oral intake of carbohydrate (CHO) may offset insulin resistance after surgery and help reduce postoperative nausea and vomiting (PONV) [6]. In cardiac surgery specifically, some randomized trials have shown that CHO loading 2 h before inducing anesthesia will reduce ICU and hospital stays while reducing the need for perioperative vasoactive drug delivery [7, 8].

In our search of the current literature, no studies to date have combined preoperative CHO loading and intraoperative infusion of ω-3 PUFA in cardiac surgery. Presuming that this combination might confer some benefit, this study was conducted to investigate the effects of these two nutrients on morbidity in ICU (POAF primarily) suffered by patients who undergo CABG with cardiopulmonary bypass (CPB).

Methods

This was a double-blind, controlled and randomized trial, examining patients subjected to CABG with CPB at General University Hospital, Cuiabá, Brazil between March, 2014 and June, 2016. The hospital's Ethics Committee granted approval in advance (Protocol No 30493514.5.000.5165; 2014), and a Clinical Trials registration (NCT: 03017001) was obtained.

Patients of both genders (age range, 18–80 years) were included, each medically diagnosed with chronic coronary heart disease and eligible for elective CABG. All patients granted written informed consent. Grounds for exclusion were insulin-dependent diabetes, hepatic or renal disorders, thrombocytopenia, critical dyslipidemia (triglycerides 3-fold greater than established normal), gastroesophageal reflux, acute coronary syndromes, allergy to fish oil, and severe malnutrition. Candidates undergoing off-pump CABG, combined heart procedures, reoperations, or blood transfusion within 3 months prior were also excluded.

Using standard software (QuickCalcs [online]; GraphPad Software Inc, San Diego, CA, USA), subjects were randomly assigned to one of four groups as follows: 1) CHO (8-h fast for solids; 2-h fast plus 200-mL oral intake of 12.5% maltodextrin [25 g] in water; no intraoperative ω-3 PUFA); 2) controls (8-fast for solids; 2-h fast plus 200-mL oral intake of water only; no intraoperative ω-3 PUFA); 3) CHO + W3 (8-h fast for solids; 2-h fast plus 200-mL oral intake of 12.5% maltodextrin [25 g] in water; intraoperative infusion of ω-3 PUFA [0.2 mcg/kg over 4 h]); and 4) W3 (8-fast for solids; 2-h fast plus 200-mL oral intake of water only; intraoperative infusion of ω-3 PUFA [0.2 mcg/kg over 4 h]).

A hospital dietitian, as sole attendant privy to charted randomization, directed preoperative intake. Drinks delivered by ward nurse were given to patients before transport to the operative suite. The anesthesiologist was also informed (by dietician) of which patients would receive intraoperative ω-3 PUFA. None of the surgical team (surgeon or assistants) was aware of patient assignments. A team of cardiologists and intensive care physicians, also blind to study design and patient randomization, collected all data.

Endpoints

Primary study endpoints were incidence of POAF and need of inotropic vasoactive drugs (dobutamine and/or noradrenalin) for weaning from CPB intraoperatively or postoperatively in ICU. As secondary endpoints, perioperative morbidity, hospital mortality, and durations of ICU and total postoperative hospitalization were analyzed.

Anesthesia and surgical technique

The same surgeon (GRF) performed all procedures. Routine anesthetic techniques were used, namely induction via infusion of etomidate (0.2 mg/kg), fentanyl citrate (5 mcg/kg), and pancuronium bromide (0.1 mg/kg). Isoflurane was administered by inhalation route in usual doses (0.6-1.8%) until end of procedure for balanced general anesthesia. As maintenance, another bolus of fentanyl (2 mcg/kg), midazolam (0.1 mg/kg), and pancuronium bromide (0.05 mg/kg) was given, serving for muscle relaxation. All patients were kept under mechanical ventilation, with oxygen (FiO2) at 60% (or higher if needed).

Surgical entry was through median sternotomy, with CPB in the allotted time. The oxygenator used was membrane type (Braile Biomédica, São José do Rio Preto, Brazil). To protect myocardium, we used hypothermic intermittent anterograde blood cardioplegia (every 15–20 min), along with mild systemic hypothermia (33°–35 °C). All patients received intravenous cefuroxime (1.5 g) 1 h before inducing anesthesia, giving another dose after CPB. Maintenance doses (750 mg) were then administered every 6 h for 48 h. A bolus of methyl prednisolone (7 mg/kg) was delivered intravenously at anesthesia induction.

Statistical analysis

The calculation of the sample size was based on the premise that the intervention with W3 + CHO protocol would reduce POAF by 50% versus controls. Assuming a β error (type II) of 20% and a α error (type I) of 5%, sample size calculations indicated 15 patients per group would be sufficient for this study. For values with Gaussian distributions, we used parametric paired (or non-paired) t-tests and analysis of variance for repeated measures, applying nonparametric tests (Friedman, Wilcoxon, and Mann-Whitney) to values with non-Gaussian distributions. Qualitative variables were assessed via chi-square and Fisher's exact tests. Descriptive analyses were undertaken in Microsoft Office Excel 2007 (Microsoft Corp, Redmond, WA, USA), and statistical computations relied on SPSS v17.0 (SPSS Inc, Chicago, IL, USA). All testing was two-tailed at 80% power, with significance set at $P < 0.05$.

Results

A study flowchart is depicted in Fig. 1. Although 96 patients were eligible, 36 were excluded for various reasons. Ultimately, 60 were randomly assigned to the four groups; and after excluding one patient each from groups CHO, W3, and controls, 57 remained for analysis (CHO + W3: $n = 15$; others: $n = 14$, each). Nutritional and demographic data are shown by group in Table 1. In Table 2, clinical data of all groups are presented. All comparisons of the above showed these groups to be homogeneous.

Intraoperative period

No patients suffered bronchial aspiration during intubation or after terminating anesthesia, and no intraoperative deaths occurred. Data from the intraoperative period are shown Table 3. There were no significant differences among the four groups.

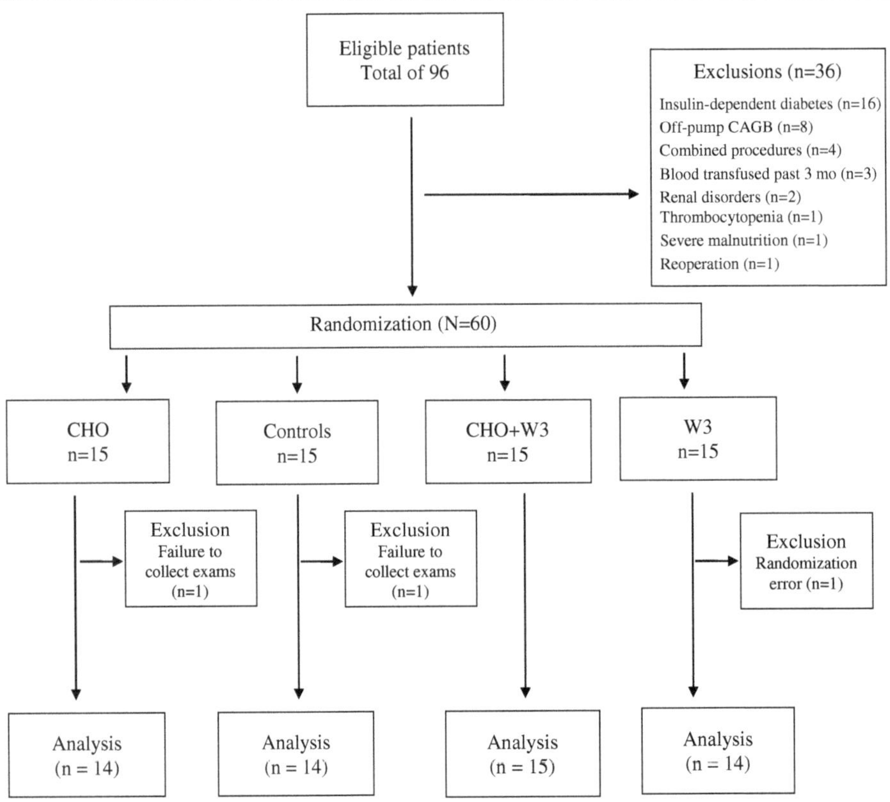

Fig. 1 Flowchart of study design

Table 1 Demographic, nutritional, and clinical data of patient population ($N = 57$) by group

	CHO ($n = 14$)	Control ($n = 14$)	CHO + W3 ($n = 15$)	W3 ($n = 14$)	*P* value
Age (y/o)	60.86 ± 10.55 (63.00)	63.43 ± 8.56 (63.50)	59.93 ± 11.77 (63.00)	62.71 ± 10.90 (65.00)	0.797[a]
Males	12 (86)	10 (71)	7 (47)	9 (64)	0.160[c]
Caucasians	7 (50)	9 (64)	8 (53)	5 (36)	0.380[c]
Body weight (kg)	72.71 ± 12.58 (71,90)	72.82 ± 11.21 (71.20)	65.95 ± 10.69 (66.00)	73.78 ± 18.66 (69.20)	0.513[b]
Height (m)	1.67 ± 0.10 (1.64)	1.63 ± 0.08 (1.62)	1.64 ± 0.07 (1.64)	1.64 ± 0.10 (1.64)	0.663[a]
BMI (kg/m^2)	26.26 ± 3.59 (26.60)	26.49 ± 3.38 (26.30)	25.27 ± 3.48 (25.40)	27.26 ± 5.64 (25.70)	0.911[b]
SGA-A (n; %)	11 (79)	13 (93)	13 (87)	13 (93)	0.617[c]

Data expressed as mean ± SD, median (in parentheses) for continuous variables, or number (%) for categorical variables
BMI body mass index, *SGA* subjective global assessment
[a]One way-ANOVA
[b]Kruskal-Wallis test
[c]Chi-square test

The number of patients needing vasoactive drugs (dobutamine and/or noradrenaline) for weaning from CPB did not differ significantly by group (CHO: 7/14, 50.0%; controls: 12/14, 85.7%; CHO + W3: 6/15, 40.0%; W3: 9/14, 64.3%), although a tendency for control subjects to require such agents was noted ($P = 0.071$). Relative to other group members (W3 and control groups), patients given preoperative CHO loads (CHO and CHO + W3 groups) were less apt to require vasoactive amines (RR = 0.60, 95% CI 0.38–0.94; $P = 0.020$).

Postoperative period

Clinical data from the postoperative period are shown in Table 4. ICU stays did not differ significantly by group ($P = 0.713$). Group means (medians) ± SD were as follows: CHO, 2.86 (2) ± 1.88 days; controls, 3.43 (2) ± 3.16 days; CHO + W3, 2.80 (3) ± 0.94 days; and W3, 3.36 (3) ± 1.55 days. Likewise, total postoperative stays did not differ significantly by group ($P = 0.998$). Group mean ± SD were as follows: CHO, 8.42 ± 7.79 days; controls, 8.07 ± 4.5 days; CHO + W3, 7.00 ± 1.51 days; and W3, 7.50 ± 2.77 days.

The number of patients needing vasoactive drugs (dobutamine and/or noradrenaline) during recovery in ICU did differ significantly by group (CHO, 3/14; 21.4%; controls, 10/14; 71.4%; CHO + W3, 3/15; 20.0%; and W3, 8/14; 57.1%) ($P = 0.008$). Notable differences were evident in both groups given preoperative CHO loads, compared with controls. No other calculations reached significance.

The overall incidence of POAF was 29.8% (17/57). However, rates differed significantly by group ($P = 0.009$). Those given ω-3 PUFA (W3 and CHO + W3 groups)

Table 2 Clinical data and risk factors of patient population ($N = 57$) by group

	CHO ($n = 14$)	Control ($n = 14$)	CHO + W3 ($n = 15$)	W3 ($n = 14$)	*P* value
LVEF	0.55 ± 0.12 (0.60)	0.57 ± 0.11 (0.60)	0.54 ± 0.13 (0.60)	0.62 ± 0.11 (0.65)	0.168[a]
Smoking	6 (43)	9 (64)	7 (47)	8 (57)	0.653[b]
Diabetes	4 (29)	3 (21)	5 (33)	6 (43)	0.666[b]
Dyslipidemia	11 (79)	12 (86)	8 (53)	11 (79)	0.204[b]
Previous AMI	7 (50)	9 (64)	6 (40)	7 (50)	0.631[b]
Beta-blocker use	9 (64)	10 (71)	6 (40)	11 (79)	0.151[b]
Statin use	11 (79)	11 (79)	9 (60)	11 (79)	0.580[b]
Fibrate use	2 (14)	2 (14)	2 (13)	3 (21)	0.930[b]
Previous PCI	1 (7)	4 (29)	4 (27)	3 (21)	0.495[b]

Data expressed as mean ± SD, median (in parentheses) for continuous variables, or number (%) for categorical variables
LVEF left ventricular ejection fraction, *AMI* acute myocardial infarction, *PCI* percutaneous coronary intervention
[a]Kruskal-Wallis test
[b]Chi-square test

Table 3 Intraoperative patient data ($N = 57$) by group

	CHO ($n = 14$)	Control ($n = 14$)	CHO + W3 ($n = 15$)	W3 ($n = 14$)	*P* value
Operative time (min)	244.64 ± 40.31 (240.00)	232.31 ± 49.27 (225.00)	249.29 ± 24.01 (240.00)	253.93 ± 40.86 (270.00)	0.532[a]
Duration of CPB (min)	77.14 ± 20.37 (82.50)	66.64 ± 24.50 (60.00)	63.53 ± 15.63 (66.00)	78.79 ± 22.93 (85.00)	0.147[a]
Duration of AC (min)	63.71 ± 17.29 (66.50)	56.86 ± 28.21 (50.50)	54.20 ± 15.52 (56.00)	61.57 ± 18.58 (68.00)	0.586[a]
Blood components transfused	7 (50)	7 (50)	7 (47)	8 (57)	0.953[b]
Number of grafts	3.00 ± 0.96 (3.00)	2.36 ± 0.93 (2.00)	2.67 ± 0.82 (3.00)	2.86 ± 0.86 (3.00)	0.266[a]
Complications	1 (7)	2 (14)	0 (0)	1 (7)	0.519[b]

Data expressed as mean ± SD, median (in parentheses) for continuous variables, or number (%) for categorical variables
CPB cardiopulmonary bypass, *AC* aortic clamping
[a]One-way ANOVA
[b]Chi-square test

experienced significantly less POAF than controls, and patients given both nutrients (CHO + W3) fared significantly better than those given CHO only ($P = 0.035$). Members of the CHO group did not differ significantly from controls ($P = 0.571$). Only 3 patients (10.3%) in the W3 and CHO + W3 groups developed POAF, compared with 14 (50.0%) in the other two groups (RR = 4.83, 95% CI 1.56–15.02; $P = 0.001$).

Infectious complications and hospital mortality

There were no instances of postoperative mediastinitis. Thirteen patients (22.8%) experienced postoperative infections, specifically pneumonia ($n = 9$; two with sepsis) and wound site infections ($n = 5$). Although differences among groups approached significance ($P = 0.069$), as seen in Table 4, groups given preoperative CHO loads (CHO and CHO + W3 groups) incurred significantly fewer infections than the others (RR = 0.29, 95% CI 0.09–0.94; $P = 0.023$).

Overall, two deaths (3.5%) were recorded, one control subject and a member of the W3 group ($P = 0.543$). These occurred during ICU recovery. The control subject was a woman diagnosed with a stroke in the immediate postoperative period. She progressed to acute renal failure (requiring hemodialysis), sepsis, and then cardiogenic and septic shock. The W3 group member was a man diagnosed with perioperative acute myocardial infarction that led to refractory cardiogenic shock and acute renal failure.

Discussion

In aggregate, these study outcomes indicate that administering preoperative CHO loads and intraoperative ω-3 PUFA is beneficial in the aftermath of CABG. Not only did fewer patients require vasoactive drugs for weaning

Table 4 Clinical data during postoperative patient recovery ($N = 57$) by group

	CHO ($n = 14$)	Control ($n = 14$)	CHO + W3 ($n = 15$)	W3 ($n = 14$)	*P* value
PONV at ICU	3 (21)	4 (29)	2 (13)	5 (36)	0.541[b]
Duration of MV (hours)	10.92 ± 11.12 (8.25)	8.47 ± 2.62 (8.50)	8.96 ± 4.01 (8.67)	8.21 ± 3.57 (7.50)	0.959[a]
Blood loss by12 h PO	353.57 ± 355.43 (300.00)	204.64 ± 99.78 (200.00)	233.33 ± 134.52 (200.00)	278.57 ± 169.52 (225.00)	0.351[a]
Vasoactive drug needed in ICU	3 (21)	10 (71)	3 (20)	8 (57)	0.008[b]
Blood components needed in ICU	6 (43)	5 (36)	3 (20)	3 (21)	0.470[b]
EVA	0 (0)	2 (14)	1 (7)	0 (0)	0.272[b]
AMI	1 (7)	0 (0)	0 (0)	1 (7)	0.557[b]
POAF	6 (43)	8 (57)	1 (7)	2 (14)	0.009[b]
Infectious complications	3 (21)	5 (36)	0 (0)	5 (36)	0.069[b]

Data expressed as mean ± SD, median (in parentheses) for continuous variable, or number (%) for categorical variables
PONV postoperative nausea and vomiting, *MV* mechanical ventilation, *PO* postoperative, *EVA* encephalic vascular accident, *POAF* postoperative atrial fibrillation, *AMI* acute myocardial infarction
[a]Kruskal-Wallis test
[b]Chi-square test

from CPB or during ICU recovery, but also instances of POAF were significantly reduced. Apparently, sparing of vasoactive drugs is a function of oral CHO intake, whereas reduced rates of POAF are attributable to intraoperative infusion of ω-3 PUFA. In addition, groups given CHO-enriched drinks experienced fewer postoperative infections.

These results are in agreement with two previous studies that document speedy recovery and less need of vasoactive drugs, if oral CHO loading is done prior to cardiac surgery [7, 8]. Curtailing of preoperative fasting, with CHO loading, is no longer a novelty approach [9]. This practice of abandoning prolonged fasts is safe and has been endorsed by anesthesiology societies around the world [10, 11]. CHO-enriched drinks may ameliorate postoperative insulin sensitivity, decrease episodes of PONV, and alleviate preoperative sensations of thirst and hunger [6]. In cardiac surgery, there is not much data on the benefits of this particular strategy, so the present findings are especially relevant. As anticipated, there were no instances of bronchial aspiration in the two groups given CHO loads, nor in the groups receiving only water.

The benefits of ω-3 PUFA have been reported for decades in several areas of medicine, but primarily in the realms of cardiology and intensive care. Intravenous ω-3 PUFA is rapidly incorporated by cell membranes [12] and may reduce the production of pro-inflammatory mediators (eg, prostaglandins, thromboxanes, leukotrienes, platelet-activating factor, and cytokines) [13, 14]. Such effects have been credited for reduced hospital stays [15] and lower rates of severe infection [16] in critically ill patients, fewer postoperative complications [17], and possibly lower mortality in acute lung injury [18]. In the field of cardiology, other benefits include declines in morbidity and mortality from congestive heart failure and in sudden death from infarction [19]. The administering of ω-3 PUFA is also linked with better control of dyslipidemia, heart rate, and chronic atrial fibrillation [20, 21]. However, data in the literature are controversial, some studies failing to confirm these benefits [22].

A number of investigations have addressed the benefits of perioperative ω-3 PUFA infusion, or even preoperative oral treatment, in the context of cardiovascular surgery. In a study by Berger et al. [1], two randomly assigned groups were compared, one a placebo (control) group. The other was given infusions of ω-3 PUFA (0.2 g/kg) 12 h and 2 h preoperatively and immediately following surgery. A significant decline in postoperative IL-6 (cytokine) was found in the ω-3 PUFA group, as well as a reduced incidence of arrhythmias, but without significant between-group differences. Our study showed a lower incidence of POAF, as reported in a meta-analysis by Langlois et al. [3]. Their efforts encompassed a systematic review of 19 randomized clinical trials, for a total of 4335 patients undergoing cardiac surgery. Similar to our study, this meta-analysis found no effect of ω-3 PUFA on duration of ICU stays and postoperative mortality rate. However, this meta-analysis showed that infusion of ω-3 PUFA was associated with shorter hospital stays and lower incidence of POAF, especially with use of CPB. The reductions of POAF seen in our patients and in the meta-analysis above perhaps reflect a dampening of inflammatory response in this setting, induced by intraoperative infusion of ω-3 PUFA.

Outcomes of the present study must be interpreted with caution, because of the small number of patients included. Indeed, further studies on this issue are warranted. Nonetheless, we may conclude that perioperative use of these two nutrients seems beneficial for recovery of patients undergoing CABG.

Abbreviations

CABG: Coronary artery bypass grafting; CHO: Carbohydrate; CPB: Cardiopulmonary bypass; ICU: Intensive care unit; POAF: Postoperative atrial fibrillation; PONV: Postoperative nausea and vomiting; ω-3 PUFA: Omega-3 polyunsaturated fatty acids

Acknowledgments

We thank the professionals of BioMed Proofreading LLC for English corrections and copyediting this manuscript.

Funding

CNPq (Conselho Nacional de Desenvolvimento Científico e Tecnológico - "National Counsel of Technological and Scientific Development" of Brazil) has partially funded the study.

Availability of data and materials

The datasets used and/or analysed during the current study available from the corresponding author on reasonable request.

Authors' contributions

GRF conception and design of the study, acquisition of data, drafting the manuscript and agrees to be accountable for all aspects of the work in ensuring that questions related to the accuracy or integrity of any part of the work are appropriately investigated and resolved; PRLL, DCB, TCS & LNB acquisition of data, and given final approval of the version to be published; LRT acquisition of data, randomization of the study, and given final approval of the version to be published; NJS Statistical analysis, and given final approval of the version to be published; JEA-N conception and design of the study, analysis and interpretation of data; drafting the manuscript and given final approval of the version to be published; agrees to be accountable for all aspects of the work in ensuring that questions related to the accuracy or integrity of any part of the work are appropriately investigated and resolved. All authors read and approved the final manuscript.

Competing interests

The authors declare that they have no competing interests.

Consent for publication

"Not applicable".

Ethics approval and consent to participate

The Ethics Committee of the General University Hospital, Cuiabá approved the study design (Protocol No 30493514.5.000.5165; 2014). The trail was registered at Clinical Trials (NCT: 03017001). All subjects have signed a consent form to participate of the study.

Publisher's Note

Author details
[1]Federal University of Mato Grosso, Cuiabá, Brazil. [2]General University Hospital, Cuiabá, Brazil. [3]UNIC - University of Cuiabá, Cuiabá, Brazil. [4]Cardiovascular Department, General University Hospital, Cuiabá, Brazil. [5]Nutrition Service, General University Hospital, Cuiaba, Brazil. [6]Department of Statistics, Federal University of Mato Grosso, Cuiabá, Brazil. [7]Federal University of Mato Grosso and UNIVAG Medical School, Varzea Grande, Brazil. [8]Rua Mal. Floriano Peixoto, 1520/503 – Duque de Caxias II, CEP:78045-395 Cuiabá, Brazil.

References

1. Berger MM, Delodder F, Liaudet L, Tozzi P, Schlaepfer J, Chiolero RL, et al. Three short perioperative infusions of n-3 PUFAs reduce systemic inflammation induced by cardiopulmonary bypass surgery: a randomized controlled trial. Am J Clin Nutr. 2013;97:246e54.
2. Albert CM, Campos H, Stampfer MJ, Ridker PM, Manson JE, Willett WC, et al. Blood levels of long-chain n-3 fatty acids and the risk of sudden death. N Engl J Med. 2002;346:1113–8.
3. Langlois PL, Hardy G, Manzanares W. Omega-3 polyunsaturated fatty acids in cardiac surgery patients: An updated systematic review and meta-analysis. Clin Nutr. 2016(16). doi: 10.1016/j.clnu.2016.05.013. [Epub ahead of print]
4. Yadava M, Hughey AB, Crawford TC. Postoperative Atrial fibrillation: incidence, mechanisms, and clinical correlates. Heart Fail Clin. 2016;12(2):299–308.
5. Perrier S, Meyer N, Hoang Minh T, Announe T, Bentz J, Billaud P, Mommerot A, Mazzucotelli JP, Kindo M. Predictors of Atrial fibrillation after coronary artery bypass grafting: a Bayesian analysis. Ann Thorac Surg. 2017;103(1):92–7. doi:10.1016/j.athoracsur.2016.05.115.
6. Pimenta GP, de Aguilar-Nascimento JE. Prolonged preoperative fasting in elective surgical patients: why should we reduce it? Nutr Clin Pract. 2014; 29(1):22–8.
7. Feguri GR, Lima PR, Lopes AM, Roledo A, Marchese M, Trevisan M, Ahmad H, Freitas BB, Aguilar-Nascimento JE. Clinical and metabolic results of fasting abbreviation with carbohydrates in coronary artery bypass graft surgery. Rev Bras Cir Cardiovasc. 2012;27(1):7–17.
8. Breuer JP, von Dossow V, von Heymann C, Griesbach M, von Schickfus M, Mackh E, Hacker C, Elgeti U, Konertz W, Wernecke KD, Spies CD. Preoperative oral carbohydrate administration to ASA III-IV patients undergoing elective cardiac surgery. Anesth Analg. 2006;103(5):1099–108.
9. Maltby JR. Fasting from midnight – the history behind the dogma. Best Pract Res Clin Anaesthesiol. 2006;20(3):363–78.
10. American Society of Anesthesiologists Committee. Practice guidelines for preoperative fasting and the use of pharmacologic agents to reduce the risk of pulmonary aspiration: application to healthy patients undergoing elective procedures: an updated report by the American society of anesthesiologists committee on standards and practice parameters. Anesthesiology. 2011;114(3):495–511.
11. Smith I, Kranke P, Murat I, Smith A, O'Sullivan G, Søreide E, Spies C, in't Veld B; European Society of Anaesthesiology. Perioperative fasting in adults and children: guidelines from the European Society of Anaesthesiology. Eur J Anaesthesiol. 2011;28(8):556–69.
12. Morlion BJ, Torwesten E, Lessire H, Sturm G, Peskar BM, Furst P, et al. The effect of parenteral fish oil on leukocyte membrane fatty acid composition and leukotriene-synthesizing capacity in patients with postoperative trauma. Metabolism. 1996;45:1208–13.
13. Mayer K, Fegbeutel C, Hattar K, Sibelius U, Kramer HJ, Heuer KU, et al. Omega-3 vs. omega-6 lipid emulsions exert differential influence on neutrophils in septic shock patients: impact on plasma fatty acids and lipid mediator generation. Intensive Care Med. 2003;29:1472–81.
14. Mayer K, Gokorsch S, Fegbeutel C, Hattar K, Rosseau S, Walmrath D, et al. Parenteral nutrition with fish oil modulates cytokine response in patients with sepsis. Am J Respir Crit Care Med. 2003;167:1321–8.
15. Pradelli L, Mayer K, Muscaritoli M, Heller AR. n-3 fatty acid-enriched parenteral nutrition regimens in elective surgical and ICU patients: a meta-analysis. Crit Care. 2012;16(5):R184.
16. Palmer AJ, Ho CK, Ajibola O, Avenell A. The role of ω-3 fatty acid supplemented parenteral nutrition in critical illness in adults: a systematic review and meta-analysis. Crit Care Med. 2013;41(1):307–16.
17. Ma YJ, Liu L, Xiao J, Cao BW. Perioperative ω-3 polyunsaturated fatty acid nutritional support in gastrointestinal cancer surgical patients: a systematic evaluation. Nutr Cancer. 2016;68(4):568–76.
18. Li C, Bo L, Liu W, Lu X, Jin F. Enteral immunomodulatory diet (omega-3 fatty acid, γ-linolenic acid and antioxidant supplementation) for acute lung injury and acute respiratory distress syndrome: an updated systematic review and meta-analysis. Nutrients. 2015;7(7):5572–85.
19. Macchia A, Levantesi G, Franzosi MG, Geraci E, Maggioni AP, Marfisi R, Nicolosi G, Schweiger C, Tavazzi L, Tognoni G, Valagussa F, Marchioli R, GISSI-Prevenzione Investigators. Left ventricular systolic dysfunction, total mortality, and sudden death in patients with myocardial infarction treated with n-3 polyunsaturated fatty acids. Eur J Heart Fail. 2005;7(5):904–9.
20. Mozaffariam D, Geelen A, Brouwer I, Geleijnse JM, Zock PL. Effect of fish Oil on heart rate in humans. A meta-analysis of randomized controlled trials. Circulation. 2005;112:1945–52.
21. Eckel RH, Jakicic JM, Ard JD, de Jesus JM, et al. 2013 AHA/ACC guideline on lifestyle management to reduce cardiovascular risk: a report of the American college of cardiology/American heart association task force on practice guidelines. J Am Coll Cardiol. 2014;63:2960–84. PMID: 24239922.
22. Avanzini F, Franzosi MG, Geraci E, Giansiracusa N, Rocchetti L. Risk and prevention study collaborative group. n-3 fatty acids in patients with multiple cardiovascular risk factors. N Engl J Med. 2013;368(19):1800–8.

Association between maternal intake of n-6 to n-3 fatty acid ratio during pregnancy and infant neurodevelopment at 6 months of age: results of the MOCEH cohort study

Hyejin Kim[1], Hyesook Kim[1], Eunjung Lee[2], Yeni Kim[3], Eun-Hee Ha[4] and Namsoo Chang[1*]

Abstract

Background & aims: Long-chain polyunsaturated fatty acids (LC-PUFAs) are essential for infant neurodevelopment. The nutritional adequacy of dietary LC-PUFAs depends not only on the LC-PUFAs intake but also on the n-6 to n-3 fatty acid ratio (n-6/n-3 PUFAs). This study aimed to identify the association between the maternal dietary n-6/n-3 PUFAs and motor and cognitive development of infants at 6 months of age.

Methods: We used data from 960 participants in the Mothers and Children's Environmental Health (MOCEH) study, which is a multi-center prospective cohort study. Dietary intake of pregnant women was assessed by a one-day 24-h recall method. Food consumption of infants was estimated based on the volume of breast milk and weaning foods. The duration of each feed was used to estimate the likely volume of milk consumed. Dietary intake of infants at 6 months was also assessed by a 24-h recall method. Cognitive and motor development of infants at 6 months of age was assessed by the Korean Bayley scales of infant development edition II (BSID-II) including the mental developmental index (MDI) and the psychomotor developmental index (PDI).

Results: Maternal intakes of n-6/n-3 PUFAs and linoleic acid (LA)-to-α-linolenic acid (ALA) ratio (LA/ALA) were 9.7 ± 6.3 and 11.12 ± 6.9, respectively. Multiple regression analysis, after adjusting for covariates, showed that n-6/n-3 PUFAs was negatively associated with both the MDI ($\beta = -0.1674$, $P = 0.0291$) and PDI ($\beta = -0.1947$, $P = 0.0380$) at 6 months of age. These inverse associations were also observed between LA/ALA and both the MDI and PDI (MDI; $\beta = -0.1567$; $P = 0.0310$, PDI; $\beta = -0.1855$; $P = 0.0367$). Multiple logistic regression analysis, with the covariates, showed that infants whose mother's LA/ALA were ranked in the 2nd, 3rd, and 4th quartile were at approximately twice the risk with more than twice the risk of delayed performance on the PDI compared to the lowest quartile (1st vs. 2nd; OR = 2.965; 95% CI = 1.376 – 6.390, 1st vs. 3rd; OR = 3.047; 95% CI = 1.374 – 6.756 and 1st vs. 4th; OR = 2.551; 95% CI = 1.160 – 5.607).

Conclusions: Both the maternal dietary n-6/n-3 PUFAs and LA/ALA intake were significantly associated with the mental and psychomotor development of infants at 6 months of age. Thus, maintaining low n-6/n-3 PUFAs and LA/ALA is encouraged for women during pregnancy.

Keywords: Bayley scales of infant development, Infants, Linoleic acid-to-α-linolenic acid ratio, Long-chain polyunsaturated fatty acids, Psychomotor development

* Correspondence: nschang@ewha.ac.kr
[1]Department of Nutritional Science and Food Management, Ewha Womans University, Seoul, South Korea
Full list of author information is available at the end of the article

Background

Long-chain polyunsaturated fatty acids (LC-PUFAs) including docosahexaenoic acid (DHA; 22:6n-3) and arachidonic acid (AA; 20:4n-6), are precursors of signaling molecules and are also essential for motor and cognitive development [1–3]. The supply of LC-PUFAs, through the maternal diet, supports maturation of the fetal brain and could enhance neurodevelopment. Neurodevelopment occurs predominantly during the last trimester of pregnancy when brain growth is most rapid and the LC-PUFAs continue to accumulate during the first 2 years after birth [2]. Earlier cohort studies have consistently reported that the maternal LC-PUFAs status can influence the cognitive and psychomotor development of infants [4–9].

It is well-established that both the intake of LC-PUFAs and the n-6-to-n-3 fatty acid ratio (n-6/n-3) are important contributing factors to nutritional adequacy of LC-PUFAs. Both linoleic acid (LA; 18:2n-6) and α-linolenic acid (ALA; 18:3n-3) are known to compete for the same desaturase enzymes in the biosynthetic pathways to AA and DHA, respectively [10]. It is generally agreed that high LA intakes result in a low n-3 fatty acid status [2]. The recommended dietary n-6/n-3 PUFAs ranges from 5:1–15:1 in Europe and from 4:1–10:1 in the United States and South Korea [11, 12].

There is some evidence that the n-6/n-3 PUFAs is associated with neurodevelopment in infants and in the child's subsequent cognitive development. Cohort studies in Seychelles [4] and France [9], reported that maternal n-6/n-3 PUFAs, in serum and in colostrum, respectively, were negatively associated with the Bayley scales of infant development edition II (BSID-II) at 9 months of age and with the ages and stages questionnaire (ASQ) at 3 years of age, respectively. A recent cohort study in the Netherlands reported that higher maternal DHA and n-3/n-6 PUFAs were associated with fewer emotional problems in children at 6 years [7]. Recent experimental studies suggested that an imbalance in the maternal n-6/n-3 PUFAs and ratio of LA-to-ALA (LA/ALA), induced impaired neocortical neurogenesis in offspring and anxiety-related behavior in adulthood [13, 14].

However, to our knowledge, no studies have evaluated the association between both maternal intake of LC-PUFAs and n-6/n-3 PUFAs and child development in the Asian population that traditionally consume considerable amounts of fish and seaweeds [15] and, hence, have a different n-6 and n-3 fatty acid intake than the Western population. Therefore, the present study aimed to determine the association between dietary intake of LC-PUFAs and their ratios in pregnant Korean women with their infants' neurodevelopment at 6 months of age.

Methods

Study design and participants

This research was conducted as part of the Mothers' and Children's Environmental Health (MOCEH) study, which is a community-based prospective birth cohort study that was established in 2006. This study was performed in three urban centers in the Republic of Korea including Seoul (metropolitan area), Ulsan (industrial area), and Cheonan (urban area). The study was approved by the three institutional review Boards at Ewha Womans University School of Medicine, Dankook University Hospital, and Ulsan University Hospital, respectively. Informed consent for participation was obtained from all participants. Details of the MOCEH study are described elsewhere, in a comprehensive review [16].

The study including recruitment to follow-up occurred between August 2006 and October 2011. The participants were followed up from delivery though the age of 5 years. Initially, the study population comprised 1751 women, who were enrolled in the MOCEH study. Of these, we excluded 31 women who were pregnant with twins, 23 who had undergone spontaneous abortions, 12 with congenital anomalies, three with intra-uterine growth retardation, and 39 with pregnancy complications (hypertension and/or diabetes). From the remaining 1643 pregnant women, we excluded 189, whose dietary intake data were not collected and seven who had a total energy consumption of <500 or >5000 kcal/day. We also excluded 448 participants, whose infants' neurodevelopment data at 6 months of age were not assessed, and 39 whose n-6/n-3 PUFAs data could not be calculated because the intake data of either the n-6 or n-3 fatty acids was not available. Therefore, 960 subjects were finally included in our analysis.

Using a structured questionnaire, trained personnel interviewed the participants to obtain sociodemographic data, such as pre-pregnancy weight (kg), height (m), family income (<USD $2000, USD $2000 – 4000, and ≥ USD $4000) and education (≤high school, ≤university, and ≤ graduate school), as well as information on health-related behaviors, such as secondhand exposure to cigarette smoke (yes/no). Pre-pregnancy BMI was calculated as weight (kg) divided by the square of height (m), using self-reported height and weight information. Data collected on pregnancy outcomes from medical records included gestational age (d), birth length (cm), and birth weight (g) of the infant. Gestational age at delivery was inferred from the last menstrual period and was also estimated by ultrasonography. Breastfeeding status at 6 months (breastfeeding, formula feeding, and combined breast and formula feeding) was collected from self-reported questionnaires at each study center.

Dietary assessment

Maternal dietary intake data during pregnancy was obtained from participants by a well-trained dietary interviewer using a 24-h recall method on the day before a blood test was administered, which occurred within 20 weeks of gestational age. Information on self-reported supplement use was collected by asking participants to list the type (vitamins, minerals, and others) and brand name of their supplements, as well as the amount and frequency of use. A fatty acids database was constructed, based on the Can-Pro 4·0 database, by incorporating the values from the United States Department of Agriculture (USDA) [17] and Korea National Fisheries Research and Development Institute [18]. We covered about 93% of the total fatty acids intake of the 24-h recall method of the subjects.

For further analysis, we defined variables for total maternal dietary intake of n-6 and n-3 fatty acids, which consisted of the sum of LA, eicosadienoic acid (20:2n-6), dihomo-γ-linolenic acid (DGLA; 20:3n-6), AA and docosapentaenoic acid (DPA n-6; 22:5n-6), for the total amount of n-6 fatty acids, and ALA, eicosatetraenoic acid (ETA; 20:4n-3), eicosapentaenoic acid (EPA; 20:5n-3), DPA n-3 (22:5n-3) and DHA, for the total amount of n-3 fatty acids. The n-6/n-3 PUFAs was calculated as the total intake of n-6 fatty acids divided by the total intake of n-3 fatty acids, and the LA/ALA was calculated as the dietary LA intake divided by the ALA intake.

Food consumption of infants at 6 months was estimated based on the volume of breast milk and weaning foods. With respect to breast milk, the duration of each feed was used to estimate the likely volume of milk consumed, based on previously validated assumptions [19]. A baseline of 100 mL was estimated for a feed lasting ≥10 min, when infants had fed only on one side; whereas, infants who had fed on both sides for ≥10 min, were assumed to have consumed 200 mL of breast milk. Infants' dietary intake data at 6 months was obtained from each mother via person-to-person interviews conducted by a well-trained dietitian using the 24-h recall method. Questionnaires were formulated regarding breastfeeding duration and timing, and formula feeding, which included the types and volumes of infant formula. Dietary intake of specific food groups and nutrients was analyzed using a computerized nutrient intake assessment software program (CAN-Pro 4.0; Korean Nutrition Society, Seoul, Korea).

Biological profiles

Blood mercury analysis in the umbilical cord samples was performed by flow injection cold vapor atomic absorption spectrometry (DMA-80, Milestone, Bergamo, Italy). The sample was initially dried in an oxygen stream passed through a quartz tube located inside a controlled heating coil. The combustion gasses were further decomposed on a catalytic column at 750 °C. Mercury vapor was collected in a gold amalgamation trap and then desorbed for quantification. The laboratory analyses were carried out using standardized quality-control procedures. Details regarding the blood mercury analysis are described elsewhere [20]. Maternal urine samples were stored frozen at −20 °C until they could be delivered to a laboratory for analysis. The urinary cotinine level was measured by high-performance liquid chromatography (HPLC)-isotope dilution tandem mass spectrometry (MS/MS) (Agilent 6410 triple Quad LCMS, Agilent Technologies, Santa Clara, CA, USA). The data were adjusted relative to the urinary creatinine level to correct for urine volume.

Assessment of infant neurodevelopment

Infant neurodevelopment was assessed at 6 months of age using the Korean version of the BSID-II [21], which is a standardized tool to assess toddler and infant development [22]. The BSID-II was conducted in a quiet room by trained examiners for 30–45 min. Each test produced developmental indices, which were expressed as an infant's mental developmental index (MDI) and psychomotor developmental index (PDI), respectively. The MDI consisted of developmental tasks to test object constancy, memory, learning, problem-solving, early verbal communication, and early abstract thinking ability. The PDI consisted of developmental tasks that gauged body control, such as fine and gross motor skills, as an indicator of an infant's psychomotor capabilities. Each index could be standardized with a mean of 100 and a standard deviation of 15, for a composite score that compared the child's develop mental performance with the norms for typically developing Korean children of the same age.

The MDI and PDI scores could be classified into four groups including 'significantly delayed performance,' 'mildly delayed performance,' 'within normal limits,' and 'accelerated performance' [22]. A standard score of ≤70, which was two standard deviations below the mean, was considered abnormal. BSID-II training was coordinated by a specialist before beginning assessments at each center. Inter-rater reliability ($\kappa > 0.8$) was confirmed annually through rater training sessions and video monitoring of the examination process. All test procedures and interpretations of results were conducted according to "The Standards for Educational and Psychological Testing", as recommended by the American Educational Research Association. Each measurement was double-checked and confirmed through feedback between the examiner and central coordinator.

Statistical analysis

Demographic and socioeconomic characteristics were expressed as numbers and percentages (categorical variables), or as means and standard deviations (continuous variables). Multivariable regression models were constructed to examine the association between either maternal fatty acid intake amounts or ratios and infants' neurodevelopment indices from the BSID-II at 6 months of age, after controlling for covariates such as maternal age (y), pre-pregnancy BMI (kg/m^2), log-transformed urinary cotinine level (μ mol/mol creatinine), residential area (Seoul, Cheonan, and Ulsan), maternal education level (≤high school, ≤university, and ≥ graduate school), use of supplements (yes/no), log-transformed maternal energy intake (kcal), gestational age (d), infant gender, breastfeeding status at 6 months of age (breastfeeding, formula feeding, and combined breast and formula feeding), log-transformed infantile PUFAs intake (g/day), and log-transformed cord blood mercury level (μ g/L). The maternal n-6/n-3 PUFAs and LA/ALA were divided into quartiles. Differences between the MDI and PDI scores, according to the dietary n-6/n-3 PUFAs and LA/ALA, were observed by dividing the MDI and PDI scores into two groups. The cut-off point for each was a score <85, which was considered significant and mildly delayed performance [22]. We also used a multivariable logistic regression analysis adjusting for confounders, to identify the odds ratios (ORs) and 95% confidence intervals (CIs) for delayed performance on the MDI and PDI (each score <85), depending on the quartiles of dietary n-6/n-3 PUFAs and LA/ALA. Statistical analyses were performed using the SAS statistical package (SAS 9.4; SAS Institute, Cary, NC, USA). Differences were considered significant at <5%.

Results

General characteristics

The participants were on average 30.1 ± 3.5 years old with a pre-pregnancy BMI of 21.3 ± 3.2 kg/m^2 (Table 1). Approximately 72% of the subjects had a university degree or higher education, and 86% of them were secondhand smokers. Gestational age at delivery was 274.9 ± 10.1 day, and birth length and weight were 50.5 ± 2.5 cm and 3268.6 ± 424.7 g, respectively. Neurodevelopmental MDI and PDI scores were 96.2 ± 11.9 and 96.0 ± 14.7, respectively.

Table 1 General characteristics of pregnant women and their babies

Characteristics	*n*	Mean ± S.D. or *n* (%)
Pregnant women		
Age, yrs	959	30.1 ± 3.5
Pre-pregnancy weight, kg	950	55.4 ± 8.9
Pre-pregnancy BMI, kg/m^2	943	21.3 ± 3.2
Residential area	960	
Seoul		223 (23.2)
Cheonan		298 (31.1)
Ulsan		439 (45.7)
Family income, US$/month	925	
<2000		250 (27.0)
2000-4000		512 (55.4)
>4000		163 (17.6)
Education	941	
≤High school		265 (28.1)
≤University		186 (19.8)
≥Graduate school		491 (52.2)
Nutritional supplements, yes	960	410 (42.7)
Secondhand smokers, yes	898	772 (86.0)
Urinary cotinine levels, μ mol/mol creatinine	905	17.4 ± 152.1
Babies		
Gestational age, d	939	274.9 ± 10.1
Birth length, cm	920	50.5 ± 2.5
Birth weight, g	959	3268.6 ± 424.7
Gender, girls	955	458 (48.0)
Umbilical cord blood mercury, μ g/L	746	5.9 ± 3.7
Breastfeeding status, yes	860	559 (65.0)
BSID-II	960	
MDI		96.2 ± 11.9
PDI		96.0 ± 14.7

S.D. standard deviation *BSID-II* Bayley Scales of Infant Development II *MDI* mental development index *PDI* psychomotor development index

Nutrient intake of pregnant women and infants

Average total daily energy intake during pregnancy was 1789.5 ± 493.7 kcal/day (Table 2). The n-6/n-3 PUFAs and LA/ALA were 9.7 ± 6.3 and 11.1 ± 6.4, respectively. On average, the study subjects consumed 10.1 ± 6.2 g of n-6 PUFAs, 9.8 ± 6.1 g of LA, and 0.1 ± 0.1 g of AA. The daily average n-3 PUFAs consumed was 1.5 ± 1.4 g, and ALA, EPA, and DHA were 1.0 ± 0.8 g, 0.1 ± 0.3 g, and 0.3 ± 0.8 g, respectively. The PUFA intake of infants at 6 months of age was 5.2 ± 1.7 g/day.

Relationship between maternal dietary fatty acid ratio and infant motor and cognitive development

We found negative correlations between maternal seaweed intake during pregnancy and the PDI of infants at 6 months ($r = -0.0946$, $P = 0.0297$), although no correlation was shown between dietary maternal fish intake and the BSID-II of the study subjects (data not shown). As shown in Table 3, neither dietary n-6 nor n-3 fatty acid intake was associated with neurobehavioral indices in a multiple regression analysis, after adjusting for maternal age, pre-pregnancy BMI, urinary cotinine level, residential area, maternal education level, use of supplements, maternal energy intake, gestational age, infant gender, breastfeeding status, infantile PUFA intake, and cord blood mercury level. There were also no associations between LA and ALA, respectively, with the neurobehavioral indices. However, negative associations were found between maternal dietary n-6/n-3 PUFAs and the MDI ($P = 0.0291$), between

Table 2 Daily nutrient intake of pregnant women and infants

Nutrient intake	*n*	Mean ± S.D.	Range
Pregnant women			
Energy, kcal/day	960	1789.5 ± 493.7	611.2 - 3935.1
Carbohydrate, g/d	960	280.6 ± 81.1	74.7 - 617.1
Protein, g/d	960	69.3 ± 25.1	21.5 -211.2
Lipid	960	46.7 ± 24.0	3.7 - 181.0
n-6 PUFAs, g/d	960	10.1 ± 6.2	0.03 - 47.57
LA		9.8 ± 6.1	0.03 -47.2
AA		0.1 ± 0.1	0 -0.8
n-3 PUFAs, g/d	960	1.5 ± 1.4	0.04 -11.74
ALA		1.0 ± 0.8	0.01 - 8.0
EPA		0.1 ± 0.3	0 -3.4
DHA		0.3 ± 0.8	0 -9.8
n-6/n-3 PUFAs	960	9.7 ± 6.3	0.1 -108.2
LA/ALA	960	11.12 ± 6.9	0.1 -108.2
Infants at 6 months of age	734		
Energy, kcal/d		604.4 ± 157.6	179.5 - 1259.5
Carbohydrate, g/d		73.9 ± 19.3	21.1 -161.7
Protein, g/d		17.5 ± 8.3	3.3 -53.0
Lipid, g/d		26.9 ± 7.6	6.5 - 51.2
PUFAs, g/d		5.2 ± 1.7	1.05 -10.58

S. D. standard deviation *PUFAs* polyunsaturated fatty acids *LA* linoleic acid *AA* arachidonic acid *ALA* α-linolenic acid, *EPA* eicosapentanoic acid; *DHA* docosahexaenoic acid *LA* (18:2n-6) eicosadienoic acid (20:2n-6), dihomo-γ-linolenic acid 28 (DGLA; 20:3n-6), *AA* (20:4n-6) and docosapentaenoic acid (DPA n-6; 22:5n-6) for the total amount of n-6 fatty acid; and *ALA* (18:3n-3), eicosatetraenoic acid (ETA; 20:4n-3), *EPA* (20:5n 3), DPA n 3 (22:5n 3) and *DHA* (22:5n-3) for the total amount of n-3 fatty acid

LA/ALA and the MDI ($P = 0.0310$), between n-6/n-3 PUFAs and the PDI ($P = 0.0380$) and between LA/ALA and the PDI ($P = 0.0367$), at 6 months of age.

Table 4 shows the results of a logistic regression analysis with the covariates, which indicates the ORs of delayed performance on the MDI and PDI (each score <85) for each n-6/n-3 PUFAs and LA/ALA quartile. There were some infants, whose mother's n-6/n-3 PUFAs and LA/ALA were ranked in the highest quartiles, who were at a respective 2.156 and 2.284 times greater risk of delayed performance on the MDI compared to the lowest quartiles (n-6/n-3 PUFAs; OR = 2.156; 95% CI = 1.025 – 4.535, LA/ALA; OR = 2.284; 95% CI = 1.042 – 5.009). Furthermore, infants whose maternal LA/ALA were ranked in the 2nd, 3rd, and 4th quartile were more than twice at risk of delayed performance on the PDI compared to the lowest quartile (1st vs. 2nd; OR = 2.965; 95% CI = 1.376 – 6.390, 1st vs. 3rd; OR = 3.047; 95% CI = 1.374 – 6.756 and 1st vs. 4th; OR = 2.551; 95% CI = 1.160 – 5.607). The number of infants with delayed performance tended to increase with increasing maternal n-6/n-3 PUFAs and LA/ALA.

Discussion

We found that both the maternal dietary n-6/n-3 PUFAs and LA/ALA during pregnancy were negatively associated with both the MDI and PDI at 6 months of age, but maternal intakes of total n-6, n-3, LA, and ALA were not associated with these development parameters. These results indicate that an adequate and balanced intake of n-6 and n-3 PUFAs, or LA and ALA, from a well-balanced diet, may be more important than the intake of these individual fatty acids, for optimal infant's neurodevelopment.

Several cohort studies reported a negative relation between maternal n-6/n-3 PUFAs status and infant and child neurodevelopment assessed by various tests [4, 7–9] and these reports partly confirmed our results. The Seychelles Child Development Nutrition Study (SCDS) [4] reported that maternal n-6/n-3 PUFAs in serum was negatively associated with the BSID-II PDI at 9 months of age but not at 30 months. The EDEN mother-child cohort in France showed that maternal dietary n-6/n-3 PUFAs intakes among never-breastfed children were negatively associated with the MacArthur Communicative Development Inventory (CDI) at 2 years of age and with the ASQ at 3 years of age [8], while the n-6/n-3 PUFAs in colostrum among breastfed children was negatively associated with the ASQ at 3 years of age [9]. Recently, the Generation R study in the Netherlands [7] demonstrated that a higher maternal plasma n-3/n-6 PUFAs was associated with fewer emotional problems in children at 6 years of age.

In the present study, no association was observed between dietary n-6 or n-3 fatty acid intakes and the MDI and PDI at 6 months of age. Similarly, Bernard et al. [8] found no association between n-3 fatty acid intake and the CDI in infants at 2 years of age and the ASQ at 3 years of age. In contrast, however, other researchers found a positive association between n-3 fatty acids in maternal serum and the PDI in infants aged 9 months [4] and a negative association between n-6 fatty acids in colostrum and the ASQ in infants at 3 years of age [9]. These disparities may be explained by the differences in assessing the fatty acid intake, in infant age at assessment and in the composition of total n-3 fatty acids (ALA, ETA, EPA, DPA, and DHA vs. ALA, EPA, and DHA), as well as potential confounders in the analysis.

PUFAs play pivotal roles in infant neurodevelopment [5, 6]. In particular, LA and ALA are regarded as nutritionally essential fatty acids because they cannot be synthesized *de novo* from macronutrients [3] and can also convert into AA and DHA, respectively [23]. LC-PUFAs, such as AA and DHA, accumulate in large amounts in the membrane phospholipids of the developing central nervous system [23]. As precursors of prostaglandins and other eicosanoids, AA and DHA play important

Table 3 Associations of maternal fatty acid intakes during pregnancy with infant neurodevelopment indices of the BSID-IIat 6 months of age

	MDI				PDI			
	n	*β*	(SE)	*P*-value	*n*	*β*	(SE)	*P*-value
n-6 PUFAs, g/d								
Model 1	960	−0.0804	(0.0621)	0.1959	960	−0.0841	(0.0769)	0.2749
Model 2	669	−0.0969	(0.0698)	0.1659	669	−0.0932	(0.0857)	0.2771
Model 3	520	−0.1299	(0.0826)	0.1165	520	−0.1611	(0.1011)	0.1116
n-3 PUFAs, g/d								
Model 1	960	0.1142	(0.2680)	0.6702	960	0.0781	(0.3317)	0.8140
Model 2	669	0.1731	(0.2961)	0.5590	669	0.2856	(0.3629)	0.4317
Model 3	520	0.1145	(0.3277)	0.7270	520	0.1701	(0.4007)	0.6714
n-6/n-3 PUFAs								
Model 1	960	−0.1354	(0.0612)	0.0271	960	−0.1840	(0.0757)	0.0152
Model 2	669	−0.1465	(0.0704)	0.0378	669	−0.2097	(0.0862)	0.0152
Model 3	520	−0.1674	(0.0765)	0.0291	520	−0.1947	(0.0936)	0.0380
LA, g/d								
Model 1	960	−0.0813	(0.0633)	0.1989	960	−0.0821	(0.0783)	0.2950
Model 2	669	−0.0991	(0.0711)	0.1642	669	−0.0920	(0.0873)	0.2924
Model 3	520	−0.1342	(0.0844)	0.1123	520	−0.1609	(0.1032)	0.1196
ALA, g/d								
Model 1	960	−0.2199	(0.4868)	0.6515	960	−0.4254	(0.6025)	0.4803
Model 2	669	−0.2555	(0.5237)	0.6258	669	−0.3763	(0.6421)	0.5581
Model 3	520	−0.3686	(0.5762)	0.5227	520	−0.7018	(0.7044)	0.3195
LA/ALA								
Model 1	960	−0.1240	(0.0601)	0.0395	960	−0.1839	(0.0744)	0.0135
Model 2	669	−0.1306	(0.0667)	0.0507	669	−0.1828	(0.0817)	0.0256
Model 3	520	−0.1567	(0.0724)	0.0310	520	−0.1855	(0.0886)	0.0367

BSID-II Bayley Scales of Infant Development II *MDI* mental development index *PDI* psychomotor development index *PUFAs* polyunsaturated fatty acids *LA* linoleic acid *AA* arachidonic acid *ALA* α-linolenic acid *EPA* eicosapentanoic acid *DHA* docosahexaenoic acid *LA* (18:2n-6) eicosadienoic acid (20:2n-6), dihomo-γ-linolenic acid (DGLA; 20:3n-6), *AA* (20:4n-6) and docosapentaenoic acid (DPA n-6; 22:5n-6) for the total amount of n-6 fatty acid; and *ALA* (18:3n-3), eicosatetraenoic acid (ETA; 20:4n-3) *EPA* (20:5n-3), *DPA* n-3 (22:5n-3) and *DHA* (22:5n-3) for the total amount of n-3 fatty acid
Model 1: Unadjusted
Model 2: Adjusted for maternal age, pre-pregnancy BMI, urinary cotinine level (log-transformed), residential area, maternal education level, use of supplements, maternal energy intake (log-transformed), gestational age, infant gender, breastfeeding status and infantile polyunsaturated fatty acid intake (log-transformed)
Model 3: Additionally adjusted for cord blood mercury level (log-transformed)

roles in regulating normal brain function [3]. Furthermore, AA can be released from the cell membrane and influence structural changes in the membrane, which affects the neuronal membrane fluidity [24]. Moreover, modifying the fatty acid composition of the brain phospholipids may influence membrane activity-bound enzymes or the number and affinity of receptors, which can directly or indirectly affect neurotransmission by influencing changes in second messenger systems, such as the eicosanoids [24]. An appropriate balance of these pathways is essential for normal brain development, whereas, an imbalance leads to impairments in neurogenesis [13].

Recent experimental studies reported that maternal n-6/n-3 PUFAs and LA/ALA imbalances induced impaired neocortical neurogenesis in offspring and anxiety-related behavior in adulthood [13, 14]. Sakayori et al. [13] reported pregnant mice fed a high n-6/n-3 PUFAs (i.e., 11.8 and 0.3% energy in the form of LA and ALA, respectively) had offspring with impaired neuronal layer formation and altered embryonic brain compared to those fed a low dietary n-6/n-3 PUFAs (i.e., 3.1 and 1.2% energy in the form of LA and ALA, respectively), as shown in a previous study [25]. More recently, Sakayori et al. [14] found that exposure to an LA/ALA imbalance during brain development resulted in offspring with enhanced anxiety during adulthood. Pregnant mice fed a higher LA/ALA (i.e., LA, 74.3% of total lipids; ALA, 0.3% of total lipids) had offspring with affected locomotor activity and anxiety-related behavior,

Table 4 Odds ratio (OR) and 95% confidence intervals (CIs) for neurodevelopment indices of BSID-II (each score below 85[a]) according to maternal fatty acids ratio

	Range	MDI				PDI			
		No. of delayed performance	OR (95% CI)			No. of delayed performance	OR (95% CI)		
			Model 1	Model 2	Model 3		Model 1	Model 2	Model 3
n-6/n-3 PUFAs									
Quartile 1	0.13-7.00	31 (12.9)[b]	1 (ref)	1 (ref)	1 (ref)	40 (16.7)	1 (ref)	1 (ref)	1 (ref)
Quartile 2	7.01-9.04	32 (13.3)	1.037 (0.611-1.762)	1.000 (0.507-1.975)	1.067 (0.477-2.384)	48 (20.0)	1.250 (0.786-1.988)	1.114 (0.619-2.002)	1.489 (0.735-3.014)
Quartile 3	9.05-11.66	35 (14.6)	1.151 (0.684-1.937)	1.468 (0.756-2.843)	1.769 (0.819-3.823)	48 (20.0)	1.250 (0.786-1.988)	1.484 (0.830-2.654)	1.819 (0.907-3.649)
Quartile 4	11.68-108.24	40 (16.7)	1.348 (0.812-2.240)	1.538 (0.806-2.936)	2.156 (1.025-4.535)	53 (22.1)	1.417 (0.898-2.237)	1.339 (0.752-2.385)	1.651 (0.820-3.321)
LA/ALA									
Quartile 1	0.13-8.20	25 (10.4)	1 (ref)	1 (ref)	1 (ref)	36 (15.0)	1(ref)	1 (ref)	1 (ref)
Quartile 2	8.21-9.69	35 (14.6)	1.468 (0.849-2.539)	1.620 (0.814-3.227)	1.507 (0.667-3.408)	52 (21.7)	1.567 (0.980-2.504)	2.111 (1.154-3.862)	2.965 (1.376-6.390)
Quartile 3	9.70-12.47	41 (17.1)	1.772 (1.039-3.021)	1.808 (0.901-3.626)	1.958 (0.867-4.423)	50 (20.8)	1.491 (0.930-2.389)	1.909 (1.016-3.588)	3.047 (1.374-6.756)
Quartile 4	12.48-108.24	37 (15.4)	1.567 (0.911-2.696)	1.707 (0.858-3.393)	2.284 (1.042-5.009)	51 (21.3)	1.529 (0.955-2.446)	1.770 (0.954-3.285)	2.551 (1.160-5.607)

BSID-II Bayley Scales of Infant Development II *MDI* mental development index *PDI* psychomotor development index *PUFAs* polyunsaturated fatty acids, *LA* linoleic acid *AA* arachidonic acid *ALA* α-linolenic acid, *EPA* eicosapentanoic acid *DHA* docosahexaenoic acid

[a]MDI and PDI can be categorized into four groups such as 'significantly delayed performance (below 70)', 'mildly delayed performance (70–84)', 'within normal limits (85–114)', and 'accelerated performance (above 114)'

[b]Values are expressed as frequency (%)

Model 1: Unadjusted

Model 2: Adjusted for maternal age, pre-pregnancy BMI, urinary cotinine level (log-transformed), residential area, maternal education level, use of supplements, maternal energy intake (log-transformed), gestational age, infant gender, breastfeeding status and infantile polyunsaturated fatty acid intake (log-transformed)

Model 3: Additionally adjusted for cord blood mercury level (log-transformed)

as measured by an open field test, compared to offspring of the mice fed a lower LA/ALA diet (i.e., LA, 20.7% of total lipids; ALA, 9.4% of total lipids). Moreover, there is experimental evidence that diets containing a high LA level inhibit n-3 fatty acid synthesis and incorporation of LC-PUFAs into tissue and blood lipids [26, 27]. When combined with our results that dietary LA/ALA during pregnancy is associated with a higher risk of delayed performance on both the MDI and PDI at 6 months of age, the results suggests that in early life, exposure to an LA/ALA imbalance, through an excessively high LA level in the maternal diet during pregnancy, may have adverse effects on infant's psychomotor and mental development. Although this finding needs replication later in childhood and in other large cohorts, it supports the current nutritional consensus that a balanced intake of n-6 and n-3 fatty acids has important health benefits, particularly during pregnancy.

Other cohort studies from England, Spain, and Japan showed that maternal seafood and fish consumption as a proxy for LC-PUFAs was associated with neuropsychological test scores in children [5, 6, 28, 29]. The dietary n-3 LC-PUFAs including ALA, are found mainly in marine products like seaweed and fish. Even though mercury is known to be a toxicant that can cause pregnant women, as well as their children, adverse health outcomes [30], an observational study showed that maternal fish consumption, as a proxy for LC-PUFAs intake, was associated with improved child neurodevelopment [31]. Our data showed that the associations between both n-6/n-3 PUFAs and the MDI and PDI, and between LA/ALA and the MDI and PDI, were still observed when umbilical cord blood mercury level was additionally included in the statistical model (model 3). Therefore, we may infer that maternal LC-PUFA intake might alleviate possible adverse effects of mercury on neurodevelopment in infants, although the exact mechanism remains unknown.

The Asian population including South Koreans, traditionally consume considerable amounts of fish and seaweeds [15], and, hence, have a different n-6 and n-3 fatty acid intake than the Western population. In our study, the mean EPA and DHA intake was higher than that reported in other countries like Australia (EPA; 0.056 g/day, DHA; 0.106 g/day) [32], Japan (EPA; 0.042 g/day, DHA; 0.064 g/day) [33], the United States (EPA; 0.049 g/day, DHA; 0.080 g/day) [34], and Costa Rica (EPA; 0.032 g/day, DHA; 0.050 g/day) [35]. The mean dietary n-6/n-3 PUFAs was 9.7 in our subjects, which was lower than that reported in Mexico (12.3) [36], India (27.5) [37], and the coastal area of Southeastern China (17.8) [38], but higher than that of pregnant women in France (approximately 8.4) [9], and those living in a river/lake (5.8) or in an inland (9.1) area of Southeastern China [38]. The recommended n-6/n-3 PUFAs range is from 5:1–15:1 in Europe, and 4:1–10:1 in the United States and South Korea [11, 12]. In contrast, 371 of the 960 (38.6%) mothers in our study had an n-6/n-3 PUFAs above 10. These differences in fatty acid intake between Korea and other countries might dissimilarly affect brain development in infants.

The present study has several limitations. A 24-h recall method might not be sufficient to assess daily nutrient intakes due to memory lapses and the day-to-day variation of intakes. However, using standard protocols, the well-trained dietitians attempted to help the subjects describe what and how much they ate each day, to minimize possible recall bias. We did not measure plasma or serum fatty acid levels, which are considered to be a more objective approach to assessing maternal fatty acid status than dietary fatty acid intake reports alone. Also, identifying the genotype of the maternal fatty acid desaturase, which can affect fatty acid metabolism, might have improved the reliability of our results. Furthermore, the intake of all supplements, rather than n-3 or n-6 fatty acid dietary supplements, was one of the covariates included in the statistical model, yet, some nutrients might not contribute to infants' neurodevelopment. Nonetheless, this study was the first to use a birth cohort to investigate the association between maternal dietary fatty acid ratios during pregnancy and neurobehavioral indices in infants, assessed by the BSID-II, at 6 months of age.

Conclusions

We found that maternal LC-PUFAs intake, particularly n-6/n-3 PUFAs and LA/ALA, during pregnancy was negatively associated with neurobehavioral outcomes in infants at 6 months of age. Therefore, an adequate and balanced intake of n-6 and n-3 fatty acids or LA and ALA, from a well-balanced diet, should be recommended for pregnant women, to promote optimal infant's neurodevelopment. The findings of the present study could help in the further development of public health policies to improve the nutritional status of LC-PUFAs during pregnancy.

Abbreviations

AA: Arachidonic acid; ALA: α-linolenic acid; ASQ: Ages and stages questionnaire; BSID-II: Bayley scales of infant development, second edition; CDI: MacArthur Communicative Development Inventory; DGLA: Dihomo-γ-linolenic acid; DHA: Docosahexaenoic acid; DPA: Docosapentaenoic acid; EPA: Eicosapentaenoic acid; ETA: Eicosatetraenoic acid; LA: Linoleic acid; LA/ALA: Linoleic acid-to-α-linolenic acid ratio; LC-PUFAs: Long-chain polyunsaturated fatty acids; MDI: Mental development index; MOCEH: Mothers' and Children's Environmental Health; n-6/n-3 PUFAs: Ratio of n-6-to-n-3 polyunsaturated fatty acids; PDI: Psychomotor development index; PUFAs: Polyunsaturated fatty acids

Acknowledgements

Not applicable.

Funding

This research was supported by the Ministry of Environment and by Brain Korean 21 Plus.

Availability of data and materials
The datasets analyzed in the current study are available from the corresponding author on reasonable request.

Author's contributions
NC and EHH designed the research protocols; HK, HK, EL, and YK conducted the research; HK and HK analyzed the data; HK and NC wrote the manuscript, and NC was primarily responsible for the final contents. All the authors read and approved the final manuscript.

Competing interests
All authors, HK, HK, EL, YK, EHH, and NC, declare that they have no competing interests.

Consent for publication
Not applicable.

Ethics approval and consent to participate
Study protocols and consent forms were approved by the Institutional Review Boards at Ewha Womans University School of Medicine, Dankook University Hospital, and Ulsan University Hospital, respectively. All participants provided informed consent to participate in the study.

Publisher's Note

Author details
[1]Department of Nutritional Science and Food Management, Ewha Womans University, Seoul, South Korea. [2]Department of Nutrition Consultation, Seoul National University Hospital, Healthcare System Gangnam Center, Seoul, South Korea. [3]Department of Child Psychiatry, National Center for Child and Adolescent Psychiatry, Seoul National University Hospital, Seoul, South Korea. [4]Department of Occupational and Environmental Medicine, Ewha Womans University, College of Medicine, Seoul, South Korea.

References

1. German JB. Dietary lipids from an evolutionary perspective: sources, structures and functions. Matern Child Nutr. 2011;7 Suppl 2:2–16.
2. Gibson RA, Muhlhausler B, Makrides M. Conversion of linoleic acid and alpha-linolenic acid to long-chain polyunsaturated fatty acids (LCPUFAs), with a focus on pregnancy, lactation and the first 2 years of life. Matern Child Nutr. 2011;7 Suppl 2:17–26.
3. Uauy R, Mena P, Rojas C. Essential fatty acids in early life: structural and functional role. Proc Nutr Soc. 2000;59:3–15.
4. Strain JJ, Davidson PW, Bonham MP, Duffy EM, Stokes-Riner A, Thurston SW, Wallace JM, Robson PJ, Shamlaye CF, Georger LA, et al. Associations of maternal long-chain polyunsaturated fatty acids, methyl mercury, and infant development in the Seychelles Child Development Nutrition Study. Neurotoxicology. 2008;29:776–82.
5. Hibbeln JR, Davis JM, Steer C, Emmett P, Rogers I, Williams C, Golding J. Maternal seafood consumption in pregnancy and neurodevelopmental outcomes in childhood (ALSPAC study): an observational cohort study. Lancet. 2007;369:578–85.
6. Julvez J, Mendez M, Fernandez-Barres S, Romaguera D, Vioque J, Llop S, Ibarluzea J, Guxens M, Avella-Garcia C, Tardon A, et al. Maternal consumption of seafood in pregnancy and child neuropsychological development: a longitudinal study based on a population with high consumption levels. Am J Epidemiol. 2016;183:169–82.
7. Steenweg-de Graaff JC, Tiemeier H, Basten MG, Rijlaarsdam J, Demmelmair H, Koletzko B, Hofman A, Jaddoe VW, Verhulst FC, Roza SJ. Maternal LC-PUFA status during pregnancy and child problem behavior: the Generation R Study. Pediatr Res. 2015;77:489–97.
8. Bernard JY, De Agostini M, Forhan A, de Lauzon-Guillain B, Charles MA, Heude B. The dietary n6:n3 fatty acid ratio during pregnancy is inversely associated with child neurodevelopment in the EDEN mother-child cohort. J Nutr. 2013;143:1481–8.
9. Bernard JY, Armand M, Garcia C, Forhan A, De Agostini M, Charles MA, Heude B. The association between linoleic acid levels in colostrum and child cognition at 2 and 3 y in the EDEN cohort. Pediatr Res. 2015;77:829–35.
10. Harnack K, Andersen G, Somoza V. Quantitation of alpha-linolenic acid elongation to eicosapentaenoic and docosahexaenoic acid as affected by the ratio of n6/n3 fatty acids. Nutr Metab (Lond). 2009;6:8.
11. Institute of Medicine. Dietary reference intakes for energy, carbohydrate, fiber, fat, fatty acids, cholesterol, protein, and amino acids. Washington D.C.: National Academies Press; 2005. p. 422–588.
12. Ministry of Health and Welfare of Korea (South Korea. The Korean Nutrition Society. Dietary reference intakes for Koreans. 2nd ed. Seoul: The Korean Nutrition Society; 2015.
13. Sakayori N, Kikkawa T, Tokuda H, Kiryu E, Yoshizaki K, Kawashima H, Yamada T, Arai H, Kang JX, Katagiri H, et al. Maternal dietary imbalance between omega-6 and omega-3 polyunsaturated fatty acids impairs neocortical development via epoxy metabolites. Stem Cells. 2016;34:470–82.
14. Sakayori N, Tokuda H, Yoshizaki K, Kawashima H, Innis SM, Shibata H, Osumi N. Maternal nutritional imbalance between linoleic acid and alpha-linolenic acid increases offspring's anxious behavior with a sex-dependent manner in mice. Tohoku J Exp Med. 2016;240:31–7.
15. Koletzko B, Boey CC, Campoy C, Carlson SE, Chang N, Guillermo-Tuazon MA, Joshi S, Prell C, Quak SH, Sjarif DR, et al. Current information and Asian perspectives on long-chain polyunsaturated fatty acids in pregnancy, lactation, and infancy: systematic review and practice recommendations from an early nutrition academy workshop. Ann Nutr Metab. 2014;65:49–80.
16. United State Department of Agriculture, Agricultural Research Service. USDA national nutrient database for standard reference, release 26 [Internet]. Washington, D.C.: Agricultural Research Service; 2013. Available from: http://www.ars.usda.gov/Services/docs.htm?docid=24936.
17. National Fisheries Research & Development Institute (KR). Fatty acid composition of fisheries products in Korea. Busan: National Fisheries Research & Development Institute; 2012.
18. Kim BM, Ha M, Park HS, Lee BE, Kim YJ, Hong YC, Kim Y, Chang N, Roh YM, Kim BN, et al. The mothers and children's environmental health (MOCEH) study. Eur J Epidemiol. 2009;24:573–83.
19. Mills A, Tyler H. Food and nutrient intakes of British infants aged 6–12 months. London: HMSO Publications Centre; 1992.
20. Kim BM, Lee BE, Hong YC, Park H, Ha M, Kim YJ, Kim Y, Chang N, Kim BN, Oh SY, et al. Mercury levels in maternal and cord blood and attained weight through the 24 months of life. Sci Total Environ. 2011;410–411:26–33.
21. Park K, Cho B. Korean Bayley scales of infant development. 2nd ed. Korea: KIDSPOP Publishing Corporation; 2006.
22. Bayley N. Bayley scales of infant development. 2nd ed. San Antonio, TX: Psychological Corporation; 1993.
23. Crawford MA, Golfetto I, Ghebremeskel K, Min Y, Moodley T, Poston L, Phylactos A, Cunnane S, Schmidt W. The potential role for arachidonic and docosahexaenoic acids in protection against some central nervous system injuries in preterm infants. Lipids. 2003;38:303–15.
24. Rustan AC, Drevon CA. Fatty acids: structures and properties. In Encyclopedia of Life Science. London: John Wiley & Sons, Ltd; 2001.
25. Zhang G, Panigrahy D, Mahakian LM, Yang J, Liu JY, Stephen Lee KS, Wettersten HI, Ulu A, Hu X, Tam S, et al. Epoxy metabolites of docosahexaenoic acid (DHA) inhibit angiogenesis, tumor growth, and metastasis. Proc Natl Acad Sci U S A. 2013;110:6530–5.
26. Smink W, Gerrits WJ, Gloaguen M, Ruiter A, van Baal J. Linoleic and alpha-linolenic acid as precursor and inhibitor for the synthesis of long-chain polyunsaturated fatty acids in liver and brain of growing pigs. Animal. 2012;6:262–70.
27. Liou YA, King DJ, Zibrik D, Innis SM. Decreasing linoleic acid with constant alpha-linolenic acid in dietary fats increases (n-3) eicosapentaenoic acid in plasma phospholipids in healthy men. J Nutr. 2007;137:945–52.
28. Mendez MA, Torrent M, Julvez J, Ribas-Fito N, Kogevinas M, Sunyer J. Maternal fish and other seafood intakes during pregnancy and child neurodevelopment at age 4 years. Public Health Nutr. 2009;12:1702–10.
29. Suzuki K, Nakai K, Sugawara T, Nakamura T, Ohba T, Shimada M, Hosokawa T, Okamura K, Sakai T, Kurokawa N, et al. Neurobehavioral effects of prenatal exposure to methylmercury and PCBs, and seafood intake: neonatal behavioral assessment scale results of Tohoku study of child development. Environ Res. 2010;110:699–704.

30. Jedrychowski W, Jankowski J, Flak E, Skarupa A, Mroz E, Sochacka-Tatara E, Lisowska-Miszczyk I, Szpanowska-Wohn A, Rauh V, Skolicki Z, et al. Effects of prenatal exposure to mercury on cognitive and psychomotor function in one-year-old infants: epidemiologic cohort study in Poland. Ann Epidemiol. 2006;16:439–47.
31. Axelrad DA, Bellinger DC, Ryan LM, Woodruff TJ. Dose–response relationship of prenatal mercury exposure and IQ: an integrative analysis of epidemiologic data. Environ Health Perspect. 2007;115:609–15.
32. Meyer BJ, Mann NJ, Lewis JL, Milligan GC, Sinclair AJ, Howe PR. Dietary intakes and food sources of omega-6 and omega-3 polyunsaturated fatty acids. Lipids. 2003;38:391–8.
33. Muramatsu K, Tsuchihashi N, Tanaka E, Yamaguchi M, Suzuki A, Ishii K, Watanabe T. Estimated intake of cholesterol and fatty acids in Japanese. Bull Chiba Coll Health Sci. 2004;23:1–25.
34. NHANES 2010: what we eat in America. NHANES 2007–2008.
35. Monge-Rojas R, Aragon MC, Chinnock A, Campos H, Colon-Ramos U. Changes in dietary intake and food sources of saturated and *cis* and *trans* unsaturated fatty acids in Costa Rican adolescents: 1996 versus 2006. Nutrition. 2013;29:641–5.
36. Parra-Cabrera S, Stein AD, Wang M, Martorell R, Rivera J, Ramakrishnan U. Dietary intakes of polyunsaturated fatty acids among pregnant Mexican women. Matern Child Nutr. 2011;7:140–7.
37. Mani I, Dwarkanath P, Thomas T, Thomas A, Kurpad AV. Maternal fat and fatty acid intake and birth outcomes in a South Indian population. Int J Epidemiol. 2016;45:523–31.
38. Zhang J, Wang C, Gao Y, Li L, Man Q, Song P, Meng L, Du ZY, Miles EA, Lie O, et al. Different intakes of n-3 fatty acids among pregnant women in 3 regions of China with contrasting dietary patterns are reflected in maternal but not in umbilical erythrocyte phosphatidylcholine fatty acid composition. Nutr Res. 2013;33:613–21.

Dietary inflammatory index and risk of first myocardial infarction; a prospective population-based study

Stina Bodén[1*], Maria Wennberg[2], Bethany Van Guelpen[1], Ingegerd Johansson[2], Bernt Lindahl[3], Jonas Andersson[4], Nitin Shivappa[5,6,7], James R. Hebert[5,6,7] and Lena Maria Nilsson[2,8]

Abstract

Background: Chronic, low-grade inflammation is an established risk factor for cardiovascular disease. The inflammatory impact of diet can be reflected by concentrations of inflammatory markers in the bloodstream and the inflammatory potential of diet can be estimated by the dietary inflammatory index (DII[TM]), which has been associated with cardiovascular disease risk in some previous studies. We aimed to examine the association between the DII and the risk of first myocardial infarction (MI) in a population-based study with long follow-up.

Method: We conducted a prospective case–control study of 1389 verified cases of first MI and 5555 matched controls nested within the population-based cohorts of the Northern Sweden Health and Disease Study (NSHDS), of which the largest is the ongoing Västerbotten Intervention Programme (VIP) with nearly 100 000 participants during the study period. Median follow-up from recruitment to MI diagnosis was 6.4 years (6.2 for men and 7.2 for women). DII scores were derived from a validated food frequency questionnaire (FFQ) administered in 1986–2006. Multivariable conditional logistic regression models were used to estimate odds ratios (OR) and 95% confidence intervals (CI), using quartile 1 (most anti-inflammatory diet) as the reference category. For validation, general linear models were used to estimate the association between the DII scores and two inflammatory markers, high sensitivity C reactive protein (hsCRP) and interleukin 6 (IL-6) in a subset ($n = 605$) of the study population.

Results: Male participants with the most pro-inflammatory DII scores had an increased risk of MI [$OR_{Q4vsQ1} = 1.57$ (95% CI 1.21–2.02) $P_{trend} = 0.02$], which was essentially unchanged after adjustment for potential confounders, including cardiovascular risk factors [$OR_{Q4vsQ1} = 1.50$ (95% CI 1.14–1.99), $P_{trend} = 0.10$]. No association was found between DII and MI in women. An increase of one DII score unit was associated with 9% higher hsCRP (95% CI 0. 03–0.14) and 6% higher IL-6 (95% CI 0.02–0.11) in 605 controls with biomarker data available.

Conclusion: A pro-inflammatory diet was associated with an elevated risk of first myocardial infarction in men; whereas for women the relationship was null. Consideration of the inflammatory impact of diet could improve prevention of cardiovascular disease.

Keywords: DII Dietary inflammatory index, MI Myocardial infarction, NSHDS Northern Sweden health and disease study, VIP Västerbotten intervention programme, MONICA Monitoring of trends and determinants in cardiovascular disease, CVD cardiovascular disease, hsCRP high-sensitivity C-reactive protein, IL-6 interleukin 6

* Correspondence: stina.boden@umu.se
[1]Department of Radiation Sciences, Oncology, Umeå University, Umeå SE-901 87, Sweden
Full list of author information is available at the end of the article

Background

Low-grade, systemic inflammation in the human body is associated with several chronic diseases and there is evidence that diet might affect the incidence of cardiovascular disease (CVD) through inflammatory mechanisms [1–5]. The impact of diet on chronic low-grade inflammation can be reflected by concentrations of inflammatory markers in the bloodstream, including cytokines, acute-phase proteins, soluble adhesion molecules and cytokine receptors [6]. A diet high in red meat, high-fat dairy, refined grains, processed meat, sweets, desserts and sugar-sweetened soft drinks has been associated with higher circulating levels of inflammatory markers in blood samples; whereas a food pattern high in fruits, vegetables and whole grains has been inversely related to inflammatory markers, such as C-reactive protein (CRP) and interleukin-6 (IL-6) [5–10]. Furthermore, a diet rich in fibre and low in fat and sugar was reported to be associated with lower systematic inflammation, which also has been suggested to have a protective role against CVD [11, 12].

The contribution of inflammation to the progression of atherosclerosis is well established, as is the association with CVD [13–17]. Atherosclerosis, characterized by accumulation of lipids, foam cell leucocytes, and fibrous elements in the large arteries, is associated with thrombosis, a complication responsible for myocardial infarction (MI) and most strokes. Multiple studies have confirmed that chronic low-grade inflammation causes an increased risk of CVD, and the risk of developing CVD rises sharply with age, particularly after long exposure to an unhealthy lifestyle involving tobacco use, excessive alcohol use, lack of physical activity, stress and consumption of a diet high in fat and red meat [1, 13, 14].

The literature-derived dietary inflammatory index (DII™) has been designed to assess the inflammatory effect of diet, in any population and independent of specific dietary assessment method [18]. A pro-inflammatory diet, as estimated by the DII, has been associated with an increased risk of CVD in several populations, [19–23]; though some conflicting results also have been published [24, 25].

The aim of this study was to examine the DII scores in relation to the risk of first myocardial infarction (MI) in a prospective study with long follow-up.

Methods

Study design and population

We performed a nested case–control study within the Northern Sweden Health and Disease Study (NSHDS). Data were collected from two NSHDS cohorts, the Västerbotten Intervention Programme (VIP) and the Northern Sweden Monitoring Trends and Determinants in Cardiovascular Disease (MONICA) Study [26, 27]. The organization, sampling procedures, availability of samples/data, ethical considerations, and quality control program of the NSHDS are described in detail elsewhere [28]. The VIP is a long-term, ongoing programme including health interventions in the northern Swedish county of Västerbotten. All residents of Västerbotten, upon turning 40, 50 and 60 years of age (also 30 year olds during the period of 1985–1996 in all municipalities and continuously on a very small scale in some municipalities), are invited to a health screening at which they fill out a questionnaire addressing health history and lifestyle factors such as tobacco use, physical activity and diet. Participants are also asked to donate a blood sample for future research (stored in a biobank at −80 °C). A health examination is conducted at the screening event, including measurement of height and weight, blood pressure, blood fats and an oral glucose tolerance test as described previously [27]. The Northern Sweden MONICA Study follows essentially the same protocol as the VIP and includes 2000 or 2500 randomly selected 25–74 year olds (25–64 years in 1986) from the counties of Västerbotten and Norrbotten, stratified for age and sex and recruited approximately every 4–5 years since 1986. Mean participation rates for the time period of this study were approximately 60% for VIP and between 74 to 81% for the Northern Sweden MONICA Study. Minor selection bias has been reported for comparisons of participants and non-participants with respect to social characteristics [29]. In the present study, 89.3% of the participants were recruited through the VIP and 10.7% through the Northern Sweden MONICA Study.

The primary endpoint in this study was incidence of first definite MI (fatal and nonfatal, ICD-10 I21.0-I21.9). Cases occurring between January 1, 1986, and December 31, 2006, were identified through linkage between the NSHDS and the essentially complete and high-quality Northern Sweden MONICA Incidence Registry [30]. Exclusion criteria for cases recruited prior to 31 Dec 1999 were previous MI or stroke, or cancer other than non-melanoma skin cancer 5 years before or 1 year after MI. Exclusion criteria for cases recruited after 31 Dec 1999 were previous MI but previous stroke or cancer were not exclusion criteria.

Figure 1 illustrates the selection and exclusion of study participants recruited from the VIP and the Northern Sweden MONICA cohort. Of 2232 eligible MI cases with food frequency questionnaires (FFQ), 843 cases were excluded due to lack of, or insufficient, dietary data, or due to extreme food intake levels (FIL) (lowest and highest 1% of the distribution as well as participants with energy intake >5000 kcal/day). Each case of first MI was matched with four control participants on sex, age (±3y), year of health examination (±3y), study cohort (VIP/MONICA), and FFQ version. Exclusion criteria for controls were the same as for cases. One control was excluded due to withdrawal of participation after the

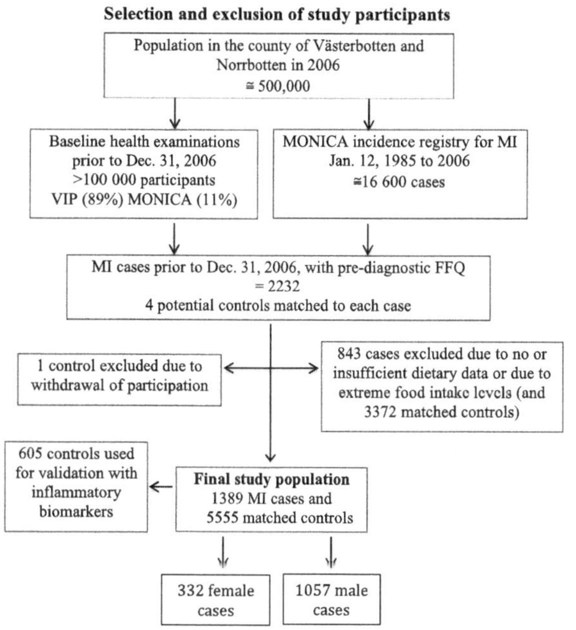

Fig. 1 Flow chart illustrating the selection and exclusion of study participants. Abbreviations: VIP, Västerbotten Intervention Programme; MONICA, Monitoring Trends and Determinants in Cardiovascular Disease; MI, myocardial infarction; FFQ, food frequency questionnaire; FIL, food intake level

matching. Thus, the final study population involved 1389 MI-cases, including 332 women and 1057 men, and a total of 5555 matched controls. Median follow-up from recruitment to MI diagnosis was 6.4 years.

Background variables

Tobacco smoking was classified as daily smokers, ex-smokers (former daily smokers) or never smokers (including occasional smokers and former occasional smokers). Total cholesterol concentrations (mmol/L) were measured in serum. Diabetes was defined as self-reported diabetes mellitus or diabetes mellitus diagnosed at the health examination (according to the WHO diagnostic criteria: fasting plasma glucose concentration ≥ 7.0 mmol/L or 2-h post-load plasma glucose concentration ≥ 11.1 mmol/L in MONICA project or ≥12.2 mmol/L in VIP, which used capillary blood). Education was dichotomized (post-secondary academic education, yes or no). Body mass index (BMI, kg/m^2) and systolic blood pressure (mmHg) were based on measurements by health care professionals. Because questions about recreational physical activity varied in the two cohorts, three different variables concerning physical activity were harmonized on a three-level scale (low, medium, high) [31].

Dietary assessment

Dietary data were collected at baseline using an optically readable, semi-quantitative FFQ, including 64 or 84 items, depending on year of measurement. Intake frequency had nine fixed alternatives (never, occasionally, 1–3 times/month, 1 time/week, 2–3 times/week, 4–6 times/week, 1 time/day, 2–3 times/day, ≥4 times/day). The frequency data, portion-size estimations and standard portion sizes were used to calculate daily intake of foods and nutrients. The FFQ has been validated and calibrated with repeated 24 h-recalls as well as biomarkers [32–34].

Dietary inflammatory index (DII^{TM})

The development of the original DII and validations using inflammatory biomarkers have been presented elsewhere [18, 35, 36]. In brief, based on a comprehensive review of the scientific literature, 45 food parameters were identified as being related to one or more of a defined set of inflammatory markers (IL-1β, IL-4, IL-6, IL-10, TNF-α and C-reactive protein), and assigned an overall inflammatory effect score based on the strength of the association and the quality of the studies. For each parameter, food consumption data from eleven populations around the world were used to calculate global mean intakes and standard deviations. The global mean standard deviation was multiplied by the overall inflammatory effect score for each food parameter, and the sum of these food-parameter-specific contributions yields the final DII score. The DII score could range from −8.87 (maximally anti-inflammatory to +7.98 (maximally pro-inflammatory).

Intakes of 30 food parameters (of a total maximum of 45) could be obtained from our FFQ and were included in our DII, including total energy, total fat, saturated fat, trans fatty acids, cholesterol, monounsaturated fat, polyunsaturated fat, omega-6 fatty acids, omega-3 fatty acids, carbohydrates, protein, fibre, alcohol, caffeine, tea, folic acid, selenium, niacin, iron, zinc, thiamin, vitamin B_2, vitamin B_6, vitamin B_{12}, vitamin A, vitamin E, vitamin C, vitamin D, magnesium and β-carotene (described with mean values and SD and compared with global mean intakes in the Additional file 1). The 15 food parameters excluded were eugenol, garlic, ginger, onion, saffron, turmeric, flanan-3-ol, flavones, flavonols, flavonones, anthocyanidins, isoflavones, pepper, thyme/oregano and rosemary. Caffeine intake was calculated as the sum of intake from coffee and tea. Tea in g/day was also kept as an independent parameter, as in the original DII.

Validation of DII using circulating inflammatory markers

In addition to the main analyses, we validated DII scores using hsCRP and IL-6, which had previously been measured in a subset of the control subjects in this study ($n = 605$ of whom 81.8% were men) with recruitment dates between 1991–1999. Enzyme-linked immunosorbent assays (ELISA) were used (IMMULITE, Diagnostic Products Corporation, USA, for hsCRP and R & D Systems, Oxford, UK, for IL-6) [37]. The data were log-transformed and included as quartiles in general linear models, with the first DII quartile (most anti-inflammatory diet) as the reference category. β-coefficients for DII in quartiles and as continuous, as well as adjusted R^2, were estimated in the general linear regression models. The first model was adjusted for total energy intake in kcal/day and for fasting duration prior to blood sample collection (classified to 0-4 h, 4–6 h, 6–8 h or >8 h). Fasting time is particularly relevant for IL-6 due to its shorter half-life (<2 h) and greater within-person variability compared to hsCRP [38]. The multivariable model was additionally adjusted for smoking, age, BMI, systolic blood pressure, diabetes, as well as the ratio between Apolipoprotein B and Apolipoprotein A1 (ApoB/ApoA1), which also was measured in these 605 controls.

Statistical analyses

Sex-specific quartiles of DII were calculated based on the distribution of the controls. ANOVA tests for continuous variables and Chi-Square tests for categorical variables were used to assess differences in baseline characteristics across the DII quartiles. Odds ratios (OR) and 95% confidence intervals (CI) for the risk of first MI were estimated using conditional logistic regression models with the first DII quartile (Q1, most anti-inflammatory diet) as the reference category. An energy-adjusted model, adjusted for total energy intake in kcal/day was first constructed. To account for potential confounders, we constructed a multivariable model in which covariates were selected if they altered any of the risk estimates by more than 10%, or for theoretical importance as confounders. The final model included the covariates total energy intake, smoking, systolic blood pressure, total serum cholesterol, diabetes, education level, BMI and recreational physical activity. Because some of the covariates, particularly cholesterol, diabetes and BMI, are potential mediating factors of the association between DII and CVD, we also tested models excluding each of these in sensitivity tests. Participants with missing values for categorical covariates were included in the conditional logistic regressions using dummy categories. Participants with missing values for the continuous variables (systolic blood pressure and total serum cholesterol) were not included in the conditional logistic regression (in total, $n = 127$). Heterogeneity in risk estimates between sexes was tested by Chi-square analysis. In order to reduce the risk of reverse causation between inflammation and CVD a sensitivity test was also carried out, excluding cases with less than two years between recruitment and incidence of MI. We also stratified the data at the median lag time from recruitment to MI.

Interaction analyses were performed between DII and some potentially important effect modifiers (smoking, BMI and diabetes). We calculated the relative excess risk due to interaction (RERI) and the synergy index (S) [39]. 95% confidence intervals were determined using the approximate variance estimator [40]. We used the likelihood ratio tests of significance comparing models including versus those excluding the interaction term, in order to evaluate the significance of the multiplicative interaction.

All analyses were performed with SPSS® statistics version 23. All P values were two-tailed and P values ≤0.05 were considered to indicate statistical significance.

Results

Table 1 presents baseline characteristics of the 5284 men and 1660 women according to sex-specific quartiles of DII. Missing values for background information, where present, are presented as frequencies. In this study, DII scores ranged from −4.16 (most anti-inflammatory) to +5.04 (most pro-inflammatory), with a mean in control subjects of 0.89 (1.66) in men and 1.08 (1.59) in women. Mean age at baseline was approximately 54 years across DII quartiles. Subjects with higher DII scores were characterized by lower education, higher smoking rates, lower physical activity and, in men, higher systolic blood pressure and higher serum total cholesterol concentrations, compared to subjects with lower DII scores. Diabetes appeared to be less common in subjects with higher DII in both men and women, though the differences did not reach statistical significance (data not shown). BMI did not vary by DII score in men, whereas obesity (BMI >30) was less common and overweight (BMI >25) more common in women with higher DII scores. The lag time from recruitment to MI was shorter in men than women, median 6.2 (25th, 75th percentile: 3.5, 9.3) and 7.2 (4.4, 10.3) years, respectively, $P = 0.001$).

We observed statistically significant associations between the most pro-inflammatory DII scores (Q4) and both higher hsCRP and higher IL-6 in a subset of the control participants with biomarker data available (Additional file 2). In the multivariable model, an increase of one DII score unit was associated with 9% higher hsCRP (95% CI 0.03–0.14, $P_{trend} = 0.003$) and 6% higher IL-6 (95% CI 0.02–0.11, $P_{trend} = 0.005$). DII explained 1.7% of elevated hsCRP and 0.7% of elevated IL-6 concentrations in the energy-adjusted model (R^2 adjusted 0.017 and 0.007 respectively).

Table 2 presents the risk associations between DII and MI. Men with the highest DII scores (Q4, most pro-inflammatory diet), had a higher risk of first MI compared to men with the lowest DII scores (Q1, most anti-inflammatory diet) (energy-adjusted OR_{Q4vsQ1} 1.57, 95% CI 1.22–2.02, $P_{trend} = 0.02$). This finding was essentially unchanged by adjusting for potential confounders, though the linear trend, using DII score as a continuous

Table 1 Baseline characteristics of participants according to sex-specific quartiles of the dietary inflammatory index[a]

	Men (n = 5284)					Women (n = 1600)				
	Q1	Q2	Q3	Q4	P[b]	Q1	Q2	Q3	Q4	P[b]
n	1266	1319	1299	1400		407	422	404	427	
DII					<0.001					<0.001
Mean	−1.38	0.43	1.60	2.90		−1.14	0.69	1.81	2.93	
SD	0.83	0.37	0.33	0.53		0.87	0.38	0.29	0.47	
Min	−4.16	−0.25	1.05	2.16		−3.86	0.00	1.29	2.31	
Max	−0.25	1.05	2.16	5.04		0.00	1.29	2.30	4.31	
Age at baseline (Y)					0.079					0.331
Mean	53.4	54.1	53.9	54.0		54.9	54.3	54.7	54.0	
SD	7.47	7.19	7.36	7.38		7.68	8.17	7.40	8.28	
Postsecondary education (%)	20.6	18.9	13.8	12.9	<0.001	22.4	16.1	16.3	10.8	<0.001
Missing (n)	11	18	17	9		8	7	9	4	
Smoking status (%)					<0.001					<0.001
Daily smokers	15.4	16.8	22.6	28.8		15.7	22.3	22.0	34.2	
Ex-smokers	30.5	31.2	30.1	29.6		19.9	19.9	17.8	20.1	
Non-smokers	52.8	50.8	45.7	40.6		63.1	55.9	58.4	45.4	
Missing (n)	16	17	20	15		5	8	7	1	
Physical activity (%)[c]					<0.001					<0.001
Medium	47.7	45.6	44.5	37.7		54.8	43.4	42.9	40.5	
High	17.5	13.2	11.1	8.6		12.0	11.0	9.9	11.3	
Missing (n)	18	7	9	9		8	9	9	10	
BMI (kg/m^2) (%)					0.944					0.017
<25	37.4	36.8	37.7	36.5		45.7	45.5	50.0	44.0	
25–29.9	51.1	50.3	49.9	50.7		32.9	35.3	36.9	40.7	
>30	11.5	12.9	12.3	12.8		21.4	19.2	13.1	15.2	
Missing (n)	1	1	3	0		0	0	0	0	
Diabetes (%)	8.2	7.5	6.2	5.9	0.054	7.1	8.1	5.4	4.9	0.211
Missing (n)	0	1	0	0		0	1	0	0	
Systolic BP (mmHg)					0.005					0.673
Mean	132.7	134.1	134.6	135.2		135.3	134.4	133.7	133.8	
SD	17.6	18.1	18.2	18.4		21.2	19.7	20.1	20.7	
Missing (n)	20	18	19	8		4	5	7	7	
S-cholesterol (mmol/L)					0.003					0.740
Mean	5.96	6.03	6.04	6.13		6.20	6.18	6.11	6.16	
SD	1.20	1.23	1.20	1.24		1.32	1.30	1.27	1.21	
Missing (n)	7	7	8	12		1	3	0	1	
Lag time (Y)[d]					0.498					0.142
Mean	6.80	6.81	6.41	6.43		6.88	7.79	8.14	6.96	
SD	4.05	3.87	4.00	4.08		3.88	3.96	4.17	4.26	

Q quartile, *DII* Dietary inflammatory index, *SD* Standard deviation, *Y* years, *BMI* Body mass index, *BP*, Blood pressure, *S-cholesterol*, Serum cholesterol, *Lag time* time from baseline to MI

[a]Quartile cutoffs for DII based on the controls

[b]P-values determined by ANOVA for continuous variables or Chi-Square tests for categorical variables

[c]Refers to recreational physical activity

[d]Years from health examination/recruitment to myocardial infarction

Table 2 The association between the dietary inflammatory index and first myocardial infarction for men and women[a]

	Q1	Q2		Q3		Q4		P trend[b]
Men								
Cases/controls (*n*)	210/1056	261/1058		242/1057		344/1056		
Range DII score	−4.16 – -0.25	−0.25 – 1.05		1.05 – 2.16		2.16 – 4.72		
	OR	OR	95% CI	OR	95% CI	OR	95% CI	
Energy-adjusted[c]	ref	1.22	0.98–1.51	1.12	0.88–1.42	1.57	1.21–2.02	0.018
Multivariable[d]	ref	1.20	0.95–1.53	1.13	0.87–1.45	1.50	1.14–1.99	0.097
Women								
Cases/controls (*n*)	75/332	90/332		72/332		95/332		
Range DII score	−3.86 – 0.00	0.00 – 1.29		1.29 – 2.31		2.31 – 4.31		
	OR	OR	95% CI	OR	95% CI	OR	95% CI	
Energy-adjusted[c]	ref	1.09	0.75–1.58	0.82	0.54–1.23	1.01	0.65–1.56	0.423
Multivariable[d]	ref	1.05	0.69–1.59	0.82	0.51–1.30	0.83	0.50–1.36	0.088

Q quartile of DII, *DII* Dietary inflammatory index, *ref* reference
[a]Conditional logistic regression models presented with odds ratio (OR) and 95% confidence interval (CI)
[b]*P* for trend when DII used as a continuous variable
[c]Adjusted for total energy intake in kcal/day
[d]Adjusted for total energy intake, body mass index, physical activity, systolic blood pressure, total serum cholesterol, diabetes, smoking, and postsecondary academic education

variable, lost statistical significance (multivariable OR_{Q4vsQ1} 1.50, 1.14–1.99, $P_{trend} = 0.10$). Excluding cholesterol, BMI or diabetes, potential mediating factors, from the multivariable model had negligible effects on the risk estimates (Additional file 3). Excluding cases with less than two years between baseline and MI diagnosis did not affect the magnitude or statistical significance of the risk estimates (multivariable OR_{Q4vsQ1} for men 1.56, 95% CI 1.16–2.10, $P_{trend} = 0.10$, Additional file 3). Stratifying at the median lag time of 6.2 years for men and 7.2 years for women also yielded largely consistent results (Additional file 3). We did not find any association between DII and MI risk in women, and the Chi-square test for heterogeneity of results between sexes was statistically significant ($P = 0.04$).

Multivariable interaction models for DII and smoking, BMI, and diabetes in relation to MI risk are presented as 3D bar graphs in Fig. 2 and Additional file 4. A positive additive interaction was found for DII and smoking in

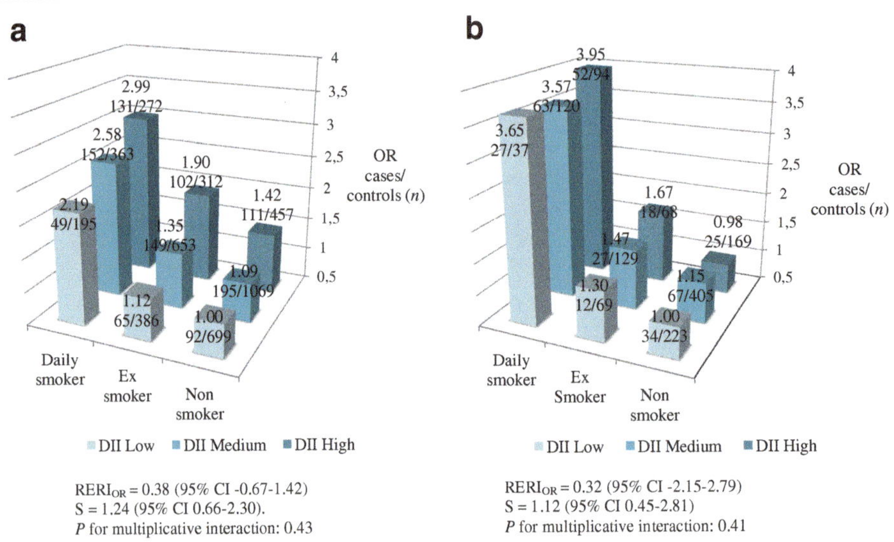

Fig. 2 Abbreviations: RERI, relative excess risk due to interaction; S, synergy index. Joint effect of dietary inflammatory index (DII) and smoking status, on the risk of first myocardial infarction (MI) in **a** men **b** women. Odds ratios (OR) were estimated from multiple regression models adjusted for total energy intake, total serum cholesterol, systolic blood pressure, body mass index (BMI), diabetes, and postsecondary academic education. The calculations of RERI and S were performed comparing daily smokers/non-smokers and low DII/high DII

men, although the RERI and S were not statistically significant (Fig. 2a, $RERI_{OR} = 0.38$ (95% CI −0.67–1.42), S = 1.24 (0.66–2.30). There was no interaction on the multiplicative scale ($P = 0.43$). In women, a small positive additive interaction was seen for DII and smoking (non-significant, Fig. 2b), Neither BMI nor diabetes interacted with DII in relation to MI risk in men or women (Additional file 4).

Discussion

In this population-based, nested case–control study, men with the highest DII scores, representing the most pro-inflammatory diet, had a higher risk of first MI. In women, no association was found. We also observed a positive, but non-significant, additive interaction between the DII and smoking in relation to MI risk in both men and women, underscoring the potential importance of evaluating pro-inflammatory lifestyle behaviors as effect modifiers of the association between DII and inflammation-related disease.

Our findings are consistent with some previous results for DII and incident CVD as well as all-cause mortality [19–23]; although null associations have also been reported [24, 25]. Effect sizes for CVD risk have generally been in the range of approximately OR 1.5 to 2, which is comparable to our results for men. The DII scores in our study population were also comparable to those of previous studies [19–22, 36], including the SEASONS study, in which DII was validated against the inflammatory marker hsCRP [36]. Also in line with previous studies [35, 36], the DII was weakly, but statistically significantly, associated with both hsCRP and the inflammatory marker IL-6 in a subset of our control participants with biomarker data available. The DII based on our FFQ and applied to our study population appears to be sufficient for this type of investigation, and for interpretation of the results in relation to previous findings.

Our finding of a significant sex difference in the association between DII and MI risk was not entirely without precedent. Null results have been reported for women in other studies of DII and CVD [21, 25], though in one of the studies the female cases were few and relatively young (mean age 35.4 years) [21]. Our study included a lower number of women than men (332 and 1057 cases, respectively), which reflects the lower incidence rate and higher age at first MI in women. Although this may explain the lack of association for women in our study, the sample size should be sufficient to detect an association. Furthermore, the OR and not just the CI and P-values, are consistent with a null association. The importance of investigating sex-related differences regarding diet and CVD risk profile has been emphasized in studies of the Mediterranean diet [41, 42]. In a 12-week dietary intervention study, men had a pronounced beneficial change in long-term, post-intervention dietary intake compared to women, as well as a greater improvement in metabolic profile [42].

Dietary changes in the northern Swedish population occurred over the study period, which might be speculated to influence our analyses. The VIP was initiated largely as a response to high CVD mortality rates in the county of Västerbotten in the mid-1980s [26, 27]. It is a strategic, population-wide programme involving both general initiatives, such as a healthy choice "key hole" label on foods, and individual health screening and lifestyle counseling. An impact of the VIP on all-cause and cardiovascular mortality has been reported [43]. However, a low-carbohydrate/high-fat dietary trend also occurred in Sweden toward the end of our study period [44]. Total fat intake (contributing essentially to a more pro-inflammatory DII score) began to increase after 2004 in both sexes, but more so in women, after decreasing during the first seven years of the VIP (1986–1992), and total serum cholesterol concentrations, after decreasing for several years, leveled off in 2004–2007 and then began to rise [45]. Although such temporal changes were probably reflected in the DII, the use of a matched case–control rather than cohort design for our study minimized the potential bias related to changes in dietary habits in the population during the data collection period.

Underreporting of dietary intake is a known problem in nutritional epidemiology. In a validation of our FFQ using repeated 24-h recalls, the prevalence and magnitude of underreporting of energy intake were directly related to BMI [46], and especially foods characterized as socially undesirable (e.g., high-fat foods and simple carbohydrates) were underreported [47, 48]. This may explain why BMI did not demonstrate an expected direct relationship with DII, and emphasizes the importance of adjusting for BMI and energy intake in studies using dietary data. Underreporting is most likely to lead to underestimation of diet-disease relations, and the null finding in women could be explained by sex-differential social desirability bias that is much more pronounced in women [48–50].

BMI has the potential to act as a mediator between diet, low-grade chronic inflammation and inflammation-related diseases, and not just as a confounder. Body fatness creates a pro-inflammatory metabolic environment, and BMI is positively related to CRP and other inflammatory markers [3, 4]. For this reason, as for the other potential mediating factors, total serum cholesterol concentrations and diabetes, we tested sequential exclusion from the multivariable model with no material effects on risk estimates. Although we excluded subjects with extreme energy intakes, underreporting is still an issue in self-reported FFQs.

Diabetes did not demonstrate the expected direct relationship with a more pro-inflammatory diet, (higher DII scores). Rather, an opposite trend was observed, though it did not reach statistical significance. This is not consistent with the causal chain, in which low-grade inflammation contributes to the development of metabolic diseases. Participants with diabetes may, speculatively, have changed their dietary patterns after advice from health care professionals.

The effect sizes observed for the DII in relation to cardiovascular endpoints are generally modest [19–23], which is not surprising, given the many other potential contributing factors to low-grade chronic inflammation. However, the general consistency of results suggests that the inflammatory impact of diet is a potential target for CVD prevention. Also, an anti-inflammatory diet, characterized by a low intake of saturated fat, high intake of vegetables and fibre, is beneficial for preventing CVD through mechanisms other than inflammation, such as lowering blood lipids and thus reducing the risk of thrombosis.

The main strengths of this study include its prospective design, which minimizes recall bias and reverse causation, and the population-based nature of the study cohorts. The sample size was large ($n = 6944$, including 1389 cases), with enough statistical power for subgroup and interaction analyses. However, there are also limitations. We were only able to include 30 of the 45 food parameters in the original DII. The 15 parameters excluded were all anti-inflammatory, which may have contributed to more pro-inflammatory DII scores. Other studies investigating the DII in relation to cardiovascular disease had similar exclusions of food parameters characterized as anti-inflammatory [21, 23]. The semi-quantitative FFQ has inherent weaknesses, particularly underreporting, but it has demonstrated validity similar to other FFQs [32–34]. Our analyses were based on a single health-screening occasion per participant, and we can, therefore, not account for intra-individual changes in dietary and lifestyle habits. Although we lacked data on aspirin use, we were able to adjust for a number of important cardiovascular risk factors. As always with observational studies, we cannot answer the question of causality, and thus a causal relationship between a predictor and the outcome cannot be confirmed.

Conclusions

In this prospective, population-based study with long follow-up, a more pro-inflammatory diet as estimated by the DII was associated with an increased risk of first MI in men. These findings support inflammation as a link between diet and cardiovascular risk as well as the usefulness of the DII for estimating the inflammatory impact of diet.

Additional files

Additional file 1: Food parameters included in the NSHDS-DII. (DOCX 113 kb)

Additional file 2: Associations between Dietary inflammatory index and the inflammatory biomarkers C-reactive protein and Interleukin 6. (DOCX 92 kb)

Additional file 3: Sensitivity and subgroup analyses for the association between the dietary inflammatory index and myocardial infarction. (DOCX 136 kb)

Additional file 4: Statistical interactions with DII-BMI and DII-diabetes. (PDF 786 kb)

Acknowledgements

The authors would like to thank the participants in the Västerbotten Intervention Programme and the Northern Sweden MONICA Study as well as the funds supporting the Northern Sweden Diet Database, the Västerbotten Intervention Project, and the MONICA project. The Swedish Research Council is acknowledged for supporting the building of the database. Thanks also to Robin Myte for statistical support and the personal at the Department of Biobank Research (EBF) for technical support, all at Umeå University, Sweden.

Funding

S.B is supported by the Cancer Research Fund in Northern Sweden (LP 16–2107) and the National Cancer Foundation in Sweden (CAN 2014/780). Drs. Shivappa, Hébert, were supported by the United States National Institute for Diabetes, Digestive and Kidney Diseases (grant no. R44DK103377). Funding sources had no role in the design, analysis or writing of this study. This study reflects the views of the authors only.

Availability of data and materials

The data that support the findings of this study are available from the Department of Biobank Research at Umeå University, Sweden, but restrictions apply to the availability of these data, which were used under license for the current study, and so are not publicly available. Data are however available from the authors upon reasonable request and with permission of the Department of Biobank Research at Umeå University, Sweden.

Authors' contributions

SB, MW, LMN, and BVG. contributed to the study concept and design; S.B. performed all data analyses and was the main author; MW, LMN, B.L, JA, and IJ contributed to the acquisition of data; MW, LMN and BVG. assisted in the data analyses; NS and JRH. designed the Dietary inflammatory index (DII^{TM}); LMN together with NS prepared the syntax for the DII in the Northern Sweden Health and Disease Study (NSHDS); all authors contributed to the interpretation of the results and drafting and/or revision of the manuscript, and all authors approved the final, submitted version of the manuscript.

Competing interests

Dr. James R. Hébert owns controlling interest in Connecting Health Innovations LLC (CHI), a company planning to license the right to his invention of the dietary inflammatory index (DII) from the University of South Carolina in order to develop computer and smart phone applications for patient counseling and dietary intervention in clinical settings. Dr. Nitin Shivappa is an employee of CHI. None of the other authors declares any competing interest.

Consent for publication

Not applicable.

Ethics approval and consent to participate

The study was approved by the Regional Ethics Review Board of Northern Sweden (Dnr 2013/332–31). All study subjects provided written informed consent at time of the recruitment into the NSHDS, and the study was conducted in accordance with the Declaration of Helsinki.

Publisher's Note

Author details

[1]Department of Radiation Sciences, Oncology, Umeå University, Umeå SE-901 87, Sweden . [2]Department of Public Health and Clinical Medicine, Nutritional Research, Umeå University, Umeå SE-901 87, Sweden. [3]Department of Public Health and Clinical Medicine, Occupational and Environmental Medicine, Umeå University, Umeå SE-901 87, Sweden. [4]Department of Public Health and Clinical Medicine, Research Unit Skellefteå, Umeå University, Umeå SE-901 87, Sweden. [5]Cancer Prevention and Control Program, University of South Carolina, 915 Greene Street, Suite 241, Columbia, SC 29208, USA. [6]Department of Epidemiology and Biostatistics, Arnold School of Public Health, University of South Carolina, Columbia, SC 29208, USA. [7]Connecting Health Innovations LLC, 1417 Gregg St., Columbia, SC 29201, USA. [8]Arctic Research Centre (Arcum), Umeå University, Umeå SE-901 87, Sweden.

References

1. Meyer J, Döring A, Herder C, Roden M, Koenig W, Thorand B. Dietary patterns, subclinical inflammation, incident coronary heart disease and mortality in middle-aged men from the MONICA/KORA Augsburg cohort study. Eur J Clin Nutr. 2011;65(7):800–7. http://www.nature.com/ejcn/journal/v65/n7/pdf/ejcn201137a.pdf. doi:10.1038/ejcn.2011.37.
2. Conti P, Shaik-Dasthagirisaeb Y. Atherosclerosis: a chronic inflammatory disease mediated by mast cells. Cent Eur J Immunol. 2015;40(3):380–6. https://www.ncbi.nlm.nih.gov/pubmed/26648785. doi:10.5114/ceji.2015.54603.
3. Egger G, Dixon J. Inflammatory effects of nutritional stimuli: further support for the need for a big picture approach to tackling obesity and chronic disease. Obes Rev. 2010;11(2):137–49. http://onlinelibrary.wiley.com/store/10.1111/j.1467-789X.2009.00644.x/asset/j.1467-789X.2009.00644.x.pdf?v=1&t=im38xo3n&s=17aed3e5528d13756684c5d91a1e5778c0382060.
4. Calder PC, Ahluwalia N, Brouns F, Buetler T, Clement K, Cunningham K, et al. Dietary factors and low-grade inflammation in relation to overweight and obesity. Br J Nutr. 2011;106(S3):S1–S78.
5. Nettleton JA, Steffen LM, Mayer-Davis EJ, Jenny NS, Jiang R, Herrington DM, et al. Dietary patterns are associated with biochemical markers of inflammation and endothelial activation in the Multi-Ethnic Study of Atherosclerosis (MESA). Am J Clin Nutr. 2006;83(6):1369–79. https://www.ncbi.nlm.nih.gov/pubmed/16762949. PMCID:PMC2933059.
6. Esmaillzadeh A, Kimiagar M, Mehrabi Y, Azadbakht L, Hu FB, Willett WC. Dietary patterns and markers of systemic inflammation among Iranian women. J Nutr. 2007;137(4):992–8. <Go to ISI>://WOS:000245230700023.
7. King DE, Egan BM, Geesey ME. Relation of dietary fat and fiber to elevation of C-reactive protein. Am J Cardiol. 2003;92(11):1335–9. http://ac.els-cdn.com/S0002914903011937/1-s2.0-S0002914903011937-main.pdf?_tid=d0a6dbe2-f015-11e5-ab14-00000aab0f01&acdnat=1458641399_0f914cef4fa1eaeb86078a37ea811479.
8. Neale EP, Batterham MJ, Tapsell LC. Consumption of a healthy dietary pattern results in significant reductions in C-reactive protein levels in adults: a meta-analysis. Nutrition Research. 2016;36(5):391–401. <Go to ISI>://WOS:000375021400001.
9. van Bussel BC, Henry RM, Ferreira I, van Greevenbroek MM, van der Kallen CJ, Twisk JW, et al. A healthy diet is associated with less endothelial dysfunction and less low-grade inflammation over a 7-year period in adults at risk of cardiovascular disease. J Nutr. 2015;145(3):532–40.
10. Smidowicz A, Regula J. Effect of nutritional status and dietary patterns on human serum C-reactive protein and interleukin-6 concentrations. Adv Nutr. 2015;6(6):738–47.
11. Dias JA, Wirfält E, Drake I, Gullberg B, Hedblad B, Persson M, et al. A high quality diet is associated with reduced systemic inflammation in middle-aged individuals. Atherosclerosis. 2015;238(1):38–44. http://ac.els-cdn.com/S002191501401569X/1-s2.0-S002191501401569X-main.pdf?_tid=caf711d0-f015-11e5-85ec-00000aab0f26&acdnat=1458641389_0f4f00b1fc201d1c078dde3ffb83ff81.
12. Hlebowicz J, Persson M, Gullberg B, Sonestedt E, Wallström P, Drake I, et al. Food patterns, inflammation markers and incidence of cardiovascular disease: the Malmö Diet and Cancer study. J Intern Med. 2011;270(4):365–76. http://dx.doi.org/10.1111/j.1365-2796.2011.02382.x.
13. Prasad S, Sung B, Aggarwal BB. Age-associated chronic diseases require age-old medicine: role of chronic inflammation. Prev Med. 2012;54 SupplS29-37. https://www.ncbi.nlm.nih.gov/pubmed/22178471. doi:10.1016/j.ypmed.2011.11.011.
14. Willeit P, Thompson SG, Agewall S, Bergstrom G, Bickel H, Catapano AL, et al. Inflammatory markers and extent and progression of early atherosclerosis: Meta-analysis of individual-participant-data from 20 prospective studies of the PROG-IMT collaboration. Eur J Prev Cardiol. 2016;23(2):194–205. https://www.ncbi.nlm.nih.gov/pubmed/25416041. doi:10.1177/2047487314560664.
15. Libby P. Inflammation in atherosclerosis. Nature. 2002;420(6917):868–74. https://www.ncbi.nlm.nih.gov/pubmed/12490960.
16. Rosenson RS, Koenig W. Utility of inflammatory markers in the management of coronary artery disease. Am J Cardiol. 2003;92(1):10–8.
17. Pearson TA, Mensah GA, Alexander RW, Anderson JL, Cannon RO, Criqui M, et al. Markers of inflammation and cardiovascular disease application to clinical and public health practice: a statement for healthcare professionals from the centers for disease control and prevention and the American Heart Association. Circulation. 2003;107(3):499–511. https://www.ncbi.nlm.nih.gov/pubmed/12551878.
18. Shivappa N, Steck SE, Hurley TG, Hussey JR, Hébert JR. Designing and developing a literature-derived, population-based dietary inflammatory index. Publ Health Nutr. 2014;17(08):1689–96.
19. O'Neil A, Shivappa N, Jacka FN, Kotowicz MA, Kibbey K, Hebert JR, et al. Pro-inflammatory dietary intake as a risk factor for CVD in men: a 5-year longitudinal study. Br J Nutr. 2015;114(12):2074–82.
20. Garcia-Arellano A, Ramallal R, Ruiz-Canela M, Salas-Salvadó J, Corella D, Shivappa N, et al. Dietary inflammatory index and incidence of cardiovascular disease in the predimed study. Nutrients. 2015;7(6):4124–38. https://www.ncbi.nlm.nih.gov/pubmed/26035241.
21. Ramallal R, Toledo E, Martinez-Gonzalez MA, Hernandez-Hernandez A, Garcia-Arellano A, Shivappa N, et al. Dietary Inflammatory Index and Incidence of Cardiovascular Disease in the SUN Cohort. PLoS One. 2015; 10(9):e0135221. https://www.ncbi.nlm.nih.gov/pubmed/26340022. doi:10.1371/journal.pone.0135221.
22. Graffouillere L, Deschasaux M, Mariotti F, Neufcourt L, Shivappa N, Hebert JR, et al. Prospective association between the Dietary Inflammatory Index and mortality: modulation by antioxidant supplementation in the SU.VI.MAX randomized controlled trial. Am J Clin Nutr. 2016;103(3):878–85. <Go to ISI>://WOS:000371650200025.
23. Shivappa N, Steck SE, Hussey JR, Ma Y, Hebert JR. Inflammatory potential of diet and all-cause, cardiovascular, and cancer mortality in National Health and Nutrition Examination Survey III Study. Eur J Nutr. 20151–10. https://www.ncbi.nlm.nih.gov/pubmed/26644215. doi:10.1007/s00394-015-1112-x
24. Alkerwi A, Shivappa N, Crichton G, Hebert JR. No significant independent relationships with cardiometabolic biomarkers were detected in the Observation of Cardiovascular Risk Factors in Luxembourg study population. Nutrition Research. 2014;34(12):1058–65. <Go to ISI>://WOS:000346113500005.
25. Vissers LE, Waller MA, van der Schouw YT, Hebert JR, Shivappa N, Schoenaker DA, et al. The relationship between the dietary inflammatory index and risk of total cardiovascular disease, ischemic heart disease and cerebrovascular disease: Findings from an Australian population-based prospective cohort study of women. Atherosclerosis. 2016,253.164–170. doi:10.1016/j.atherosclerosis.2016.07.929. Epub 2016 Jul 30.
26. Stegmayr B, Lundberg V, Asplund K. The events registration and survey procedures in the Northern Sweden MONICA Project. Scand J Public Health. 2003;31(61 suppl):9–17.
27. Norberg M, Wall S, Boman K, Weinehall L. The Västerbotten Intervention Programme: background, design and implications. Glob Health Action. 2010;3:4643. doi:10.3402/gha.v3i0.4643.
28. Hallmans G, Ågren Å, Johansson G, Johansson A, Stegmayr B, Jansson J-H, et al. Cardiovascular disease and diabetes in the Northern Sweden Health and Disease Study Cohort-evaluation of risk factors and their interactions. Scand J Public Health. 2003;31(61 suppl):18–24.
29. Weinehall L, Hallgren C-G, Westman G, Janlert U, Wall S. Reduction of selection bias in primary prevention of cardiovascular disease through involvement of primary health care. Scand J Prim Health Care. 1998;16(3):171–6.
30. Tunstall-Pedoe H, Kuulasmaa K, Amouyel P, Arveiler D, Rajakangas AM, Pajak A. Myocardial infarction and coronary deaths in the world health organization MONICA project. Registration procedures, event rates, and

case-fatality rates in 38 populations from 21 countries in four continents. Circulation. 1994;90(1):583–612.
31. Wennberg P, Lindahl B, Hallmans G, Messner T, Weinehall L, Johansson L, et al. The effects of commuting activity and occupational and leisure time physical activity on risk of myocardial infarction. Eur J Cardiovasc Prev Rehabil. 2006;13(6):924–30.
32. Johansson I, Hallmans G, Wikman Å, Biessy C, Riboli E, Kaaks R. Validation and calibration of food-frequency questionnaire measurements in the northern Sweden health and disease cohort. Publ Health Nutr. 2002;5(03):487–96.
33. Johansson I, Van Guelpen B, Hultdin J, Johansson M, Hallmans G, Stattin P. Validity of food frequency questionnaire estimated intakes of folate and other B vitamins in a region without folic acid fortification. Eur J Clin Nutr. 2010;64(8):905–13.
34. Wennberg M, Vessby B, Johansson I. Evaluation of relative intake of fatty acids according to the Northern Sweden FFQ with fatty acid levels in erythrocyte membranes as biomarkers. Public Health Nutr. 2009;12(9):1477–84.
35. Tabung FK, Steck SE, Zhang J, Ma Y, Liese AD, Agalliu I, et al. Construct validation of the dietary inflammatory index among postmenopausal women. Ann Epidemiol. 2015;25(6):398–405. http://ac.els-cdn.com/S1047279715001192/1-s2.0-S1047279715001192-main.pdf?_tid=dd706ef6-f015-11e5-aa82-00000aab0f02&acdnat=1458641420_c36a7b706956d723a7909a0e540a1742.
36. Shivappa N, Steck SE, Hurley TG, Hussey JR, Ma Y, Ockene IS, et al. A population-based dietary inflammatory index predicts levels of C-reactive protein in the seasonal variation of blood cholesterol study (SEASONS). Publ Health Nutr. 2014;17(08):1825–33.
37. Oellerich M. Enzyme-immunoassay: a review. J Clin Chem Clin Biochem. 1984;22(12):895–904. https://www.ncbi.nlm.nih.gov/pubmed/6396369.
38. Danesh J, Kaptoge S, Mann AG, Sarwar N, Wood A, Angleman SB, et al. Long-term interleukin-6 levels and subsequent risk of coronary heart disease: two new prospective studies and a systematic review. PLoS Med. 2008;5(4):e78. https://www.ncbi.nlm.nih.gov/pubmed/18399716. doi:10.1371/journal.pmed.0050078
39. VanderWeele TJ, Knol MJ. A tutorial on interaction. Epidemiol Methods. 2014;3(1):33–72.
40. Hosmer DW, Lemeshow S. Confidence interval estimation of interaction. Epidemiology. 1992;3(5):452–6.
41. Bedard A, Riverin M, Dodin S, Corneau L, Lemieux S. Sex differences in the impact of the Mediterranean diet on cardiovascular risk profile. Br J Nutr. 2012;108(8):1428–34.
42. Leblanc V, Begin C, Hudon AM, Royer MM, Corneau L, Dodin S, et al. Gender differences in the long-term effects of a nutritional intervention program promoting the Mediterranean diet: changes in dietary intakes, eating behaviors, anthropometric and metabolic variables. Nutr J. 2014; 13107. https://www.ncbi.nlm.nih.gov/pubmed/25416917. doi:10.1186/1475-2891-13-107.
43. Blomstedt Y, Norberg M, Stenlund H, Nystrom L, Lonnberg G, Boman K, et al. Impact of a combined community and primary care prevention strategy on all-cause and cardiovascular mortality: a cohort analysis based on 1 million person-years of follow-up in Vasterbotten County, Sweden, during 1990–2006. BMJ open. 2015;5:12:e009651. https://www.ncbi.nlm.nih.gov/pubmed/26685034.
44. Mann J, Nye ER. Fad diets in Sweden, of all places. Lancet. 2009;374(9692):767–9.
45. Johansson I, Nilsson LM, Stegmayr B, Boman K, Hallmans G, Winkvist A. Associations among 25-year trends in diet, cholesterol and BMI from 140,000 observations in men and women in Northern Sweden. Nutr J. 2012; 1140. https://www.ncbi.nlm.nih.gov/pubmed/22686621.
46. Johansson G, Wikman Å, Åhrén A-M, Hallmans G, Johansson I. Underreporting of energy intake in repeated 24-h recalls related to gender, age, weight status, day of interview, educational level, reported food intake, smoking habits and area of living. Publ Health Nutr. 2001;4(04):919–27.
47. Hebert JR, Clemow L, Pbert L, Ockene IS, Ockene JK. Social desirability bias in dietary self-report may compromise the validity of dietary intake measures. Int J Epidemiol. 1995;24(2):389–98. https://www.ncbi.nlm.nih.gov/pubmed/7635601.
48. Hebert JR, Ma Y, Clemow L, Ockene IS, Saperia G, Stanek 3rd EJ, et al. Gender differences in social desirability and social approval bias in dietary self-report. Am J Epidemiol. 1997;146(12):1046–55. https://www.ncbi.nlm.nih.gov/pubmed/9420529.
49. Hebert JR, Ebbeling CB, Matthews CE, Hurley TG, Ma Y, Druker S, et al. Systematic errors in middle-aged women's estimates of energy intake: comparing three self-report measures to total energy expenditure from doubly labeled water. Ann Epidemiol. 2002;12(8):577–86.
50. Hebert JR, Peterson KE, Hurley TG, Stoddard AM, Cohen N, Field AE, et al. The effect of social desirability trait on self-reported dietary measures among multi-ethnic female health center employees. Ann Epidemiol. 2001; 11(6):417–27. <Go to ISI>://WOS:000170274300008.

21

Effects of whole grain rye, with and without resistant starch type 2 supplementation, on glucose tolerance, gut hormones, inflammation and appetite regulation in an 11–14.5 hour perspective; a randomized controlled study in healthy subjects

Jonna C. Sandberg*, Inger M. E. Björck and Anne C. Nilsson

Abstract

Background: The prevalence of obesity is increasing worldwide and prevention is needed. Whole grain has shown potential to lower the risk of obesity, cardiovascular disease and type 2 diabetes. One possible mechanism behind the benefits of whole grain is the gut fermentation of dietary fiber (DF), e.g. non-starch polysaccharides and resistant starch (RS), in whole grain. The purpose of the study is to investigate the effect of whole grain rye-based products on glucose- and appetite regulation.

Method: Twenty-one healthy subjects were provided four rye-based evening test meals in a crossover overnight study design. The test evening meals consisted of either whole grain rye flour bread (RFB) or a 1:1 ratio of whole grain rye flour and rye kernels bread (RFB/RKB), with or without added resistant starch (+RS). White wheat flour bread (WWB) was used as reference evening meal. Blood glucose, insulin, PYY, FFA, IL-6 as well as breath H_2 and subjective rating of appetite were measured the following morning at fasting and repeatedly up to 3.5 h after a standardized breakfast consisting of WWB. *Ad libitum* energy intake was determined at lunch, 14.5 h after evening test and reference meals, respectively.

Results: The evening meal with RFB/RKB + RS decreased postprandial glucose- and insulin responses (iAUC) ($P < 0.05$) and increased the gut hormone PYY in plasma the following morning 0–120 min after the standardized breakfast, compared to WWB ($P = 0.01$). Moreover, RFB increased subjective satiety and decreased desire to eat, and both RFB and RFB/RKB decreased feeling of hunger (AUC 0–210 min). All rye-based evening meals decreased or tended to decrease fasting FFA ($P < 0.05$, RFB/RKB: $P = 0.057$) and increased breath hydrogen concentration (0–120 min, $P < 0.001$). No effects were noted on energy intake at lunch or inflammatory marker IL-6 (0 + 180 min) after the rye-based evening meals, compared to WWB.
(Continued on next page)

* Correspondence: jonna.sandberg@food-health-science.lu.se
Food for Health Science Centre, Lund University, SE-221 00 Lund, Sweden

(Continued from previous page)

Conclusion: Whole grain rye bread has the potential to improve cardiometabolic variables in an 11–14.5 h perspective in healthy humans. The combination RFB/RKB + RS positively affected biomarkers of glucose- and appetite regulation in a semi-acute perspective. Meanwhile, RFB and RFB/RKB improved subjective appetite ratings. The effects probably emanate from gut fermentation events.

Trial registration: The study was registered at: ClinicalTrials.gov, register number NCT02347293 (www.clinicaltrials.gov/ct2/show/NCT02347293). Registered 15 January 2015.

Keywords: Rye, Glucose regulation, Dietary fiber, Whole grain, Dietary prevention, Gut hormones, Appetite regulation, Gut fermentation, Type 2 diabetes, Obesity

Background

The worldwide increase in prevalence of obesity-related metabolic diseases such as the metabolic syndrome, cardiovascular disease and type 2 diabetes is predicted to continue [1]. These diseases are lifestyle-related and therefore to a large extent preventable. In this respect, increased intake of whole grain (WG) has shown health benefits. Thus epidemiological data show that WG intake is associated with reduced risk of type 2 diabetes [2], cardiovascular disease [3], and also a decreased risk of obesity and weight gain [4]. At least parts of the beneficial effects of WG are suggested to emanate from mechanisms originating from gut fermentation of indigestible carbohydrates, i.e. dietary fiber (DF) components such as non-starch polysaccharides (NSP) and resistant starch (RS). Previously it was shown that intake of whole kernel barley or rye products improved markers of glucose regulation [5–9], and increased gut hormones involved in appetite- and metabolic regulation (GLP-1 and/or PYY) [5–7], 11–14 h after ingestion in healthy subjects. The effects were suggested to originate from gut fermentation of the DF components.

WG flour based products are usually rich in NSP, whereas the RS level is lower in comparison to WG kernel based products, making the total amounts of DF inferior in flour based products. It has previously been suggested that products made from WG flour with a low content of RS did not beneficially affect metabolic variables as oppose to WG kernel based products rich in RS. Consequently, opposite to what was observed after kernel based barley products, it was shown that barley flour porridge did not result in beneficial effects on glucose regulation in a 10.5–12.5 h perspective [10]. The lower concentrations of RS in WG flour may be compensated for e.g. by adding ungelatinized RS (RS2) from high-amylose maize (HAMRS2). RS2 is a fermentable source of DF previously shown to lower acute insulin response (0–420 min after intake) in healthy humans when added to a standardized breakfast and lunch [11]. In addition, adding RS2 to a barley DF supplemented white wheat bread (WWB) improved glucose tolerance at breakfast, 10.5–12.5 h after intake, compared to WWB without supplementation [7]. However, to the best of our knowledge, there is no information regarding the effect of supplementation of RS2 to WG rye products on metabolic parameters in healthy subjects within a short time frame. Rye is a rich source of indigestible carbohydrates mainly in the form of arabinoxylans, fructans, cellulose, β-glucan and lignin [12] but depending on the botanical integrity, i.e. proportion of kernels to flour, the RS content may vary.

The aim of this study was to investigate the potential impact of WG rye products (bread), varying in botanical structure of rye and RS content, on cardiometabolic risk markers and appetite regulation, in a time perspective of 11–14.5 h after intake. For this purpose, four WG rye breads with different flour to kernel ratio and supplementation of commercial RS2 were provided to healthy subjects as evening meals. A white wheat bread was included as a reference evening meal. The rye-based test products and the reference product were consumed in the evening, in a randomized crossover study design, and test markers in blood were determined the next morning prior and following a standardized breakfast to measure glucose regulation (glucose and insulin), gut hormones (peptide YY (PYY)), blood lipids (free fatty acids (FFA)) and inflammatory tonus (interleukin 6 (IL-6)). Additionally, breath hydrogen (H_2) excretion was measured as a marker of gut fermentation, and subjective appetite ratings (hunger, satiety, and desire to eat) were registered. Finally, *ad libitum* energy intake was registered at a lunch provided 3.5 h after the standardized breakfast.

Materials and methods

Ethical statement

The study was registered at ClinicalTrials.gov (NCT02347293). Approval of the study was given by the Regional Ethical Review Board in Lund, Sweden (Reference 2013/241).

Subjects

Twenty-four healthy volunteers, 11 men and 13 women were enrolled in the study. Three of the subjects, 1 man and 2 women, did not complete all five visits. The twenty-one volunteers that completed the study and were included in the statistical evaluation were aged 25.3 ± 3.9 years (mean ± standard deviation (SD)), with normal body mass indices (BMI) (mean ± SD = 22.7 ± 2.3 kg/m^2). The inclusion criteria were age between 20 – 35 years, BMI between 19 and 25 kg/m^2, non-smoker and no known metabolic disorders, food allergies or consumption of any specific diet (e.g. vegetarian or vegan diet). Recruitments of test subjects were ongoing between January 21 to March 3, 2015, and the experimental work was finished by May 22, 2015. Prior inclusion, each subject was given a full written as well as an oral explanation of the purpose and procedure of the study, and written informed consent was obtained from each subject. All test subjects were informed of the possibility of withdrawing from the study at any time they desired.

Test products and reference product

The study included four different rye-based test products, presented as cereal dry matter (DM): 100% whole grain (WG) rye flour based bread (**RFB**), 50% WG rye flour and 50% rye kernel based bread (**RFB/RKB**), 75% WG rye flour based bread with 25% added high-amylose maize flour (Hi-Maize® 260, including 60% RS2) (**RFB + RS**), and 43% WG rye flour and 43% rye kernel based bread with 14% added Hi-Maize® 260 (**RFB/RKB + RS**). A 100% DM white wheat flour based bread (**WWB**) was included as reference product. The proportions of ingredients in the rye-based test products and reference product WWB are displayed in Table 1. The size of the test portions, to be consumed in the evening, was based on 50 g available starch. Both the rye flour and rye kernels (separate commercial blends) were generously provided by Lantmännen Cerealia (Järna, Sweden), Hi-Maize® 260 (60% RS2 and 40% digestible starch) was kindly provided by Kåkå (Lomma, Sweden) and commercial white wheat flour was obtained from Kungsören AB (Järna, Sweden).

RFB

600 g whole grain rye flour, 6 g yeast (Jästbolaget AB, Sollentuna, Sweden) and 6 g NaCl were mixed for 1 min in a food processor (Electrolux Assistent AKM3110W) and then 400 g lukewarm water was added and an additional 4 min of mixing was done. The dough was proofed at room temperature in a bread pan for 30 min. Baking was performed in a house-hold oven at 200 °C with steam the first 15 min and then the bread was covered with aluminum foil the last 45 min (total baking time 60 min).

RFB/RKB

300 g rye kernels were boiled in 250 g salted water (6 g NaCl) for 30 min and then set to cool in room temperature for 30 min. All water was absorbed into the kernels when cooked. 300 g whole grain rye flour and 6 g yeast (Jästbolaget AB, Sollentuna, Sweden) were added to the kernels and were mixed for 4 min in a food processor (Electrolux Assistent AKM3110W). The dough was proofed at room temperature in a bread pan for 30 min. Baking was performed in a house-hold oven at 200 °C with steam the first 15 min and then the bread was covered with aluminum foil the last 45 min (total baking time 60 min).

RFB + RS

The bread was baked according to the same procedure as RFB, except that 200 g Hi-Maize was mixed together with the other dry ingredients (600 g whole grain rye flour, 6 g yeast and 6 g NaCl).

RFB/RKB + RS

The bread was baked according to the same procedure as RFB/RKB, except that 100 g Hi-Maize was mixed together with the 300 g cooled rye kernels along with the other dry ingredients (300 g whole grain rye flour and 6 g yeast).

After baking, the bread was cooled for 3 h, then placed in a plastic bag overnight. In the morning the bread was sliced into portions, wrapped in aluminum foil, put into plastic bags and stored in a freezer (−20 °C). Portion sizes are presented in Table 2.

Table 1 The proportions of cereal ingredients in the rye-based test- and WWB reference evening meals[1]

	Test products				
	RFB	RFB/RKB	RFB + RS	RFB/RKB + RS	WWB
			% dry matter		
Whole grain rye flour	100	50	75	43	-
Rye kernels	-	50	-	43	-
HAMRS2	-	-	25	14	-
White wheat flour	-	-	-	-	100

[1] Data presented as % dry matter. *RFB* rye flour based bread, *RFB/RKB* rye flour and kernel based bread, *RS* resistant starch, *RFB + RS* RFB with added RS, *RFB/RKB + RS* RFB/RKB with added RS, *WWB* white wheat flour based reference bread, *HAMRS2* high-amylose maize resistant starch type 2

Table 2 Portion size and carbohydrate composition of the test- and reference products respectively[1]

Product	Portion size	Starch			NSP		Total DF	DF components	
		Total	Available	RS	Insoluble	Soluble		Fructan	Arabinoxylan
					% dry matter				
RFB		59.3	56.0	3.4	13.9	5.1	22.4	3.3	7.3
RFB/RKB		58.2	51.2	6.9	14.6	4.4	25.9	3.9	7.0
RFB + RS		67.4	54.2	13.2	15.9	3.5	32.6	2.5	5.0
RFB/RKB + RS	-	71.5	58.9	12.7	14.3	4.1	31.1	3.2	6.3
WWB	-	80.2	78.5	1.7	3.4	0.9	6.0	0.5	0.5
					g/portion				
RFB	187.2	53.0	50.0	3.0	11.0	4.1	18.1	3.0	6.5
RFB/RKB	184.0	56.8	50.0	6.8	12.5	3.7	23.0	3.8	6.8
RFB + RS	168.4	62.1	50.0	12.1	11.9	2.9	26.9	2.3	4.6
RFB/RKB + RS	157.9	60.8	50.0	10.8	9.9	3.1	23.8	2.7	5.3
WWB	122.0	51.0	50.0	1.1	2.0	0.5	3.6	0.3	0.3

[1] Data are presented as means. Available starch is calculated as difference between total starch [14] and RS [15]. Values of total starch are based on means of 2 replicates, RS means of 6 replicates and DF are based on means of 2 replicates. Insoluble and soluble DF were determined gravimetrically according to Asp et al. (1983) [16]. The fructan content was analyzed in duplicates using the enzymatic/spectrophotometric AOAC method 999.03 [17]. Analysis of arabinoxylans was performed in duplicates using the Uppsala method [18] and was corrected for the amount of arabinogalactan present by assuming 0.69 ratio between arabinose and galactose [19]. Total DF include RS, and insoluble and soluble NSP. *RFB* rye flour based bread, *RFB/RKB* rye flour and kernel based bread, *RS* resistant starch, *RFB + RS* RFB with added RS, *RFB/RKB + RS* RFB/RK with added RS, *DF* dietary fiber, *NSP* non-starch polysaccharides, *WWB* white wheat flour based reference bread

WWB

The WWB was baked in a home baking machine (Tefal home bread model nr. 573102; Menu choice, program 2 [white bread, 1000 g, quick (time2:32)]) according to a standardized procedure. The bread ingredients consisted of 540 g white wheat flour, 360 g water, 4.8 g dry yeast and 4.8 g NaCl. After cooling, the crust was removed and the bread was sliced and portions were wrapped in aluminum foil, put into plastic bags and stored in a freezer (−20 °C). Portion sizes are presented in Table 2. WWB was used both as reference evening meal and included in the standardized breakfast, see below.

The test subjects stored the bread products in their freezer during the study period. At the day of consumption, they were instructed to take a portion from the freezer in the morning and thaw it at ambient temperature, still wrapped in aluminum foil and in the plastic bag. Optional amounts of water, coffee or tea (without milk and/or sugar) were allowed to be consumed with the test- and reference products.

Standardized breakfast

The standardized breakfast consisted of 122.0 g WWB, corresponding to 50 g available starch, and 200 ml of water. The breakfast bread was baked according the same standardized procedure as WWB, reference product.

Ad libitum lunch

To evaluate *ad libitum* energy intake, the test subjects were instructed to serve themselves with lunch consisted of fried Swedish hash, i.e. diced potato, meat and onion (Felix Krögarpytt Klassisk), from an oven sheet. The lunch was generously provided by Orkla Foods Sverige AB (Malmö, Sweden). According to previous analysis by Johansson et al. (2013) the nutritional content is 234 kcal/100 g of Swedish hash, whereof the proportion of macronutrients (% DM) is 38.5% carbohydrates, 13.9% protein and 27.5% fat [6]. 100 ml of water was provided just before the lunch was served.

Study design and procedure

The study included five bread products: four test products (RFB, RFB/RKB, RFB + RS and RFB/RKB + RS) and one reference product (WWB) which were consumed as evening meals (09.00 pm) in a randomized cross-over study design, with approximately 1 week in between each test product. After this meal, the test subjects were fasting until the standardized breakfast was served the following morning at the research unit Food for Health Science Centre, Lund University. Number of participants ($n = 21$, subjects including in the statistical evaluation) starting with respective product: RFB ($n = 4$), RFB/RKB ($n = 5$), RFB + RS ($n = 3$), RFB/RKB + RS ($n = 5$) and WWB ($n = 4$).

During the day prior to each experimental day, the subjects were encouraged to standardize their meal pattern and to maintain their regular eating habits with the exception to avoid food rich in DF. They were also instructed to avoid alcohol and excessive physical exercise during the day prior to the experimental day. No antibiotics or probiotics were allowed within 2 weeks before or during the study period. To facilitate the standardization of meal patterns prior to each experimental day during the study period, the test subjects were requested to provide a meal record from the day before each experimental day. The test subjects were in addition given a list of foods rich in DF to simplify the instructions regarding avoidance of DF the day before the experimental day. At the experimental days, the subjects arrived to the research unit at 0730 am. Fasting capillary blood samples were collected, and appetite and breath H_2 excretion were registered before the breakfast. A standardized breakfast was served at 0800 am and finished within 15 min. At time point 210 min after commencement of the breakfast, *ad libitum* lunch was served. The test subjects served themselves food from an oven sheet with a surplus of food and were instructed to eat until they felt pleasantly full and to obtain the same degree of induced satiation (i.e. the process that results in termination of eating [13]) at every experimental day. To attain this, they were informed that they were allowed to have a second serving and also to leave food on their plate if necessary. The amount (weight) of lunch consumed was registered. The test subjects were told to sustain a low physical activity during the experimental day (4.5 h).

Chemical analyses of evening meals and standardized breakfast

The test products and breakfast were analyzed with respect to total starch [14], RS [15], NSP (soluble and insoluble) [16], fructans [17] and arabinoxylans [18]. Information regarding the characterization of carbohydrates in the test and reference meals is provided in Table 2. Before analysis of total starch and NSP, the bread products were air dried and milled (IKA A11 basic mixer model A11 B, Germany). RS in all test products were analyzed on products as eaten. The available starch content was calculated by subtracting RS from total starch. The enzymatic/spectrophotometric AOAC method 999.03 was performed to analyze the fructo-oligosaccharides and inulin (in the following referred to as fructans) content, in duplicate, in the test products using the enzyme assay kit K-FRUC (Megazyme, Bray, Ireland). To avoid possible interference of raffinose-series oligosaccharides the analysis included treatment with α-galactosidase [17]. Arabinoxylans were determined by analyzing the monomeric composition in the isolated dietary fiber residue from the test products using the Uppsala method [18]. The amount of arabinoxylan content was calculated from the xylose, galactose and arabinose, and corrected for the amount of arabinogalactan present by assuming ratio 0.69 between arabinose and galactose [19].

Physiological test parameters

Fasting and postprandial measurements were performed at all five visits. Finger-prick capillary blood samplings were applied for determination of blood glucose (HemoCue®B-glucose, HemoCue AB, Ängelholm, Sweden). Additional capillary blood samples were collected to determine serum (s-) insulin, s-FFA, s-IL-6 and plasma (p-) PYY. Breath hydrogen was measured as an indicator of gut fermentation activity, using an EC 60 gastrolyzer (Bedfont EC60 Gastrolyzer, Rochester, England). Pre- and post-breakfast subjective appetite sensations (satiety, hunger and desire to eat) were obtained using a 100 mm Visual Analogue Scale (VAS). Breath H_2 and VAS ratings for subjective appetite (hunger, satiety and desire to eat) were obtained at fasting (time 0 min) and at 15, 30, 45, 60, 90, 120, 180 and 210 min after commencing the breakfast. Blood glucose was determined on similar times points, excluding 210 min, and s-insulin was collected at all time points except 15 and 210 min. Plasma PYY was determined at time 0 min and at 120 min after breakfast. Serum IL-6 was obtained at time 0 min and at 180 min. Serum FFA was determined at time 0 min.

Serum insulin was determined with a solid phase two-site enzyme immunoassay kit (Insulin ELISA 10-1113-01, Mercodia AB, Uppsala, Sweden), *s-FFA* concentrations with an enzymatic colorimetric method using a 96 well microplate (NEFA C, ACS-ACOD method, WAKO Chemicals GMbH, Germany). The quantitative determination of *s-IL-6* was performed with an enzyme immunoassay (Human IL-6 HS600B, R&D Systems, Abingdon, UK) and the concentrations of *PYY*, both PYY (3–36) and PYY (1–36), in plasma were determined with a competitive enzyme immunoassay (Human PYY EIA YKO8O, Yanaihara Institute Inc. Shizuoka, Japan).

Calculations and statistical methods

Data are expressed as means ± SEM. Statistical evaluations involving glucose and insulin concentrations are based on incremental changes from fasting concentrations. The absolute values are used in the statistical calculations of the rest of the test variables. The incremental area- and area under the curve (iAUC and AUC, respectively) were calculated for each subject and evening meal, using the trapezoid model. iAUC or AUC were used in the statistical evaluation of results regarding blood glucose, insulin and parameters for appetite sensations. Incremental peak (iPeak) concentrations were calculated for glucose and insulin as individual maximum postprandial increase from the baseline. GraphPad Prism (version 6, GraphPad Software, San Diego, CA, USA) was used for graph plotting and calculation of AUC.

Investigations with respect to significant differences in test variables depending on the different evening meals were assessed with ANOVA (general linear model) followed by Dunnett's multiple comparison procedure, using results after the reference product WWB as a control. The data was analyzed in MINITAB Statistical Software (release 17; Minitab, Minitab Inc, State College, PA, USA). The significance level was set at *P*-values < 0.05. In the cases of unevenly distributed residuals (tested with Anderson-Darling and considered unevenly distributed when $P < 0.05$), a Box Cox transformation was performed on the data prior to the ANOVA analysis. Differences between the products at different time points during the experimental day were evaluated using a mixed model (PROC MIXED in SAS release 9.4; SAS Institute Inc, Cary, NC, USA) with repeated measures and an autoregressive covariance structure. Randomization of the consumption order of test products was performed using a random number function in Microsoft Excel 2013 (Washington, USA). If a result of a test variable from a test subject was missing for the reference product, the test subject was excluded from the statistical calculations of that specific test variable. If a result of a test variable from a test subject was missing for one of the test products, the test subject's results for the remaining products will be included in the statistical calculations of that specific test variable. For breath H_2, where the variation in the concentration changed scarcely over time, a weighted mean was produced by calculating a mean for equal time intervals (one mean per hour) over the test period, and then a mean for the different hours was calculated and used in the statistical analysis.

Power calculation

Primary outcome measure was change in blood glucose incremental area under the curve (iAUC) 0–120 min after the standardized breakfast. Number of participants required for the study was determined in MINITAB, using previous results from a study including single evening test meals consisting of rye kernels and the effects the following morning on glucose incremental area under the curve 0–120 min (iAUC) [5]. Assuming a 44 mmol · min/L (25%) difference between consumption of WWB compared to rye-based test products the previous evening, and a SD of 60 mmol · min/L, with $\alpha = 0.05$ and $1 - \beta = 0.8$, a minimum number of 17 participants were required (two-tailed test). However, due to lack of information from previous similar study designs including different rye flour based products and including drop-out margin, we recruited 24 test subjects. Three of the subjects dropped out of the study, which resulted in 21 subjects remaining in the statistical evaluation.

Results

Glucose and insulin

Compared to the WWB reference evening meal, the evening meal consisting of RFB/RKB + RS decreased (iAUC 0–120 min) responses for glucose (−27%) and insulin (−21%) in the morning following the standardized breakfast, see Table 3 and Fig. 1. A strong tendency to decrease glucose iPeak concentrations was observed after the standardized breakfast following intake of RFB/RKB + RS evening meal (−17%, $P = 0.057$), compared to WWB, see Table 3 and Fig. 1. The evening meal with RFB, in comparison to the WWB evening meal, resulted in a non-significant trend towards a decrease (−19%, $P = 0.100$) in postprandial glucose responses (iAUC 0–120 min) to the standardized breakfast. There were no significant differences in fasting values after test products compared to reference product for neither glucose nor insulin concentrations.

Table 3 B-glucose, s-insulin, s-FFA, p-PYY and s-IL-6 concentrations 11–14 h following test- and reference evening meals[1]

	WWB	RFB		RFB/RKB		RFB + RS		RFB/RKB + RS	
			%Δ[2]		%Δ[2]		%Δ[2]		%Δ[2]
Glucose, Fasting[3] *(mmol/l)*	5.4 ± 0.1	5.3 ± 0.1	−1	5.4 ± 0.1	0	5.4 ± 0.1	1	5.3 ± 0.1	−2
Glucose, iAUC 0–120 min[3] *(mmol · min/l)*	153.0 ± 13.2	123.6 ± 10.8	−19	140.2 ± 13.8	−8	138.8 ± 15.0	−9	112.1 ± 10.6	−27*
Glucose, iPeak [3] *(mmol/l)*	2.9 ± 0.2	2.6 ± 0.2	−11	2.8 ± 0.2	−3	2.8 ± 0.2	−2	2.4 ± 0.2	−17†
Insulin, Fasting[3] *(nmol/l)*	0.034 ± 0.002	0.038 ± 0.003	13	0.037 ± 0.003	10	0.036 ± 0.003	6	0.033 ± 0.002	−3
Insulin, iAUC 0–120 min[3] *(nmol · min/l)*	9.88 ± 1.21	8.50 ± 0.91	−14	9.52 ± 1.13	−4	9.40 ± 1.00	−5	7.86 ± 0.78	−21*
Insulin, iPeak[3] *(nmol · min/l)*	0.16 ± 0.02	0.16 ± 0.02	0	0.16 ± 0.02	0	0.17 ± 0.02	1	0.15 ± 0.02	−8
FFA, Fasting *(mmol/l)*	0.65 ± 0.04[3]	0.54 ± 0.04[4]	−17*	0.54 ± 0.04[4]	−17†	0.54 ± 0.04[3]	−17*	0.54 ± 0.03[3]	−17*
PYY, Fasting[4] *(ng/ml)*	0.50 ± 0.09	0.54 ± 0.10	7	0.53 ± 0.09	6	0.53 ± 0.10	6	0.59 ± 0.09	17*
PYY, Mean 0 + 120 min[4] *(ng/ml)*	0.50 ± 0.09	0.53 ± 0.10	5	0.52 ± 0.09	5	0.53 ± 0.09	6	0.58 ± 0.09	15**
IL-6, Fasting *(pg/ml)*	1.08 ± 0.21[3]	0.81 ± 0.06[3]	−25	0.93 ± 0.12[3]	−15	1.00 ± 0.12[4]	−7	0.82 ± 0.09[3]	−25
IL-6, Mean 0 + 180 *(pg/ml)*	1.33 ± 0.22[4]	1.04 ± 0.15[5]	−22	1.02 ± 0.14[4]	−23	1.20 ± 0.16[5]	−9	1.02 ± 0.12[4]	−23

[1] Data are presented as means ± SEM. *Different from WWB $P < 0.05$; **$P = 0.01$, †$P = 0.057$ (ANOVA followed by Dunnett's test). [2] The percentage change is calculated as the difference from the WWB. [3] $n = 21$, [4] $n = 20$, [5] $n = 19$ healthy subjects. *RFB* rye flour bread, *RFB/RKB* 50/50 rye flour and rye kernel bread, + *RS* added resistant starch, *iAUC* incremental area under curve, *iPeak* incremental peak

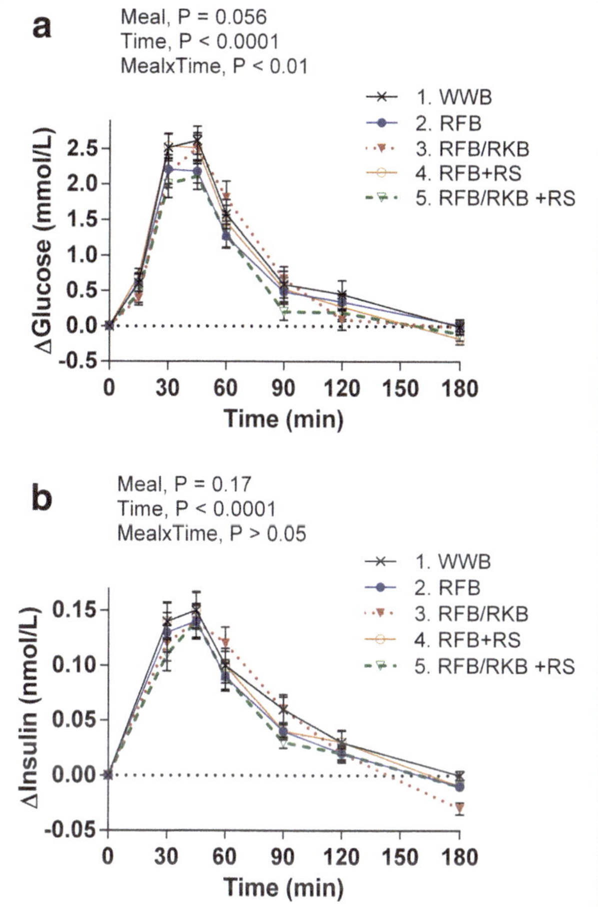

Fig. 1 Incremental blood glucose- and serum insulin concentrations after a standardized breakfast following the evening meals Changes (Δ) in mean incremental concentrations of blood glucose (**a**) and serum insulin (**b**) from fasting concentrations in the morning after a standardized breakfast, 11–14 h following the rye-based test- or WWB reference evening meals. Values are means ± SEM. Repeated measures; mixed model in SAS. RFB, rye flour bread; RFB/RKB, 50/50 rye flour and rye kernel bread; + RS, added resistant starch; WWB, white wheat bread

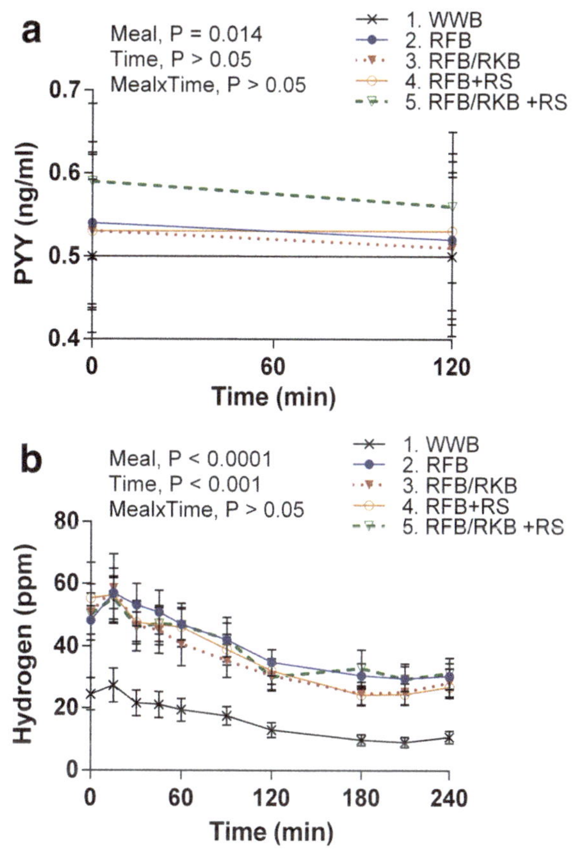

Fig. 2 Concentrations of plasma PYY and breath hydrogen after a standardized breakfast following the evening meals Mean concentrations of plasma PYY (**a**) and breath hydrogen excretion (**b**) in the morning after a standardized breakfast, 11–13 h respectively 11–14.5 h following the rye-based test- or WWB reference evening meals. Values are means ± SEM. Repeated measures; mixed model in SAS. RFB, rye flour bread; RFB/RKB, 50/50 rye flour and rye kernel bread; + RS, added resistant starch; WWB, white wheat bread

s-FFA

The fasting concentrations of FFA are presented in Table 3 and were significantly decreased after test evening meals with RFB, RFB + RS and RFB/RKB + RS, compared to WWB (−17% for all, $P < 0.05$). Additionally, a tendency towards decreased FFA concentrations was shown after RFB/RKB (−17%, $P = 0.057$).

s-IL-6

No differences were observed in the concentrations of IL-6 depending on the evening meal, see Table 3.

p-PYY

P-PYY response at the standardized breakfast is presented in Table 3 and Fig. 2. In comparison with the reference WWB, the evening meal comprising RFB/RKB + RS resulted in an increased p-PYY concentration at fasting (+17%, $P < 0.05$) as well as an increased postprandial mean concentration including time points 0 and 120 min (+15%, $P = 0.01$).

Breath H_2

The response in breath H_2 is presented in Table 4 and Fig. 2. In comparison to WWB, all rye-based evening meals resulted in increased breath H_2 levels at fasting, that remained increased after the standardized breakfast ($P < 0.001$).

Subjective appetite ratings and energy intake

The data for subjective appetite ratings are shown in Table 4 and Fig. 3. The RFB evening meal significantly increased the feeling of satiety (21%, $P < 0.01$) and decreased feelings of hunger (−15%, $P < 0.05$) and desire to eat (−20%, $P < 0.01$) during the experimental day, 0–210 min after the standardized breakfast (AUC),

Table 4 Breath hydrogen excretion, subjective appetite ratings and voluntary energy intake (lunch), following the evening meals[1]

	WWB	RFB		RFB/RKB		RFB + RS		RFB/RKB + RS	
			%Δ[2]		%Δ[2]		%Δ[2]		%Δ[2]
Hydrogen, Fasting[3] *(ppm)*	24.5 ± 5.3	48.3 ± 4.5	97***	50.8 ± 9.0	107***	55.3 ± 11.5	126***	50.2 ± 6.6	105***
Hydrogen, Mean 0–210 min *(ppm)*	16.2 ± 2.9[3]	40.4 ± 4.0[3]	150***	35.9 ± 5.5[3]	122***	37.6 ± 4.3[3]	133***	34.8 ± 4.5[4]	115***
Satiety, Fasting[3] *(mm)*	29.2 ± 4.5	35.0 ± 5.3	20	37.9 ± 5.9	30	29.6 ± 4.3	2	33.3 ± 6.1	14
Satiety, AUC 0-210 min *(mm · min)*	9590 ± 930[5]	11640 ± 950[5]	21**	11390 ± 1110[6]	19	10070 ± 930[5]	5	10400 ± 910[6]	8
Hunger, Fasting[3] *(mm)*	61.2 ± 4.4	52.5 ± 6.4	−14	51.7 ± 6.0	−15	58.6 ± 5.7	−4	58.3 ± 5.7	−5
Hunger, AUC 0–210 min *(mm · min)*	10400 ± 950[5]	8800 ± 880[7]	−15*	8680 ± 1070[4]	−17*	10090 ± 910[5]	−3	9340 ± 840[6]	−10
Desire to eat, Fasting[3] *(mm)*	67.1 ± 5.0	62.9 ± 5.8	−6	58.7 ± 5.7	−13	68.3 ± 5.5	2	63.4 ± 6.7	−6
Desire to eat, AUC 0–210 min *(mm · min)*	11360 ± 1020[5]	9070 ± 1030[5]	−20**	9750 ± 1170[4]	−14	11110 ± 1020[5]	−2	11450 ± 1090[6]	1
Energy intake, Lunch[3] *(kcal)*	689 ± 87	657 ± 74	−5	644 ± 73	−7	649 ± 61	−6	667 ± 70	−3

[1] Data are presented as means ± SEM. *Different from WWB $P < 0.05$; **$P < 0.01$, ***$P < 0.001$ (ANOVA followed by Dunnett's test). [2] The percentage change is calculated as the difference from the WWB. [3] $n = 21$, [4] $n = 18$, [5] $n = 20$, [6] $n = 17$, [7] $n = 19$ healthy subjects. *RFB* rye flour bread, *RFB/RKB* 50/50 rye flour and rye kernel bread, + *RS* added resistant starch, *AUC* area under curve

compared to WWB. In addition, the evening meal RFB/RKB decreased the hunger sensation during the experimental day (AUC 0–210 min, −17%, $P < 0.05$). No significant differences were seen in the energy intake at lunch depending on the evening meal.

Discussion

It has previously been shown that certain kernel based cereal products, e.g. barley kernel products, and more recently also rye kernel products, beneficially affected cardiometabolic test variables 11–16 h [6] or 10.5–13.5 h [5] after intake, in comparison to a flour based product (WWB). The effects were proposed to emanate from gut fermentation of the mixture of DF in the intact kernels, i.e. NSP and RS. In the present study, it was hypothesized that similar metabolic benefits could be achieved also with bread containing rye flour or rye flour mixed with rye kernels by simulating the DF composition and amount in the intact kernels, through supplementation with commercial RS (HAMRS2) to compensate for the loss of RS (RS1) in the milling process. Previous inclusion of HAMRS2 in the diet was shown to beneficially impact insulin demand up to 7 h after ingestion in healthy humans and to reduce energy intake during 24 h, compared to a low-RS diet [11]. RS has also been shown to stimulate secretion of GLP-1 and PYY in rats fed a RS diet for 10 days [20].

The hypothesis was confirmed, with respect to the RFB/RKB product with and without RS supplementation. Consequently, postprandial glucose regulation was improved and plasma PYY levels increased in a time perspective of 11–13 h after intake of the RFB/RKB + RS, compared to WWB. No such effects were seen after the RFB/RKB without RS supplementation. The results are thus in support of the importance of RS components, and/or the specific mixture of NSP and RS in kernels on metabolic regulation. However, independently of the RS content, all rye-based test products resulted in a decrease in fasting FFA concentrations the following morning compared to the WWB evening meal, with potential benefits on insulin sensitivity. An improved glucose regulation and decreased concentrations of FFA were recently observed in the morning when rye kernel based bread was included as an evening meal [5]. Increased levels of FFA have been observed in type 2 diabetes patients compared to those with normal glucose tolerance [21] and were associated with impaired insulin signaling [22]. Hence, the present results indicate that rye kernels have beneficial semi-acute effects on glucose regulation and insulin sensitivity.

Previously, intake of rye kernels were shown to increase plasma levels of SCFA 10.5 h after intake [5], and as judged from the increased levels of breath H_2 following the rye-based evening meals, the metabolic benefits seen in the present work are most likely emanating from gut fermentation. Substrate-induced increase in SCFA concentrations in the gut may potentially have beneficial implications on appetite- and metabolic regulation since SCFA has been suggested to stimulate the L-cells to secrete GLP-1 and PYY [23], and in addition increase the uptake of circulating FFA [24]. In the present study, plasma levels of SCFA were not determined. However, RFB/RKB + RS significantly increased the concentrations of plasma PYY 11 and 13 h after intake. In fact, the other rye-based products also tended to increase the PYY concentrations in plasma. It has previously been shown that intravenous infusion with PYY in lean or obese subjects decreased the food intake with 31% respectively 30%, at an *ad libitum* buffet served after 2 h, compared to infusion with saline [25], indicating an anti-obesogenic potential of PYY. A rye kernel based evening meal has previously shown to increase both PYY and GLP-1 the following morning [5]. In this context, although GLP-1 concentrations were not measured

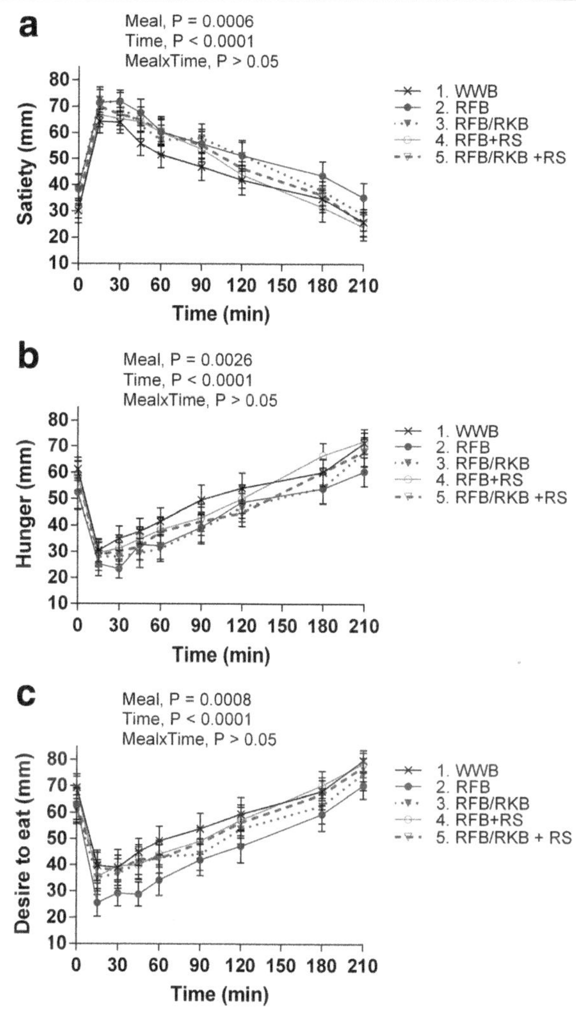

Fig. 3 Subjective appetite ratings after a standardized breakfast following rye-based test- or WWB reference evening meal Data is presented as mean ± SEM of subjective appetite ratings (VAS) of satiety (**a**), hunger (**b**) and desire to eat (**c**) during the following 3.5 h after standardized breakfast in the morning, 11–14.5 h after intake of a rye-based evening meal or a WWB reference evening meal. Repeated measures; mixed model in SAS. RFB, rye flour bread; RFB/RKB, 50/50 rye flour and rye kernel bread; + RS, added resistant starch; WWB, white wheat bread

in this study due to small quantities of plasma via capillary sampling, it might be anticipated that an increase in PYY would indicate a potential increase also in GLP-1 since PYY is co-released together with GLP-1 after a meal [26]. These gut hormones have been shown to have anti-diabetic properties [27] and could partially explain the improved glucose regulation after intake of the rye-based test products.

Despite the significantly increased PYY levels in the present study, the effects on appetite variables and energy intake at lunch did not reach statistical significance after intake of RFB/RKB + RS. Instead, the non-supplement products, i.e. 100% flour based rye bread (RFB) and the RFB/RKB bread, which induced less increased PYY levels compared to RFB/RKB + RS, showed the most pronounced beneficial effects on subjective appetite ratings. In accordance, it has been reported that PYY levels do not always correlate with subjective appetite [28]. However, this does not preclude the potential role of PYY in the appetite regulation but that the mechanisms remain to be elucidated.

Although no significant effects on energy intake at lunch depending on the previous evening meals could be detected in this study, there was a non-significant decrease in energy intake after RFB/RKB evening meal (−7%) in comparison to the WWB. Consequently, this is in accordance with results after boiled rye kernels in a previous study with similar study design [29]. A decrease in energy intake (−12%) in this time perspective has previously been shown also after intake of barley kernel based products [6], indicating potential anti-obesogenic properties of certain fermentable DF. The energy content at the standardized breakfast in the current study, 273 kcal, can be considered to be low (kcal content obtained from [30]), and it can be speculated that, at least for some of the test subjects, the low energy content at breakfast could have interfered with the possibility to differentiate voluntary energy chosen at the subsequent lunch. The previous over-night studies ([6, 29]), including barley or rye as an evening meal, showed effects on voluntary energy intake at lunch after a more realistic and high caloric breakfast composed of either an *ad libitum* breakfast [6] or a breakfast with e.g. butter, cheese, jam (and a pastry) [29]. In this context it is worth to consider that these breakfasts probably closer resemble the test subjects' normal diets compared to the breakfast included in the current study (WWB and water).

It has previously been shown that an evening meal including WWB supplemented with a mix of RS (similar to the RS product used in the present study) and NSP (from barley) in proportions similar to the composition and content of indigestible carbohydrates in intrinsic barley kernels, significantly lowered the glucose response the following morning. Further it was observed that supplementation of a WWB with RS or DF separately did not improve glucose tolerance the next morning, compared to un-supplemented WWB [7, 9]. This indicates that the combination of RS and NSP is necessary to mediate benefits on glucose tolerance in a time perspective of approximately 10–14 h, such as from the evening meal to a subsequent standardized breakfast. As expected, based on the chemical analysis it was confirmed that RFB and RFB/RKB contained less RS compared to the RS supplemented products. In the present study the RS supplementation of the RFB/RKB product seems to be important with respect to effects on glucose regulation and release of PYY. However, supplement with RS in the form of HAMRS2 did not improve other test variables included in the study. Probably both the total amounts- and composition of DF components are important. The rye portion in the RFB + RS was replaced with 25% HAMRS2 flour (DM), and in the RFB/RKB + RS the replacement with HAMRS2 flour was 14%. The HAMRS2 flour product included, in addition to RS (60%), a considerable proportion of available starch (40%). Thus, the lack of benefits with the HAMRS2 supplement to RFB, i.e. RFB + RS, can possibly be due to an important loss of rye DF due to dilution of the rye dry matter when replacing rye flour with HAMRS2. A loss of DF was confirmed in the chemical analysis and showed that both RFB + RS and RFB/RKB + RS contained lower concentrations of soluble DF, and decreased levels of fructans and arabinoxylans, compared to the breads without RS supplementation. Thus, since the only known difference between the ingredients in rye-based products is the addition of RS, it can be suggested that the comparatively high concentrations of soluble fiber in the un-supplemented RFB and RFB/RKB could have contributed to the beneficial effects observed on appetite ratings after these products. This is to the best of our knowledge the first study that observes significant difference in appetite ratings 11–14.5 h after intake of WG rye flour product. These effects have previously only been observed in acute studies when serving WG rye flour bread as breakfast [31, 32].

A limitation in the study was the small volumes of blood samples obtained, due to capillary blood sampling instead of venous blood sampling. Consequently, it was not possible to investigate additional parameters of inflammatory variables and gut hormones. Another potential study limitation was the relative low number of subjects and the low energy intake at breakfast when investigating subjective appetite sensations during the experimental day and voluntary food intake at lunch. Nevertheless, the appetite ratings and energy registration from the present study indicate that rye-based products, in particular the combination of WG rye flour and rye kernels (RFB/RKB), have the potential to lower energy intake at the subsequent day, but further studies are necessary to confirm this.

Conclusion

The present study showed that addition of RS to a rye bread based on 50% intact kernels and 50% WG flour (DM) beneficially impact metabolic parameters in an 11–14 h perspective, as demonstrated by improved postprandial glucose regulation, decreased concentration of FFA at fasting and increased levels of PYY. In addition, it was shown that WG rye flour bread contributed to increased sensation of satiety and that WG rye flour bread solely or combined with rye kernels lowered perceived hunger sensations, 11–14.5 h after intake. The findings suggest that WG rye has anti-diabetic and anti-obesogenic potential. More studies are needed to further evaluate the metabolic effects of inclusion of commercially available RS fractions in different food matrices.

Abbreviations

AUC: Area under curve; b-: Blood-; BMI: Body mass index; DF: Dietary fiber; DM: Dry matter; f-: Fasting-; FFA: Free fatty acids; GLP-1: Glucagon-like peptide-1; H_2: Breath hydrogen; HAMRS2: High-amylose maize resistant starch type 2; iAUC: Incremental area under curve; IL-6: Interleukin-6; iPeak: Incremental peak; NSP: Non-starch polysaccharides; PYY: Peptide YY; RFB: Rye flour bread; RKB: Rye kernel bread; RS: Resistant starch; RS2: Resistant starch type 2; SCFA: Short chain fatty acids; SD: Standard deviation; SEM: Standard error mean; VAS: Visual analogue scale; WG: Whole grain; WWB: White wheat bread

Acknowledgement

This project has been funded by grants from the VINNOVA Excellence Centre Antidiabetic Food Centre, Lund University, Lund, Sweden. Rye flour and rye kernels were provided by Lantmännen Cerealia (Järna, Sweden), Hi-Maize® 260 was provided by Kåkå (Lomma, Sweden) and Felix Krögarpytt Klassisk was provided by Orkla Foods Sverige AB (Malmö, Sweden). Funders and companies providing study supplies had no role in study design, data collection and analysis, decision to publish, or preparation of the manuscript.

Funding

This study was funded by the Lund University Antidiabetic Food Centre, a VINNOVA VINN Excellence Centre.

Availability of data and materials

The datasets analyzed during this study are available from the corresponding author on reasonable request.

Authors' contributions

The authors' responsibilities were as follows: ACN, IMEB and JCS designed the study; JCS coordinated the study, performed the majority of the experimental work and the statistical calculations. ACN, IMEB and JCS evaluated the data, wrote the paper and had primary responsibility for the final content. All authors read and approved the final manuscript.

Competing interests

The authors declare that they have no competing interests.

Consent for publication

Not applicable

Ethics approval and consent to participate

Approval of the study was given by the Regional Ethical Review Board in Lund, Sweden (Reference 2013/241). Prior to inclusion, each subject got a full written and oral explanation of the purpose and procedure of the study and written informed consent was obtained from each subject.

Publisher's Note

References

1. World Health Organization. World Health Statistics 2012. 2012. [cited 2016 7 June]; Available from: http://apps.who.int/iris/bitstream/10665/44844/1/9789241564441_eng.pdf.
2. Yao B, et al. Dietary fiber intake and risk of type 2 diabetes: a dose–response analysis of prospective studies. Eur J Epidemiol. 2014;29(2):79–88.
3. Threapleton DE, et al. Dietary fibre intake and risk of cardiovascular disease: systematic review and meta-analysis. BMJ. 2013;347:f6879.
4. Ye EQ, et al. Greater whole-grain intake is associated with lower risk of type 2 diabetes, cardiovascular disease, and weight gain. J Nutr. 2012;142:1304–13.

5. Sandberg JC, Björck IME, Nilsson AC. Rye-based evening meals favorably affected glucose regulation and appetite variables at the following breakfast; a randomized controlled study in healthy subjects. PLoS One. 2016;11(3):e0151985.
6. Johansson EV, et al. Effects of indigestible carbohydrates in barley on glucose metabolism, appetite and voluntary food intake over 16 h in healthy adults. Nutr J. 2013;12:46.
7. Nilsson AC, et al. Including indigestible carbohydrates in the evening meal of healthy subjects improves glucose tolerance, lowers inflammatory markers, and increases satiety after a subsequent standardized breakfast. J Nutr. 2008;138(4):732–9.
8. Priebe MG, et al. Factors related to colonic fermentation of nondigestible carbohydrates of a previous evening meal increase tissue glucose uptake and moderate glucose-associated inflammation. Am J Clin Nutr. 2010;91(1):90–7.
9. Nilsson AC, et al. Effect of cereal test breakfasts differing in glycemic index and content of indigestible carbohydrates on daylong glucose tolerance in healthy subjects. Am J Clin Nutr. 2008;87(3):645–54.
10. Nilsson A, et al. Effects of GI vs content of cereal fibre of the evening meal on glucose tolerance at a subsequent standardized breakfast. Eur J Clin Nutr. 2008;62(6):712–20.
11. Bodinham CL, Frost GS, Robertson MD. Acute ingestion of resistant starch reduces food intake in healthy adults. Br J Nutr. 2010;103(6):917–22.
12. Frolich W, Aman P, Tetens I. Whole grain foods and health - a Scandinavian perspective. Food Nutr Res. 2013;57(1):18503.
13. Blundell J, et al. Appetite control: methodological aspects of the evaluation of foods. Obes Rev. 2010;11(3):251–70.
14. Björck IME, Siljeström MA. In-vivo and in-vitro digestibility of starch in autoclaved pea and potato products. J Sci Food Agric. 1992;58(4):541–53.
15. Akerberg AK, et al. An in vitro method, based on chewing, to predict resistant starch content in foods allows parallel determination of potentially available starch and dietary fiber. J Nutr. 1998;128(3):651–60.
16. Asp NG, et al. Rapid enzymatic assay of insoluble and soluble dietary fiber. J Agric Food Chem. 1983;31(3):476–82.
17. McCleary BV, Murphy A, Mugford DC. Measurement of total fructan in foods by enzymatic/spectrophotometric method: collaborative study. J AOAC Int. 2000;83(2):356–64.
18. Theander O, et al. Total dietary fiber determined as neutral sugar residues, uronic acid residues, and Klason lignin (the Uppsala method): collaborative study. J AOAC Int. 1995;78(4):1030–44.
19. Loosveld A-MA, Grobet PJ, Delcour JA. Contents and structural features of water-extractable arabinogalactan in wheat flour fractions. J Agric Food Chem. 1997;45(6):1998–2002.
20. Zhou J, et al. Dietary resistant starch upregulates total GLP-1 and PYY in a sustained day-long manner through fermentation in rodents. Am J Physiol Endocrinol Metab. 2008;295(5):E1160–6.
21. Reaven GM, et al. Measurement of plasma glucose, free fatty acid, lactate, and insulin for 24 h in patients with NIDDM. Diabetes. 1988;37(8):1020–4.
22. Belfort R, et al. Dose-response effect of elevated plasma free fatty acid on insulin signaling. Diabetes. 2005;54(6):1640–8.
23. Tolhurst G, et al. Short-chain fatty acids stimulate glucagon-like peptide-1 secretion via the G-protein-coupled receptor FFAR2. Diabetes. 2012;61(2):364–71.
24. Canfora EE, Jocken JW, Blaak EE. Short-chain fatty acids in control of body weight and insulin sensitivity. Nat Rev Endocrinol. 2015;11(10):577–91.
25. Batterham RL, et al. Inhibition of food intake in obese subjects by peptide YY3–36. N Engl J Med. 2003;349(10):941–8.
26. De Silva A, Bloom SR. Gut hormones and appetite control: a focus on PYY and GLP-1 as therapeutic targets in obesity. Gut Liver. 2012;6(1):10–20.
27. Tan T, Bloom S. Gut hormones as therapeutic agents in treatment of diabetes and obesity. Curr Opin Pharmacol. 2013;13(6):996–1001.
28. Cooper JA. Factors affecting circulating levels of peptide YY in humans: a comprehensive review. Nutr Res Rev. 2014;27(1):186–97.
29. Ibrugger S, et al. Second meal effect on appetite and fermentation of wholegrain rye foods. Appetite. 2014;80:248–56.
30. Ekstrom LM, Bjorck IM, Ostman EM. On the possibility to affect the course of glycaemia, insulinaemia, and perceived hunger/satiety to bread meals in healthy volunteers. Food Funct. 2013;4(4):522–9.
31. Rosen LA, et al. Postprandial glycemia, insulinemia, and satiety responses in healthy subjects after whole grain rye bread made from different rye varieties. 1. J Agric Food Chem. 2011;59(22):12139–48.
32. Isaksson H, et al. Rye kernel breakfast increases satiety in the afternoon - an effect of food structure. Nutr J. 2011;10:31.

Diverse characteristics of the urinary excretion of amino acids in humans and the use of amino acid supplementation to reduce fatigue and sub-health in adults

R. H. Dunstan[1*], D. L. Sparkes[1], M. M. Macdonald[1], X. Janse De Jonge[2], B. J. Dascombe[3], J. Gottfries[4], C.-G. Gottfries[5] and T. K. Roberts[1]

Abstract

Background: The excretion of amino acids in urine represents an important avenue for the loss of key nutrients. Some amino acids such as glycine and histidine are lost in higher abundance than others. These two amino acids perform important physiological functions and are required for the synthesis of key proteins such as haemoglobin and collagen.

Methods: Stage 1 of this study involved healthy subjects ($n = 151$) who provided first of the morning urine samples and completed symptom questionnaires. Urine was analysed for amino acid composition by gas chromatography. Stage 2 involved a subset of the initial cohort ($n = 37$) who completed a 30 day trial of an amino acid supplement and subsequent symptom profile evaluation.

Results: Analyses of urinary amino acid profiles revealed that three groups could be objectively defined from the 151 participants using k-means clustering. The amino acid profiles were significantly different between each of the clusters (Wilks' Lambda = 0.13, $p < 0.0001$). Cluster 1 had the highest loss of amino acids with histidine being the most abundant component. Cluster 2 had glycine present as the most abundant urinary amino acid and cluster 3 had equivalent abundances of glycine and histidine. Strong associations were observed between urinary proline concentrations and fatigue/pain scores ($r = .56$ to .83) for females in cluster 1, with several other differential sets of associations observed for the other clusters.

Conclusions: Different phenotypic subsets exist in the population based on amino acid excretion characteristics found in urine. Provision of the supplement resulted in significant improvements in reported fatigue and sleep for 81% of the trial cohort with all females reporting improvements in fatigue.

Trial registration: The study was registered on the 18th April 2011 with the Australian New Zealand Clinical Trials Registry (ACTRN12611000403932).

Keywords: Sub-health, Fatigue, Amino acids, Nutritional supplement, Collagen turnover, Urine

* Correspondence: hugh.dunstan@newcastle.edu.au
[1]School of Environmental and Life Sciences, University of Newcastle, Callaghan, Australia
Full list of author information is available at the end of the article

Background

The amino acids derived from ingested proteins are used as substrates for the biosynthesis of structural and functional proteins in the body. These digested amino acids can be used for oxidative phosphorylation and gluconeogenesis [1, 2] as well as the facilitation of numerous physiological functions including acting as precursors for the biosynthesis of neurotransmitters [3], hormones, phosphoglycerols, glycolipids and nucleic acids [4, 5]. It has been estimated that the skeletal muscles in the human body comprise 40–60% of body mass and thus represent the major repository of the body's protein [6]. The body does not maintain specific protein stores, but when it is not possible to obtain sufficient protein via ingestion during exercise, ill health or trauma, the body accesses amino acids via the process of proteolysis where the non-myofibrillar proteins display a high turnover rate to meet demands [7]. The amino acids released from this turnover of protein can enter the blood circulation for metabolism as required and can also be lost in sweat and urine [1, 2]. Healthy resting human adults can achieve nitrogen balance by taking in around 0.8 g/Kg/day of protein [6]; humans synthesise approximately 3 g/Kg/day of new protein [8], indicating that reutilisation of amino acids released during protein turnover is critical to health.

High levels of exercise activity would increase the requirement for protein intake and for protein turnover in order to offset the increased losses of free amino acids arising from demands for energy metabolism, tissue repair and recovery processes [8, 9] as well as excretory losses via sweating [10, 11]. Similar increased demands for amino acids would be seen during illness and recovery from trauma. Increased losses of amino acids were observed in breast cancer patients who suffered fatigue during and following radiation therapy, with evidence for altered amino acid homeostasis [12]. Significantly depleted amino acid levels have also been associated with long-term fatigue [13] leading to the proposal that the nitrogen balance in these patients was less than optimal. A negative nitrogen balance may arise if the supply of amino acids is inadequate as a result of insufficient protein ingestion or impaired digestion such that the body's requirements for protein synthesis cannot be met. The demand for amino acids is met via proteolysis of non-myofibrillar muscle proteins. A prolonged state of negative nitrogen balance could result in proteolysis of myofibrillar proteins which would in turn lead to muscle wasting and damage. Increased metabolic activities to support exercise, mount host defences against infection, or support recovery from illness and injury, place additional demands on protein turnover within the body [6–8].

It has been shown that the levels of several key amino acids including serine, glycine, histidine, alanine and ornithine are present in sweat at much higher concentrations than occur in the plasma [10, 11, 14, 15]. It was proposed that these levels of amino acids in sweat, as has been found to be the case with sweat electrolytes [16], could be achieved by a process of leaching of the amino acids from the natural moisturising factor in the stratum corneum of the skin to combine with the quantities excreted in sweat [10, 11, 15]. The majority of amino acids which constitute the natural moisturising factor are thought to be derived from the protein filaggrin which is primarily composed of glutamine/glutamic acid, arginine/ornithine, serine, proline, glycine, histidine, and aspartic acid/alanine [17]. Loss of amino acids via sweating as a result of exercise, living in a hot climate, or night sweats associated with illness could exacerbate the requirement for proteolysis when the body cannot obtain proteins via ingestion. It is proposed that subjects experiencing a net negative nitrogen balance with depleted amino acid resources would experience fatigue and pain [1, 18, 19]. If a net negative nitrogen balance is associated with fatigue then it would follow that amino acid supplementation would have the potential to assist in restoring nitrogen balance. Provision of free amino acids removes the requirement for digestion of proteins; amino acids can be directly absorbed into the circulation making them rapidly available to the body's tissues and organs including striated muscle. The development of an amino acid supplement is not straightforward as considerations of solubility, palatability, composition and dosage need to be addressed [20]. A pilot study on healthy male subjects from the general population experiencing non-debilitating fatigue, demonstrated that a 30 day period of daily supplementation with a complex formulation of amino acids resulted in significantly improved scores for fatigue as well as associated alterations in urinary excretion of amino acids [21].

An early study from our laboratory revealed that amino acid excretion profiles could delineate human subjects suffering fatigue into population subgroups [22]. The basis for differentiation was thought to involve genetic differences in kidney reabsorption mechanisms, metabolic efficiencies, skin moisturisation and sweating processes as well as environmental factors such as dietary influences and infective history. The proposal that different human phenotypes exist on the basis of amino acid homeostasis may explain why some subjects are more susceptible to developing chronic fatigue or are better able to cope with different types of exercise challenge. Fatigue illness is highly prevalent in Western society and significant fatigue is a common feature of many medical conditions [23]. Sub-health is a state that falls between health and disease and involves psychological, physical and medical components believed to increase the risk of illness [24].

Methods

The current study aimed to determine whether healthy individuals could be separated into discrete subgroups based on the makeup of their urinary excretion profiles. Analyses of a broad range of symptoms were assessed to build a symptom index evaluation of general fatigue, general body pains, gastrointestinal function, sleep and vitality for evaluating sub-health in the general healthy population. Following the initial recruitment and urine analysis, healthy subjects that reported non-debilitating levels of fatigue were provided with a complex amino acid supplement to assess whether supplementation for 30 days would alleviate fatigue. Memberships of population subgroups based on amino acid excretion profiles were tested to determine whether subgroup membership influenced the efficacy of the supplement.

The study involved recruiting healthy adults who were reportedly free from any significant medical or psychological condition. The project was divided into two stages; 172 subjects were initially recruited to supply urine samples for analyses and complete general health and fatigue questionnaires as summarised in Fig. 1. Recruits were not included if they did not provide urinary samples or they did not complete the questionnaires for evaluation of general health symptoms and fatigue. The standardised timing of the urine sample collection was aimed at assessing the profile composition of amino acids representing homeostasis without contributions of the dietary intake associated with the 24 h collection of urine [25]. Participants therefore provided a fasted first of the morning urine sample which was transported in a Urine-Monovette® 10 ml boric acid tube (Sarstedt, Germany). Amino acid analysis of the urine samples was performed using the commercial EZ: Faast™ derivatisation method (esterification of amino acids) followed by gas chromatography/flame ionisation detection (GC/FID) as previously described [25].

The Chalder fatigue scale questionnaire (total 11 items, seven items related to physical symptoms of fatigue and four items related to mental symptoms of fatigue, Likert scored) was used to assess levels of fatigue; the scale has been validated for use in both a healthy population free from any known medical conditions as well as patients with various forms of chronic fatigue [26]. The current general health of the participants was also assessed using an 86 item questionnaire which was based on a questionnaire previously used by our research team [27–29] which included symptoms covering fatigue, pain, gastrointestinal (GIT), cognitive, neurological and infection related symptoms. Participants were required to report how much they had been affected by these symptoms during the previous 7 days. The questionnaire was Likert scored with responses ranging from 0 "not at all" to 4 "extremely". Five symptom indices were compiled from symptoms pertaining to the categories of general fatigue, general body pain, GIT function, sleep and vitality in order to evaluate the potential influence of supplementation on general health as shown in Table 1. General body pain and GIT symptoms were monitored to determine whether any adverse side effects were associated with the amino acid supplement. Correlation and factor analyses were carried out to select the minimum number of optimal symptoms required to define each symptom index and to remove any redundant items.

Eligible subjects were enrolled in stage 2 ($n = 73$) of the program to receive the Fatigue Reviva™ amino acid

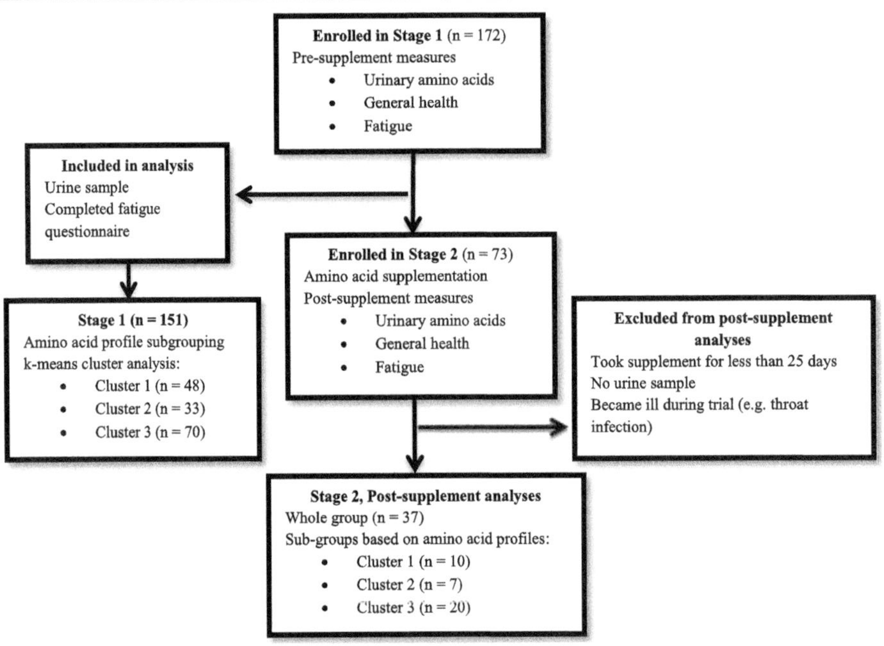

Fig. 1 Study design including statistical analyses for the amino acid supplement trial

Table 1 Symptom indices based on selected items from an 86-item general health questionnaire

General Fatigue Index	Pain Index	Gastrointestinal Index	Sleep Index	Vitality Index
Individual scale items				
Low in energy	Muscle cramps	Abdominal pain	Prolonged Sleep	Libido
Trouble concentrating	Face pain	Diarrhoea	Trouble falling asleep	Night sweats
Muscle weakness	Neck Pain	Constipation	Trouble awakening	Cravings
Forgetfulness	Shoulder pain	Irritable bowel	Disturbed sleep	
Everything an effort	Arm pain	Gastric reflux	Mental fatigue	
Mental confusion	Muscle soreness			
	Heavy limbs			

supplement for a 30 day period. Participants were required to take 20 g of the amino acid based dietary supplement dissolved in 100 ml of water daily. The commercially available nutritional supplement, Fatigue Reviva™ (Top Nutrition Pty Ltd) was comprised of 20 L-amino acids (glycine, proline, glutamine, carnitine, threonine, lysine, alanine, valine, taurine, serine, cysteine, arginine, histidine, isoleucine, phenylalanine, leucine, methionine, glutamic acid, aspartic acid, tyrosine), fructo-oligosaccharide (FOS), malic acid, citric acid, succinic acid, ribose, 13 minerals and 13 vitamins. Production of the supplement Fatigue Reviva™ was carried out according to the restrictions of the NSW Food Regulation 2010 [30], the NSW Food Act 2003 [31] and the Foods Standards Code (FSANZ) [32] whilst the dosages were governed by restrictions of the NSW Food Authority.

At the end of the 30 days, participant data were excluded from the analyses if they had either not taken the supplement for a minimum of 25 days, reported having developed an infection or did not provide a urine sample and completed questionnaires. The data generated from the remaining subjects' urine samples and questionnaires were included in the analyses. The study was carried out as part of an initial phase of product assessment to determine whether population subgroups exist and if so, does membership of a subgroup influence the efficacy of the supplement. The determination of population subgroups was deemed critical in preparation for future studies in terms of integrating placebo treatments. Participants were also asked to indicate whether they felt the supplement improved their health and whether they would continue to take the supplement if given the opportunity. All participants provided written consent. The trial was registered with the Australian New Zealand Clinical Trials Registry (ACTRN12611000403932) and approved by the University of Newcastle Human Research Ethics Committee (H-2010-1313).

Chalder fatigue scale scores were analysed using Wilcoxon signed-rank test. The general health questionnaire data were assessed by correlation and factor analyses to construct symptom indices appropriate for assessing the impact of amino acid supplementation on general health and wellbeing. Amino acid data were assessed for normality using Shapiro-Wilks W test. Univariate analysis of amino acid data included ANOVA, Wilcoxon matched pairs test and Mann-Whitney *U* test. Multivariate analysis of amino acid data included standard and forward stepwise function analysis of arcsine transformed data. Comparisons were made between the amino acid profiles, general health and levels of fatigue pre- and post-supplementation for a cohort of participants ($n = 37$) who had both successfully completed the amino acid trial and for whom both pre-supplement and post-supplement urine samples were assessed for amino acid content. K-means cluster analysis was used to separate the data collected pre-supplement from 151 participants into three groups based upon their amino acid profiles (relative abundance data). Comparisons were then made between the amino acid profiles pre- and post-supplementation of the three sub-groups based upon the results of the cluster analysis. Statistical analyses were carried out using Dell Statistica (data analysis software system), version 13, software.dell.com, Dell Inc. (2015). Levels of statistical significance were set at $p < 0.05$.

Results

Initial evaluation of urinary excretion patterns

Initially, 172 participants (aged 18 years or older) were recruited from the general public for stage 1 of the study. A final study group of 151 subjects provided urine samples and full responses to questionnaires and were reportedly free from any significant medical conditions. The participant group comprised 99 males with an average age of 29.5 ± 11.8 (mean ± SD) and 52 females with an average age of 35 ± 13.7. The first stage of the investigation involved appraising the pre-supplementation urine excretion profiles of the 151 recruits. The amino acid compositions were determined by GC-FID analyses and used to generate a dataset of relative percentage abundances of 29 amino acids and amino acid derivatives. These data were assessed by k-means clustering techniques to determine that the study participants could be partitioned into three clusters based the amino acid relative abundances with a minimum cluster membership of $n > 10$. Standard discriminant function analysis was then applied to determine whether each of the clusters had significantly different amino acid profiles (Wilks' Lambda = 0.13, $F(46,252) = 9.85$, $p < 0.0001$) as shown in the canonical plot (Fig. 2) with glycine and histidine levels providing the major discrimination between the groups. The members in each cluster were tightly grouped based upon their urinary excretion profiles and each subgroup was clearly resolved from the other subgroups with minimal overlap.

Seventeen amino acids contributed towards differentiating the composition profiles of the clusters by displaying significant differences in relative abundances for the subgroups and the concentrations of the key components have been summarised in Table 2. Histidine and glycine were the most abundant amino acids in the urinary profiles and displayed different relative abundances for each of the three clusters. Cluster 1 was characterised by a high histidine to glycine ratio of 2.0, cluster 2 displayed a low ratio of 0.4 and cluster 3 had equivalent levels resulting in a ratio of 1.0. Cluster 1 had the highest total urinary concentration of excreted amino acids where histidine levels were 2.4 – 3.6 times those in clusters 3 and 2 respectively. Cluster 1 also had significantly higher concentrations of glutamine, tyrosine and the branch chain amino acids compared with both clusters 2 and 3. In addition, serine and alanine were higher in cluster 1 compared with cluster 3 (Table 2). Cluster 2 was equivalent to cluster 3 in these parameters but was clearly distinguished by the high level of glycine excretion in the urine.

The objective partitioning by k-means clustering of subjects based on similarities in their urinary excretion profile removed user-bias in group allocation. Cluster 3 had the highest frequency of membership (46%) followed by cluster 1 (32%) and then cluster 2 (22%) as shown in Table 2. The three subgroups within the study cohort had similar BMI values and were primarily Caucasian. Clusters 1 and 3 had similar mean ages but cluster 2 had a significantly higher mean age than both clusters 1 and 3. Gender was not equally balanced across the three groups where cluster 2 contained predominantly females ($p < 0.05$). Sixteen out of 27 males who identified themselves as athletes were assigned to cluster 1, ten to cluster 3 and only one to cluster 2. There were no significant differences in total amino acid concentrations between the genders in the whole study cohort where males ($n = 99$) had a mean level of 5185 ± 290 μmol/L (mean ± SEM) and females ($n = 52$) 4955 ± 452 μmol/L. Comparisons between the urinary compositions of amino acids in males and females revealed significant differences for glutamic acid (males 16.7 ± 2 vs females 25.0 ± 3 μmol/L, $p < 0.05$), glycine-proline dipeptide (78.0 ± 5 vs 54.7 ± 6 μmol/L, $p < 0.01$), proline-hydroxyproline dipeptide (234.3 ± 15 vs 154.7 ± 19 μmol/L, $p < 0.01$) and tyrosine (96.8 ± 7 vs 72.8 ± 9 μmol/L, $p < 0.05$).

Levels of fatigue were assessed using the Chalder fatigue scale [26] where the average total fatigue score was calculated to be 13.6 ± 5.9 (mean ± SD) for the whole group. However, evaluation of the clusters revealed that cluster 2 had a significantly higher level of total fatigue compared with cluster 1, while clusters 1 and 3 had similar scores (Table 2). The results of the Chalder fatigue scale were mirrored by the fatigue index results derived from the general health questionnaire. Cluster 2 also reported higher levels of symptoms assessed by the sleep index compared with cluster 1.

Correlation analyses were performed to evaluate potential associations between the levels of urinary metabolites and the various symptom indices for each of the clusters. There were distinctive arrays of correlations noted for each of the clusters with some strong positive associations ($r > .50$) noted for cluster 1 females (Table 3). It was evident for females belonging to cluster 1 ($n = 13$) that higher urinary concentrations of glutamic acid, hydroxylysine, methionine, ornithine, proline and valine were all positively correlated with values of the Chalder physical fatigue score ($r > .55$, $p < 0.05$). In the same group, increasing scores in the gastrointestinal index were very strongly associated with higher urinary levels of proline ($r = .92$), methionine ($r = .82$) and valine ($r = .70$). These amino acids were also correlated with a range of other symptoms as shown in Table 3. Females in Cluster 2 only exhibited positive correlations for two amino acids, where the urinary concentration for asparagine was associated with the gastrointestinal index and proline was associated with all four fatigue measures and the gastrointestinal index. In contrast, Cluster 3 females displayed

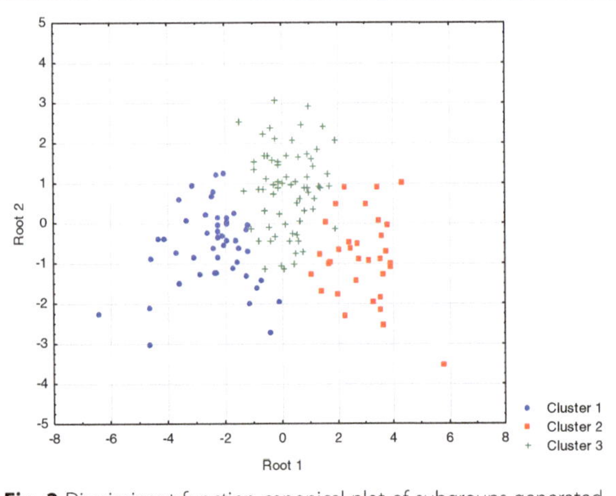

Fig. 2 Discriminant function canonical plot of subgroups generated via k-means clustering

Table 2 Characteristics of participant groups by amino acid profile cluster: significant differences in amino acid levels and symptom indices

Characteristic	Pre-supplement large cohort ($n = 151$)			
	Cluster 1 $n = 48$	Cluster 2 $n = 33$	Cluster 3 $n = 70$	p value
Mean Age[a]	26.0 (1.2)	37.8 (2.3)	31.9 (1.6)	C1 < C2 = C3 $p < 0.001$
Mean BMI[a]	24.8 (0.4)	24.2 (0.7)	25.4 (0.4)	ns
Proportion Males (number)[a]	75% (36)	30.3% (10)	75.7% (53)	C2 < C1 = C3 $p < 0.001$
Caucasian (%)[a]	95.1%	100%	93.8%	ns
Urine Amino Acids				
Total amino acids µmole/L	6,609 (495)	4,339 (462)	4,425 (306)	C1 > C2 = C3 $p < 0.01$[‡]
Histidine	2,152 (185)	599 (76)	886 (74)	C1 > C2 = C3 $p < 0.0001$
Glycine	1,077 (86)	1,412 (157)	861 (68)	C2 > C3 $p < 0.001$
Glutamine	626 (63)	443 (46)	480 (29)	C1 > C2 = C3 $p < 0.05$
Serine	411 (49)	320 (34)	279 (16)	C1 > C3 $p < 0.05$
Alanine	313 (29)	232 (25)	236 (18)	C1 > C3 $p < 0.05$
Tyrosine	129 (13)	57 (8)	77 (5)	C1 > C2 = C3 $p < 0.0001$
Branched chain amino acids	106 (7)	62 (7)	84 (6)	C1 > C2 = C3 $p < 0.001$
Proline	5.0 (1.9)	9.1 (2.0)	10.7 (1.5)	ns
Symptom Indices				
Chalder total fatigue	12.8 (0.7)	16.0 (1.0)	13.4 (0.8)	C2 > C1 $p < 0.05$
Chalder mental fatigue	4.5 (0.3)	5.9 (0.4)	4.6 (0.3)	C2 > C1 = C3 $p < 0.05$
General fatigue index	3.2 (1.0)	11.2 (1.6)	8.3 (1.1)	C2 > C1 $p < 0.05$
Pain index	5.1 (0.8)	8.1 (1.3)	5.3 (0.7)	ns
Gastrointestinal index	1.7 (0.7)	3.8 (1.0)	2.0 (0.4)	ns
Sleep index	8.2 (1.0)	14.0 (1.9)	11.5 (1.2)	C2 > C1 $p < 0.05$
Vitality index	6.5 (1.2)	9.1 (1.3)	5.5 (0.8)	ns

Statistical tests: ANOVA, Tukey's HSD for unequal sample sizes, *Chi square; mean (SEM)

negative associations between general fatigue and alanine, aspartic acid, isoleucine, phenylalanine, and tyrosine. The males in cluster 1 displayed nine negative correlations between amino acids and symptoms, where seven of these involved associations with the gastrointestinal index (Table 4). The males from cluster 2 had positive associations between α-aminobutyric acid and the four fatigue indices. The males from cluster 3 had six symptom indices (all four fatigue measures, pain and vitality) positively associated with β-aminoisobutyric acid and showed no negative correlations.

Evaluation of amino acid supplementation

Compliance for the supplementation trial was 51% where 37 participants successfully completed the trial by taking the amino acid supplement for a period of 25–30 days as well as returning general health questionnaires and providing post-supplement urine samples. The supplement trial cohort ($n = 37$) comprised 10 females and had an average age of 33.8 years ranging from 19 to 65 years.

Levels of fatigue were assessed using both the Chalder fatigue scale [26] and a general fatigue index developed by the current research team, where lower scores were indicative of a lower level of fatigue for both measures. After completion of the supplement trial, 30 out of the group of 37 participants (81%) reported an improvement in their levels of fatigue. A significant reduction in the mean total fatigue scores for the entire cohort was observed from 13.4 ± 0.8 (mean ± SEM) to 8.8 ± 0.6 (Wilcoxon matched pairs test, $p < 0.0001$) following supplementation. General health and wellbeing was also assessed using an 86 item questionnaire from which several indices were generated (Table 1). Scores were standardised to values out of 40, where a score of "0" indicated that the subject was not affected by any of the symptoms comprising that index, and a score of "40" indicating that the subject experienced all of the symptoms in the index group to a high degree. Following supplementation, significant reductions in questionnaire scores representing potential improvements were seen in the fatigue,

Table 3 Correlations between urinary concentrations of amino acids and symptom index scores for each of the three clusters defined by k-means clustering of urinary amino acid profiles for the female participants

Females: Amino Acid versus Symptom Index	Cluster 1 $n = 13$	Cluster 2 $n = 21$	Cluster 3 $n = 17$
ALA vs General fatigue	ns	ns	$r = -.56$
ASN vs GIT	ns	$r = 0.50$	ns
ASP vs General fatigue	ns	ns	$r = -.50$
GLU vs Chalder total fatigue	$r = .59$	ns	ns
GLU vs Chalder physical fatigue	$r = .63$	ns	ns
HYL vs Chalder physical fatigue	$r = .57$	ns	ns
HYP vs Pain	$r = .56$	ns	ns
ILE vs General fatigue	ns	ns	$r = -.49$
MET vs Pain	$r = .66$	ns	ns
MET vs GIT	$r = .82$	ns	ns
MET vs Sleep	$r = .59$	ns	ns
MET vs Chalder physical fatigue	$r = .60$	ns	ns
ORN vs GIT	$r = .66$	ns	ns
ORN vs Vitality	$r = .58$	ns	ns
ORN vs Chalder total fatigue	$r = .59$	ns	ns
ORN vs Chalder physical fatigue	$r = .56$	ns	ns
PHE vs General fatigue	ns	ns	$r = -.50$
PRO vs General fatigue	$r = .63$	$r = .48$	ns
PRO vs Pain	$r = .83$	ns	ns
PRO vs GIT	$r = .92$	$r = .45$	ns
PRO vs Sleep	$r = .70$	ns	ns
PRO vs Vitality	$r = .74$	ns	ns
PRO vs Chalder total fatigue	$r = .56$	$r = .52$	ns
PRO vs Chalder physical fatigue	$r = .63$	$r = .49$	ns
PRO vs Chalder mental fatigue	ns	$r = .44$	ns
TYR vs General fatigue	ns	ns	$r = -.49$
VAL vs Pain	$r = .60$	ns	ns
VAL vs GIT	$r = .70$	ns	ns
VAL vs Sleep	$r = .61$	ns	ns
VAL vs Chalder total fatigue	$r = .60$	ns	ns
VAL vs Chalder physical fatigue	$r = .67$	ns	ns
Total BCAA vs Chalder physical fatigue	$r = .59$	ns	ns

Table 4 Correlations between urinary concentrations of amino acids and symptom index scores for each of the three clusters defined by k-means clustering of urinary amino acid profiles for the male participants

Males: Amino Acid versus Symptom Index	Cluster 1 $n = 35$	Cluster 2 $N = 21$	Cluster 3 $N = 49$
ALA vs GIT	$r = -.34$	ns	ns
ABA vs General fatigue	ns	$r = .47$	ns
ABA vs Chalder total fatigue	ns	$r = .56$	ns
ABA vs Chalder physical fatigue	ns	$r = .46$	ns
ABA vs Chalder mental fatigue	ns	$r = .60$	ns
BAIB vs General fatigue	ns	ns	$r = .50$
BAIB vs Pain	ns	ns	$r = .37$
BAIB vs Vitality	ns	ns	$r = .38$
BAIB vs Total fatigue	ns	ns	$r = .32$
BAIB vs Chalder physical fatigue	ns	ns	$r = .28$
BAIB vs Chalder mental fatigue	ns	ns	$r = .33$
ASN vs General fatigue	$r = .34$	ns	ns
GLY vs GIT	$r = -.41$	ns	ns
HYP vs Vitality	ns	ns	$r = .37$
LEU vs GIT	$r = -.49$	ns	ns
ORN vs Chalder mental fatigue	ns	ns	$r = .33$
PHE vs GIT	$r = -.40$	ns	ns
PHE vs Chalder physical fatigue	$r = .35$	ns	ns
PHP vs Vitality	$r = -.37$	ns	ns
PHP vs Chalder physical fatigue	$r = -.38$	ns	ns
TYR vs Chalder physical fatigue	$r = .38$	ns	ns
VAL vs GIT	$r = -.39$	ns	ns
Total BCAA vs GIT	$r = -.47$	ns	ns
Total AA vs GIT	$r = -.36$	ns	ns

sleep and vitality indices (Table 5). In response to the questions regarding their experience using the supplement, 25 responders (68%) indicated that they felt the supplement had improved their health and 28 (76%) stated that they would continue to take the supplement if given the opportunity.

The seven participants who did not report any improvements in fatigue were all males and had an average Chalder total fatigue score of 10.0 ± 1.4 (mean ± SEM) prior to supplementation whereas the remainder of the cohort (n = 30) had a significantly higher mean Chalder fatigue score of 14.2 ± 0.8 (Mann-Whitney U test, $p < 0.02$). The participants that showed improvements in fatigue thus had a higher level of fatigue prior to commencing the supplementation. The larger group who reported having

Table 5 Reported improvements in general health indices following amino acid supplementation

Symptom index	Pre-supplement Mean (SE)	Post-supplement Mean (SE)	p value
Chalder Total Fatigue	13.4 (0.8)	8.8 (0.6)	<0.0001
Chalder Physical fatigue	8.3 (0.6)	5.5 (0.4)	<0.001
Chalder Mental Fatigue	5.1 (0.3)	3.3 (0.2)	<0.0001
General Fatigue index	6.9 (1.2)	3.7 (1.0)	<0.01
Pain index	4.7 (1.1)	3.9 (1.0)	ns
Gastrointestinal index	2.0 (0.6)	2.7 (0.8)	ns
Sleep index	10.4 (1.5)	6.6 (1.0)	<0.01
Vitality index	6.5 (1.2)	2.2 (0.7)	<0.001

Statistical test: Wilcoxon matched pairs test

experienced relief from fatigue ultimately reported post-supplementation fatigue scores that were significantly lower (8.1 ± 0.6, mean ± SEM) than those who did not report improved fatigue (11.7 ± 1.4, $p < 0.04$). Six out of the seven males who did not respond to the amino acid supplementation were classified by their pre-supplementation urinary profile as belonging to cluster 3 and the seventh non-responder was assigned to cluster 1.

Discussion

Analyses of the urine samples collected from the pre-supplement cohort of 151 healthy participants revealed that it was possible to delineate three clear clusters based upon urinary amino acid profiles. Cluster 3 was the most prevalent of the clusters with its membership totalling 46% of the total cohort with the next largest, cluster 1, comprising 32% of the cohort. An earlier study appraised the amino acid composition of 1993 patient urine samples referred by general practitioners to generate 6 subgroups with a minimum membership of n > 50 [22]. It was thus argued that evidence from this study of the healthy general population and the earlier study of referral patients [22] supported the hypothesis that within the Australian context, phenotypic subgroups exist within the general population based on amino acid excretion characteristics found in urine. It is very likely that with more subjects, a greater number of proportionally smaller subgroups would emerge using k-means clustering techniques. The additional clusters may be relevant to certain lower frequency population phenotypes which could be associated with congenital metabolic anomalies or predispositions to certain medical conditions. Phenotypic membership may also represent epigenetic outcomes where responses by the body to environmental conditions (nutrition, exercise, temperature) or responses to pathogenic challenge which have resulted in alterations in amino acid homeostasis and nitrogen balance.

The objective of measuring the first of the morning fasted urine samples was to minimize confounding from dietary intake in order to assess potential differences in body homeostasis between individuals. Cluster 1 had the highest average concentration of amino acids in the fasted urine samples at approximately 1.5 times the levels measured for clusters 2 and 3. Although total amino acid losses were not determined from 24 h urine samples, the higher first of the morning urinary concentrations suggested that this group may have a greater potential to lose amino acids via urinary excretion suggesting the operation of less efficient mechanisms for kidney reabsorption processes. Histidine was the major component in urine from cluster 1 at 2.4 – 3.6 times the concentrations observed in the other clusters. Histidine has been demonstrated to be an essential amino acid in adults on the basis that histidine deficient diets in both animal models and human studies have led to a negative nitrogen balance with reduced haemoglobin and haematocrit levels [33]. On provision of histidine, the subjects' nitrogen balances were restored and haemoglobin and haematocrit levels were returned to normal [34]. Haemoglobin protein contains 10% histidine and insufficient supply of this amino acid can lead to anaemia [34]. If a particular human phenotype was more susceptible to histidine loss then there may be a need to compensate for such losses via an increased intake of appropriate protein sources or a negative nitrogen balance would slowly develop with resultant sub-optimal haemoglobin production and associated fatigue. In a previous study carried out by the current research team, amino acid levels were investigated in breast cancer radiotherapy patients who developed fatigue following radiotherapy treatment [12]. Those women who developed significant fatigue had higher levels of urinary histidine excretion prior to treatment compared with those women who remained fatigue free, while their plasma histidine levels dropped below detectable levels following radiotherapy. Cluster 1 from the current study also displayed elevated output of tyrosine, serine and alanine as well as the branch chained amino acids. The excretion of tyrosine in the urine can be indicative of higher non-myofibrillar protein turnover [6, 35, 36] which could further contribute towards fatigue.

Cluster 2 was characterised by glycine as the major excretory product and a predominance of females (70%). Comparison of the male and female urinary amino acid levels for the entire cohort did not reveal any significant differences in the concentrations of histidine, glycine, glutamine, serine or alanine. Glycine is a non-essential amino acid that is primarily derived from serine and is a vital component of human metabolism. Glycine is a major component of collagen (33%) which is the most abundant family of proteins in the body providing structure and form for tissues and organs. Excessive losses of glycine may negatively impact on collagen turnover which has been shown to be higher in females [37]. In addition to protein synthesis it has numerous metabolic functions such the biosynthesis of heme, creatine and nucleic acids [38]. It also has important roles in metabolic regulation, bile secretion and neurological function [38]. As glycine is utilised in so many essential pathways and has high demands in protein synthesis, it has often been referred to as a "conditionally essential" amino acid in reference to situations where *de novo* synthesis can no longer meet demands [38].

A major feature of cluster 3 was a set of positive correlations for the males for β-aminoisobutyric acid (BAIB) with the symptom indices for vitality, pain and all four fatigue measures. This non-protein amino acid exists as two enantiomers, one as a catabolic product of the pyrimidine base thymine found exclusively in urine and the other enantiomer derived from valine is found in plasma [39]. In certain forms of anaemia and in thalassaemia BAIB has been shown to be excreted [40] and has also been negatively associated with haemoglobin levels and erythrocyte count [41]. The vitality index was comprised of the symptoms of night sweats, libido and food cravings, which were grouped together by factor analysis of the symptom profiles. Reduced testosterone levels have been associated with night sweats [42] as well as reduced libido [43] and insulin resistance [44]. Changes in the vitality index in the males may point to reductions in testosterone levels which have previously been associated with fatigue, muscle weakness, reduced muscle protein synthesis and anaemia [44].

The correlation analyses of amino acids with symptom expression measured by the various indices revealed further differences between the three clusters. Although the associations between urinary amino acids and symptoms cannot be interpreted as providing a direct cause and effect mechanism, the data suggested that increased outputs of certain metabolites contributed towards symptom expression in sub-health. The presence or absence of correlations also demonstrated differences between males and females in each of the clusters. Proline for example displayed a number of very strong correlations for females in cluster 1, to a lesser extent in cluster 2 and finally no associations at all in cluster 3. In contrast to the females, there were no associations with proline recorded for males regardless of the cluster membership. Proline together with alanine, glycine, glutamine and valine represented 52% of the amino acid components in resting human plasma [15] which indicates their importance as a circulatory reservoir to meet the body's demands. The positive associations of urinary proline concentration and symptoms in females relating to fatigue and pain may point to an increased demand in females due to the turnover of non-myofibrillar protein to maintain plasma homeostasis. Proline is the second major component of collagen (after glycine) comprising around 13% of the protein with a further 9% of collagen containing hydroxyproline. The hydroxyproline is formed via post-translational modification of pro-collagen where residues of proline (and lysine) are hydroxylated to form the final collagen product. Hydroxyproline is primarily found in collagen, and the appearance of it in urine can be used as a measure of collagen turnover [45, 46]. It was thus proposed that females from cluster 1 were susceptible to experiencing higher levels of fatigue and pain if they had higher urinary levels of the collagen components hydroxyproline, hydroxylysine and proline. Collagen turnover is generally thought to be higher in females due to the influence of oestrogen on the maintenance of joint flexibility [47]. Chronic fatigue syndrome is reportedly more prevalent in women [48, 49]. The same cluster 1 also had a significantly higher urinary concentration of tyrosine which can also be indicative of an elevated turnover of non-myofibrillar proteins [35, 36]. Higher rates of collagen turnover and losses of proline in urine could therefore have significant implications for meeting the demand for collagen synthesis in a broad range of body tissues and organ systems.

The supplement trial was completed successfully, but only 51% of the recruits were considered to have complied sufficiently by completing a minimum of 25 days of supplementation, completing the questionnaires and providing a final urine sample. Low compliance with trials of this nature is recognised as a common problem [50]. The group that completed the supplementation trial had a similar distribution of gender and cluster membership as observed in the first study survey. The low numbers made it impossible to evaluate differences between the males and females within the subgroups and so the majority of the analyses were focussed on the whole study group with references as appropriate to the incidence of non-responders to the supplement in the various clusters.

The trial group reported experiencing improvements in wellbeing following the supplementation period as evidenced by reductions in the Chalder fatigue scores as well as the general health indices for fatigue, sleep and vitality. The Chalder fatigue scale has been validated for use in the general population as well as those suffering ill health [51]. In the current study, substantial reductions in fatigue were reported with 81% of the cohort indicating an improvement in fatigue and all female participants reporting an improvement in fatigue after taking the supplement. The formulation of the amino acid supplement was such that it would have provided a direct source of amino acids capable of reducing the requirement for non-myofibrillar catabolism and therefore it had the potential to relieve fatigue. The higher levels of urinary histidine (cluster 1) and glycine (cluster 2) could have contributed to limitations in haemoglobin production and collagen turnover respectively and provision of both histidine and glycine in the supplement may have led to enhancements in the synthesis of these proteins [33, 34, 38, 45] and a reduction in associated symptoms such as fatigue and pain.

The seven participants who did not show any improvement following supplementation were all males, six of whom belonged to cluster 3. Cluster 3 had no obvious anomalies of high level excretions of amino acids such as those observed for histidine (cluster 1) and glycine (cluster 2). In addition, the males that did not respond to amino acid support had low Chalder fatigue scores at the beginning of the supplementation period and were therefore not experiencing problematic levels of fatigue in need of treatment. Thus it was concluded that males primarily assigned to cluster 3 via initial urine analysis and who also had low Chalder fatigue scores would be unlikely to achieve improved levels of fatigue from supplementation with amino acids. These subjects would appear to have been free from the symptoms that characterise sub-health. The combined use of the urinary amino acid profiling and the Chalder fatigue scale could be effectively utilised in future testing of amino acid supplementation by allowing selection of those individuals most likely to be experiencing a negative nitrogen balance and fatigue, and who would therefore potentially be more likely to benefit from amino acid support. The use of the general health questionnaire indices provided a framework for appraising the symptoms of sub-health which could be used for monitoring improvements in wellbeing. On this basis, future clinical trials could be developed with appropriate screening for inclusion of significant sub-health issues associated with fatigue, sleep and vitality.

Conclusions

Using urine excretion profiles of amino acids, it was possible to define three major phenotypic clusters of adult human subjects. Cluster 1 had the highest concentration of amino acids in urine with histidine present at 2.4–3.6 times the concentrations observed in the other clusters while cluster 2 was characterised by a high level of urinary glycine. The three clusters thus had differential excretion characteristics and sets of sub-health symptom profiles, where the females within the three clusters had different associations between nutrient losses and symptom expression compared with the corresponding males. Evidence suggested that collagen/non-myofibrillar muscle protein turnover rates were higher in the females and were associated with the experience of more intense sub-health symptom presentation compared with the males. Provision of the amino acid supplement for 30 days resulted in significant improvements in reported fatigue and sleep for 81% of the trial cohort. It was concluded that people suffering fatigue, assessed as a Chalder fatigue scale score > 13, would be likely to experience significant benefits from amino acid supplementation.

Abbreviations

AA: Amino acid; ABA: Alpha-aminobutyric acid; ALA: Alanine; ASN: Asparagine; ASP: Aspartic acid; BAIB: Beta-aminoisobutyric acid; BCAA: Branched-chain amino acid; FOS: Fructo-oligosaccharide; GIT: Gastrointestinal tract; GLU: Glutamate; GLY: Glycine; HYL: Hydroxylysine; HYP: Hydroxyproline; ILE: Isoleucine; LEU: Leucine; MET: Methionine; ORN: Ornithine; PHE: Phenylalanine; PHP: Proline-hydroxyproline; PRO: Proline; SEM: Standard error of the mean; TYR: Tyrosine; VAL: Valine

Acknowledgements

Anthony Martin is thanked for analyses of samples and assistance in coordinating distribution of supplements and receipt of samples. Marcus Crompton and Grace Murphy are also thanked for their assistance in sample processing.

Funding

This work was funded by a research contract from TOP Nutrition Pty Ltd. The product being assessed, Fatigue Reviva™, was donated by TOP Nutrition Pty Ltd. The funding body played no role in the design of the study, analysis or interpretation of data and had no part in writing the manuscript.

Availability of data and materials

It has not been possible to make the project's raw data available as ethics approval was only obtained for the publication of aggregated results.

Authors' contributions

RHD and TR conceived the study, were responsible for the study design and the formulation of the dietary supplement. DLS and MM contributed to the study design and performed the statistical analysis along with RHD. RHD and DLS drafted the manuscript. BD and XJDJ were involved in coordinating the study and recruiting participants. JG and C-GG gave advice on data analysis, interpretation and clinical relevance. All authors were involved in interpretation of data, developing the content of the manuscript. All authors read and approved the final manuscript.

Competing interests

Hugh Dunstan and Tim Roberts have previously worked as consultants for the company Top Nutrition Pty Ltd to oversee a program of development for the amino acid supplement Fatigue Reviva™ trialled in the current study. Diane Sparkes has previously worked as a data-processing consultant for Top Nutrition Pty Ltd. The authors declare that they have no competing interests.

Consent for publication

Not applicable.

Ethics approval and consent to participate

The study was approved by the University of Newcastle Human Research Ethics Committee (H-2010-1313). All participants provided informed written consent before taking part in the trial.

Publisher's Note

Springer Nature remains neutral with regard to jurisdictional claims in published maps and institutional affiliations.

Author details

[1]School of Environmental and Life Sciences, University of Newcastle, Callaghan, Australia. [2]School of Environmental and Life Sciences, University of Newcastle, Ourimbah, Australia. [3]Latrobe University, Melbourne, Australia. [4]Department of Chemistry and Molecular Biology, University of Gothenburg, Gothenburg, Sweden. [5]Department of Neuroscience, University of Gothenburg, Gothenburg, Sweden.

References

1. Boirie Y. Physiopathological mechanism of sarcopenia. J Nutr Health Aging. 2009;13:717–23.
2. Jagoe RT, Engelen MPKJ. Muscle wasting and changes in muscle protein metabolism in chronic obstructive pulmonary disease. Eur Respir J. 2003;22: 52s–63s.
3. Oehler R, Roth E. Glutamine metabolism. In: Cynober LA, editor. Metabolic and therapeutic aspects of amino acids in clinical nutrition. Secondth ed. New York: CRC Press; 2004. p. 169–82.
4. Udenfriend S, Wyngaarden JB. Precursors of adrenal epinephrine and norepinephrine in vivo. Biochim Biophys Acta. 1956;20:48–52.
5. de Koning TJ, Snell K, Duran M, Berger R, Poll-The B-T, Surtees R. L-Serine in disease and development. Biochem J. 2003;371:653–61.
6. Poortmans JR, Carpentier LO, Pereira-Lancha LO, Lancha Jr A. Protein turnover, amino acid requirements and recommendations for athletes and active populations. Braz J Med Biol Res. 2012;45:875–90.
7. Phillips SM. Protein requirements and supplementation in strength sports. Nutrition. 2004;20:689–95.
8. Waterlow JC, Jackson AA. Nutrition and protein turnover in man. Br Med Bull. 1981;37:5–10.
9. Corsetti R, Barassi A, Perego S, Sansoni V, Rossi A, Damele CAL, d'Eril GM, Banfi G, Lombardi G. Changes in urinary amino acids excretion in relationship with muscle activity markers over a professional cycling stage race: in search of fatigue markers. Amino Acids. 2016;48:183–92.
10. Dunstan RH, Sparkes DL, Dascombe BJ, Evans CA, Macdonald MM, Crompton MJ, Franks J, Murphy G, Gottfries J, Carlton B. Sweat facilitated losses of amino acids in Standardbred horses and the application of

supplementation strategies to maintain condition during training. Comp Exercise Physiol. 2015;11:201–12.
11. Dunstan RH, Sparkes DL, Dascombe BJ, Macdonald MM, Evans CA, Stevens CJ, Crompton MJ, Gottfries J, Franks J, Murphy G, et al. Sweat facilitated amino acid losses in male athletes during exercise at 32-34 °C. PLoS One. 2016;11:1–16.
12. Dunstan RH. Altered amino acid homeostasis and the development of fatigue by breast cancer radiotherapy patients: A pilot study. Clin Biochem. 2011;44:208–15.
13. Niblett SN. Hematologic and urinary excretion anomalies in patients with chronic fatigue syndrome. Exp Biol Med. 2007;232:1041–9.
14. Liappis N, Hungerland H. Quantitative study of free amino acids in human eccrine sweat during normal conditions. Am J Clin Nutr. 1972;25:661–3.
15. Armstrong MD, Stave U. A study of plasma free amino acid levels. II. Normal values for children and adults. Metabolism. 1973;22:561–9.
16. Weschler LB. Sweat electrolyte concentrations obtained from within occlusive coverings are falsely high because sweat itself leaches skin electrolytes. J Appl Physiol. 2008;105:1376–7.
17. Scott IR, Harding CR, Barrett JG. Histidine-rich protein of the keratohyalin granules. Source of the free amino acids, urocanic acid and pyrrolidone carboxylic acid in the stratum corneum. Biochim Biophys Acta. 1982;719:110–7.
18. Kingsbury KJ, Kay L, Hjelm M. Contrasting plasma free amino acid patterns in elite athletes: association with fatigue and infection. Br J Sports Med. 1998;32:25–32.
19. Paddon-Jones D. Atrophy and impaired muscle protein synthesis during prolonged inactivity and stress. J Clin Endocrinol Metabol. 2006;91:4836–41.
20. Dunstan RH, Sparkes DL, Roberts TK, Crompton MJ, Gottfries J, Dascombe BJ. Development of a complex amino acid supplement, fatigue reviva™, for oral ingestion: initial evaluations of product concept and impact on symptoms of sub-health in a group of males. Nutr J. 2013;12:115.
21. Dunstan RH, Sparkes DL, Roberts TK, Dascombe BJ. Preliminary evaluations of a complex amino acid supplement, fatigue Reviva™, to reduce fatigue in a group of professional male athletes and a group of males recruited from the general public. Food Nutr Sci. 2014;5:231–5.
22. Dunstan RH, McGregor NR, Butt HL, Roberts TK, Klineberg IJ, Niblett SN, Rothkirch TB, Buttfield I. Characterization of differential amino acid homeostasis amongst population subgroups: a basis for determining specific amino acid requirements. J Nutr Environ Med. 2000;10:211–23.
23. Watanabe N, Stewart R, Jenkins R, Bhugra DK, Furukawa TA. The epidemiology of chronic fatigue, physical illness, and symptoms of common mental disorders: a cross-sectional survey from the second British national survey of psychiatric morbidity. J Psychosom Res. 2008;64:357–62.
24. Li G, Xie F, Yan S, Hu X, Jin B, Wang J, Wu J, Yin D, Xie Q: Subhealth: definition, criteria for diagnosis and potential prevalence in the central region of China. BMC Public Health. 2013;13.
25. Evans C, Dunstan RH, Rothkirch T, Roberts TK, Reichelt KL, Cosford R, Deed G, Ellis EB, Sparkes DL. Altered amino acid excretion in children with autism. Nutr Neurosci. 2008;11:9–17.
26. Chalder T, Berelowitz G, Pawlikowska T, Watts L, Wessely S, Wright D, Wallace EP. Development of a fatigue scale. J Psychosom Res. 1993;37:147–53.
27. McGregor NR, Dunstan RH, Zerbes M, Butt HL, Roberts TK, Klineberg IJ. Preliminary determination of the association between symptom expression and urinary metabolites in subjects with chronic fatigue syndrome. Biochem Mol Med. 1996;58:85–92.
28. Dunstan RH, McGregor NR, Butt HL, Roberts TK. Biochemical and microbiological anomalies in chronic fatigue syndrome: the development of laboratory based tests and the possible role of toxic chemicals. J Nutr Environ Med. 1999;9:97–108.
29. Richards RS, Roberts TK, McGregor NR, Dunstan RH, Butt HL. Blood parameters indicative of oxidative stress are associated with symptom expression in chronic fatigue syndrome. Redox Rep. 2000;5:35–41.
30. Australian New Zealand Food Standards Codes [http://www.comlaw.gov.au/Search/Australia%20New%20Zealand%20Food%20Standards]. Accessed 13 Jun 2013.
31. Food Act 2003 No 43 [http://www.legislation.nsw.gov.au/viewtop/inforce/act+43+2003+FIRST+0+N/]. Accessed 13 Jun 2013.
32. Food Regulation 2010 [http://www.legislation.nsw.gov.au/viewtop/inforce/subordleg+250+2010+cd+0+N]. Accessed 13 Jun 2013.
33. Clemens RA, Kopple JD, Swendseid ME. Metabolic effects of histidine-deficient diets fed to growing rats by gastric tube. J Nutr. 1984;114:2138–46.
34. Cooperman JM, Lopez R. The role of histidine in the anemia of folate deficiency. Exp Biol Med. 2002;227:998–1000.
35. Viru A, Viru A. Biochemical monitoring of sport training. 1st ed. Champaign: Human Kinetics Publishers; 2001.
36. Haralambie G, Berg A. Serum urea and amino nitrogen changes with exercise duration. Eur J Phys Occup Physiol. 1976;36:39–48.
37. Hedges REM, Clement JG, Thomas DL, O'Connell TC. Collagen turnover in the adult femoral mid-shaft: modeled from anthropogenic radiocarbon tracer measurements. Am J Phys Anthropol. 2007;133:808–16.
38. Wang W, Wu Z, Dai Z, Yang Y, Wang J, Wu G. Glycine metabolism in animals and humans: implications for nutrition and health. Amino Acids. 2013;45:463–77.
39. Cory JG. Purine and pyrimidine nucleotide metabolism. In: Devlin TM, editor. Textbook of biochemistry with clinical correlations. 3rd ed. New York: Wiley-Liss; 1992. p. 529–73.
40. Fessas PH, Koniavitis A, Zeis A. Urinary beta-aminoisobutyric acid excretion in thalassaemia. J Clin Pathol. 1969;22:154–7.
41. Enkhjargal T, Tserennadmid C. Urinary excretion of beta-aminoisobutyric acid in hematological diseases (abstract). Rinsho Byori Jpn J Clin Pathol. 2004;52:17–21.
42. Matsumoto AM. Andropause: clinical implications of the decline in serum testosterone levels with aging in men. J Gerontol. 2002;57A:M76–99.
43. Novak A, Brod M, Elbers J. Andropause and quality of life: findings from patient focus groups and clinical experts. Maturitas. 2002;43:231–7.
44. Bain J. Testosterone replacement therapy for aging men. Can Fam Physician. 2001;47:91–7.
45. Nogueira Ade C, Vale RG, Gomes AL, Dantas EH. The effect of muscle actions on the level of connective tissue damage. Res Sports Med. 2011;19:259–70.
46. Prockop DJ, Sioerdsma D. Significance of urinary hydroxyproline in man. Clin Invest. 1961;40:843–9.
47. Kjaer M, Hansen M. The mystery of female connective tissue. J Appl Physiol. 2008;105:1026–7.
48. Jason LA, Richman JA, Rademaker AW, Jordan KM, Plioplys AV, Taylor RR, McCready W, Huang C-F, Plioplys S. A community-based study of chronic fatigue syndrome. Arch Intern Med. 1999;159:2129–37.
49. Wessely S. The epidemiology of chronic fatigue syndrome. Epidemiologic Rev. 1995;17:139–51.
50. Boudes P. Drug compliance in therapeutic trials: a review. Control Clin Trials. 1998;19:257–68.
51. Cella M, Chalder T. Measuring fatigue in clinical and community settings. J Psychosom Res. 2010;69:17–22.

PERMISSIONS

All chapters in this book were first published in Nutrition, by BioMed Central; hereby published with permission under the Creative Commons Attribution License or equivalent. Every chapter published in this book has been scrutinized by our experts. Their significance has been extensively debated. The topics covered herein carry significant findings which will fuel the growth of the discipline. They may even be implemented as practical applications or may be referred to as a beginning point for another development.

The contributors of this book come from diverse backgrounds, making this book a truly international effort. This book will bring forth new frontiers with its revolutionizing research information and detailed analysis of the nascent developments around the world.

We would like to thank all the contributing authors for lending their expertise to make the book truly unique. They have played a crucial role in the development of this book. Without their invaluable contributions this book wouldn't have been possible. They have made vital efforts to compile up to date information on the varied aspects of this subject to make this book a valuable addition to the collection of many professionals and students.

This book was conceptualized with the vision of imparting up-to-date information and advanced data in this field. To ensure the same, a matchless editorial board was set up. Every individual on the board went through rigorous rounds of assessment to prove their worth. After which they invested a large part of their time researching and compiling the most relevant data for our readers.

The editorial board has been involved in producing this book since its inception. They have spent rigorous hours researching and exploring the diverse topics which have resulted in the successful publishing of this book. They have passed on their knowledge of decades through this book. To expedite this challenging task, the publisher supported the team at every step. A small team of assistant editors was also appointed to further simplify the editing procedure and attain best results for the readers.

Apart from the editorial board, the designing team has also invested a significant amount of their time in understanding the subject and creating the most relevant covers. They scrutinized every image to scout for the most suitable representation of the subject and create an appropriate cover for the book.

The publishing team has been an ardent support to the editorial, designing and production team. Their endless efforts to recruit the best for this project, has resulted in the accomplishment of this book. They are a veteran in the field of academics and their pool of knowledge is as vast as their experience in printing. Their expertise and guidance has proved useful at every step. Their uncompromising quality standards have made this book an exceptional effort. Their encouragement from time to time has been an inspiration for everyone.

The publisher and the editorial board hope that this book will prove to be a valuable piece of knowledge for researchers, students, practitioners and scholars across the globe.

LIST OF CONTRIBUTORS

Mostafa Goud and Laila Hussein
Department of Nutrition & Food Sc, National Research Center, Giza, Dokki, Egypt

Amr Moustafa
Department of Biochemistry, Faculty of Agriculture, Cairo University, Giza, Egypt

Mohamed Hamza
Department of Agronomy, Faculty of Agric, Cairo University, Giza, Egypt

Amely M. Verreijen, Mariëlle F. Engberink, Robert G. Memelink and Suzanne E. van der Plas
Department of Nutrition and Dietetics, Faculty of Sports and Nutrition Amsterdam University of Applied Sciences, Dr. Meurerlaan 8, 1067 SM Amsterdam, Netherlands

Marjolein Visser
Department of Health Sciences, Faculty of Earth and Life Sciences, VU University Amsterdam, De Boelenlaan 1085, 1081 HV Amsterdam, Netherlands
Department of Nutrition and Dietetics, Internal Medicine, VU University Medical Center, De Boelenlaan 1117, 1081 HV Amsterdam, Netherlands

Peter J. M. Weijs
Department of Nutrition and Dietetics, Faculty of Sports and Nutrition, Amsterdam University of Applied Sciences, Dr. Meurerlaan 8, 1067 SM Amsterdam, Netherlands
Department of Nutrition and Dietetics, Internal Medicine, VU University Medical Center, De Boelenlaan 1117, 1081 HV Amsterdam, Netherlands

Subin Park
Department of Research Planning, Mental Health Research Institute, National Center for Mental Health, Seoul, South Korea

Yeeun Lee
Department of psychology, Korea University, Seoul, South Korea

Junghyun H. Lee
Department of Psychiatry, National Center for Mental Health, 127, Yongmasan-ro, Gwangjin-gu, Seoul 04933, South Korea

L. H. Jomaa
Lamis Jomaa, Faculty of Agricultural and Food Sciences, American University of Beirut, Beirut, Lebanon

N. C. Hwalla
Nahla Hwalla, Faculty of Agricultural and Food Sciences, American University of Beirut, Beirut, Lebanon

J. M. Zidek
Jeremy Zidek, Futura Food, 113 Creekside Drive, State College, PA 16801, USA

Jing Chen, Jianhua Piao, Lichen Yang and Xiaoguang Yang
Department of Trace Element Nutrition, National Institute of Nutrition and Health, Chinese Center for Disease Control and Prevention, Room 103, Nanwei Road No. 29, Xicheng District, Beijing 100050, People's Republic of China

Chunfeng Yun
Institute of Population Research, Peking University, Beijing 100871, People's Republic of China

Yuna He
Department of Nutrition Surveillance, National Institute of Nutrition and Health, Chinese Center for Disease

Jennifer McGuire and and Rima Kleiner
1National Fisheries Institute, 7918 Jones Branch Dr #700, McLean, VA 22102, USA

Jason Kaplan and John Lapolla
inVentiv Medical Communications, 450 West 15th Street, Suite 405, New York, NY 10011, USA

Yanni Papanikolaou
Nutritional Strategies Inc., 59 Marriott Place, Paris, ON N3L 0A3, Canada

Julie Miller Jones
Distinguished Scholar and Professor Emerita of Food and Nutrition, Department of Foods and Nutrition, St. Catherine University, 4030 Valentine Ct. Arden Hills, Minnesota, MN 55112, USA

Victor L. Fulgoni III
Nutrition Impact, LLC, 9725 D Drive North, Battle Creek, MI, USA

Antje R. Weseler and Aalt Bast
Department of Pharmacology and Toxicology; Faculty of Health, Medicine and Life Sciences, P.O. Box 6166200, MD, Maastricht, The Netherlands

Mindy Patterson Maziarz
Department of Nutrition and Food Sciences, Institute of Health Sciences, Texas Woman's University, 6700 Fannin Street, Houston, TX 77030, USA

Sara Preisendanz, Shanil Juma, Victorine Imrhan and Parakat Vijayagopal
Department of Nutrition and Food Sciences, Texas Woman's University, P.O Box 425888, Denton, TX 76204, USA

Chandan Prasad
Department of Nutrition and Food Sciences, Texas Woman's University, P.O Box 425888, Denton, TX 76204, USA
Department of Medicine (Endocrinology), Louisiana State University Health Science Center, New Orleans, LA 70112, USA

S. Nicole Fearnbach, Travis D. Masterson and Haley A. Schlechter
Department of Nutritional Sciences, The Pennsylvania State University, 110 Chandlee Laboratory, University Park, PA 16802, USA

Amanda J. Ross, Michael J. Rykaczewski and Danielle S. Downs
Department of Kinesiology, The Pennsylvania State University, 276 Recreation Building, University Park, PA 16802, USA

Eric Loken
Department of Human Development and Family Studies, The Pennsylvania State University, 119 Health and Human Development Building, University Park, PA 16802, USA
Department of Educational Psychology, University of Connecticut, 328 Charles B. Gentry Building, Storrs, CT 06269, USA

David Thivel
Laboratory of the Metabolic Adaptations to Exercise under Physiological and Pathological Conditions (AME2P), Clermont Auvergne University, EA 3533 Clermont-Ferrand, France
CRNH-Auvergne, 58 Rue Montalembert, 63009 Clermont-Ferrand, France

Kathleen L. Keller
Department of Nutritional Sciences, The Pennsylvania State University, 110 Chandlee Laboratory, University Park, PA 16802, USA
Department of Food Science, The Pennsylvania State University, 202 Rodney A. Erickson Food Science Building, University Park, PA 16802, USA

Sangmi Kim, Joohee Kim, Yeni Lim, You Jin Kim and Oran Kwon
Department of Nutritional Science and Food Management, Ewha Womans University, Seoul 03760, Republic of Korea

Ji Yeon Kim
Department of Food Science and Technology, Seoul National University of Science and Technology, Seoul 01811, Republic of Korea

Colin D. Rehm and Adam Drewnowski
Center for Public Health Nutrition, University of Washington, Seattle, WA 98195-3410, USA

Jianhua Su
Department of Geriatric Intensive Care Unit, The First Affiliated Hospital, Nanjing Medical University, Guangzhou road 300, Nanjing 210029, China
Department of Geriatric Medicine, Wuxi NO.2 People's Hospital, Nanjing Medical University, Zhongshan road 68, Wuxi 214002, China

Jin Geng
Department of Cardiology, Huai'an First People's Hospital, Nanjing Medical University, Beijingxi road 6, Huai'an 223300, China

Jisheng Bao, Yin Tang, Menglan Liu, Haibin Yu and Wei Huang
Department of Geriatric Medicine, Wuxi NO.2 People's Hospital, Nanjing Medical University, Zhongshan road 68, Wuxi 214002, China

Yi Han and Suming Zhou
Department of Geriatric Intensive Care Unit, The First Affiliated Hospital, Nanjing Medical University, Guangzhou road 300, Nanjing 210029, China

Hilary J. Powers, Mark Stephens and Marilyn H. Hill
Human Nutrition Unit, University of Sheffield, Sheffield, UK

Jean Russell
Corporate Information and Computing Services, University of Sheffield, Sheffield, UK

Da-Li Sun
Department of General Surgery, Wuhan Clinical School of Southern Medical University/Wuhan General Hospital of Guangzhou Military Command, Wuhan 430070, China
Department of Gastrointestinal Surgery, Second Affiliated Hospital of Kunming Medical University, Kunming 650101, China
Research Center for Surgical Clinical Nutrition in Yun-Nan Province, Kunming 650101, China

Wei-Ming Li
Department of Gastrointestinal Surgery, Second Affiliated Hospital of Kunming Medical University, Kunming 650101, China

Shu-Min LiYun-Yun Cen , Qing-Wen Xu , Yi-Jun Li , Yan-Bo Sun ,Yu-xing Qi, Yue-ying Lin and Ting Yang, and Peng-Yuan Xu
Department of Gastrointestinal Surgery, Second Affiliated Hospital of Kunming Medical University, Kunming 650101, China Research Center for Surgical Clinical Nutrition in Yun-Nan Province, Kunming 650101, China

Tsuyoshi Chiba, Yoko Sato, Etsuko Kobayashi and Keizo Umegaki
Information Center, National Institute of Health and Nutrition, National Institutes of Biomedical Innovation, Health and Nutrition, 1-23-1 Toyama, Shinjuku-ku, Tokyo 162-8636, Japan

Kazuki Ide and Hiroshi Yamada
Department of Drug Evaluation & Informatics, Graduate School of Pharmaceutical Sciences, University of Shizuoka, 52-1 Yada, Suruga-ku, Shizuoka 422-8526, Japan

Gibran Roder Feguri
Federal University of Mato Grosso, Cuiabá, Brazil
General University Hospital, Cuiabá, Brazil
UNIC - University of Cuiabá, Cuiabá, Brazil
Rua Mal. Floriano Peixoto, 1520/503 - Duque de Caxias II, CEP:78045-395 Cuiabá, Brazil

Paulo Ruiz Lúcio de Lima
Cardiovascular Department, General University Hospital, Cuiabá, Brazil

Danilo de Cerqueira Borge, Larissa Nadaf Batista and Thaís Carvalho e Silva
General University Hospital, Cuiabá, Brazil

Laura Ramos Toledo
Nutrition Service, General University Hospital, Cuiaba, Brazil

Neuber José Segri
Department of Statistics, Federal University of Mato Grosso, Cuiabá, Brazil

José Eduardo de Aguilar-Nascimento
Federal University of Mato Grosso and UNIVAG Medical School, Varzea Grande, Brazil

Qi-Ping Lu
Department of General Surgery, Wuhan Clinical School of Southern Medical University/Wuhan General Hospital of Guangzhou Military Command, Wuhan 430070, China

Hyejin Kim, Hyesook Kim, and Namsoo Chang
Department of Nutritional Science and Food Management, Ewha Womans University, Seoul, South Korea

Eunjung Lee
Department of Nutrition Consultation, Seoul National University Hospital, Healthcare System Gangnam Center, Seoul, South Korea

Yeni Kim
Department of Child Psychiatry, National Center for Child and Adolescent Psychiatry, Seoul National University Hospital, Seoul, South Korea

Eun-Hee Ha
Department of Occupational and Environmental Medicine, Ewha Womans University, College of Medicine, Seoul, South Korea

Stina Bodén and Bethany Van Guelpen
Department of Radiation Sciences, Oncology, Umeå University, Umeå SE-901 87,
Sweden

Maria Wennberg and Ingegerd Johansson
Department of Public Health and Clinical Medicine, Nutritional Research, Umeå University, Umeå SE-901 87, Sweden

Bernt Lindahl
Department of Public Health and Clinical Medicine, Occupational and Environmental Medicine, Umeå University, Umeå SE-901 87, Sweden

Jonas Andersson
Department of Public Health and Clinical Medicine, Research Unit Skellefteå, Umeå University, Umeå SE-901 87, Sweden

Nitin Shivappa and James R. Hebert
Cancer Prevention and Control Program, University of South Carolina, 915 Greene Street, Suite 241, Columbia, SC 29208, USA.
Department of Epidemiology and Biostatistics, Arnold School of Public Health, University of South Carolina, Columbia, SC 29208, USA
Connecting Health Innovations LLC, 1417 Gregg St., Columbia, SC 29201, USA

Jonna C. Sandberg, Inger M. E. Björck and Anne C. Nilsson
Food for Health Science Centre, Lund University, SE-221 00 Lund, Sweden

R. H. Dunstan, D. L. Sparkes, M. M. Macdonald and T. K. Roberts
School of Environmental and Life Sciences, University of Newcastle,
Callaghan, Australia

X. Janse De Jonge
School of Environmental and Life Sciences, University of Newcastle, Ourimbah, Australia

B. J. Dascombe
Latrobe University, Melbourne, Australia

J. Gottfries
Department of Chemistry and Molecular Biology, University of Gothenburg, Gothenburg, Sweden

C.-G. Gottfries
Department of Neuroscience, University of Gothenburg, Gothenburg, Sweden

Lena Maria Nilsson
Department of Public Health and Clinical Medicine, Nutritional Research, Umeå University, Umeå SE-901 87, Sweden
Arctic Research Centre (Arcum), Umeå University, Umeå SE-901 87, Sweden

Index